Arrhythmia Treatment and Therapy

Arrhythmia Treatment and Therapy

Evaluation of Clinical Trial Evidence

edited by

Raymond L. Woosley

Georgetown University Medical Center
Washington, D.C.

Steven N. Singh

Georgetown University Medical Center and
Veterans Affairs Medical Center
Washington, D.C.

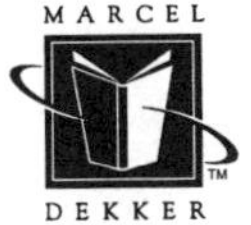

MARCEL DEKKER, INC.　　　　　NEW YORK · BASEL

ISBN: 0-8247-8164-3

This book is printed on acid-free paper.

Headquarters
Marcel Dekker, Inc.
270 Madison Avenue, New York, NY 10016
tel: 212-696-9000; fax: 212-685-4540

Eastern Hemisphere Distribution
Marcel Dekker AG
Hutgasse 4, Postfach 812, CH-4001 Basel, Switzerland
tel: 41-61-261-8482; fax: 41-61-261-8896

World Wide Web
http://www.dekker.com

The publisher offers discounts on this book when ordered in bulk quantities. For more information, write to Special Sales/Professional Marketing at the headquarters address above.

We dedicate this book to the memory of one of the
leaders in this field and a beloved colleague,
Ronald W. F. Campbell, M.D., F.R.C.P.

Introduction

For a specific patient, one must consider the response both of the patient and of the arrhythmia to the drug; the actual plasma concentration of the drug is often of secondary importance. Low drug concentration can exert a therapeutic or toxic effect in some patients, while drug concentrations higher than the normal range may be needed and tolerated in other patients (1).

Douglas P. Zipes, M.D.

It is difficult to imagine a statement that would better illustrate the complexity of treating dysrhythmia. In addition to considering the responses of both the patient and the arrhythmia to any given drug, one must also consider the type and severity of arrhythmia. Thus, it is not surprising that so much attention and effort have been devoted to developing different classes of antiarrhythmic medication as well as interventional procedures. During the past two decades, each newly developed drug, as well as different indications for already existing medications, has led to major clinical trials that have greatly helped in the treatment of patients suffering from dysrhythmia. Nonetheless, the specific indications, dosages, and combination therapies remain very complex.

This book brings together in one volume the results of the most influential clinical trials. Each is discussed by an expert on the specific medication under study. This compilation of the major studies of antiarrhythmic agents is designed to assist those involved in the care of patients with arrhythmia. But, in addition, it also poses challenges to the biomedical community engaged in research in this area.

The roster of editors and authors who contributed to this volume is a list of ''Who's Who'' in the field. A great deal of research has been conducted in the past, and much is now under way. Fortunately, it is successful and therefore very valuable research. However, its true value comes only from its application and use in clinical practice.

This volume facilitates this translation from the bench to the bedside.

Claude Lenfant, M.D.
Bethesda, Maryland

REFERENCE

1. Zipes, DP. Management of Cardiac Arrhythmias. In: Braunwald E, ed. Pharmacological, Electrical and Surgical Treatments in Heart Disease: A Textbook of Cardiovascular Medicine, 5th ed. Philadelphia: W.B. Saunders Co, 1997.

Preface

The treatment of arrhythmias, especially ventricular arrhythmias, has changed dramatically over the last 50 years. More than in any other field of medicine, the advances in the practice of cardiology, especially in the treatment of arrhythmias, have been the direct result of controlled clinical trials. The reliance on science-based therapeutics serves as a model for other disciplines to emulate and for the future of medicine.

For over 30 years, the presence of ventricular arrhythmias in postmyocardial infarction patients has been well accepted as a powerful risk factor for sudden cardiac death (1). Because of the experience with other risk factors, such as cholesterol and blood pressure, in which control of the risk factor was associated with improved clinical outcome, it was only natural for practicing physicians to assume that suppression of ventricular arrhythmias would prevent sudden cardiac death. In the 1980s, nine antiarrhythmic drugs were in regular use and another ten were in development. Two very different modes of arrhythmia management had evolved and these were compared in the Electrophysiology Study Versus Electrocardiographic Monitoring (ESVEM) Trial (2).

During the 1980s, 70% of cardiologists surveyed reported that they routinely prescribed antiarrhythmic drugs for asymptomatic ventricular arrhythmias (3). Few doubted the wisdom of suppressing ventricular arrhythmias, but the scientific leaders of the National Heart, Lung and Blood Institute were convinced that the practice should be based on scientific fact and called for a clinical trial to evaluate the effects of antiarrhythmic drugs on mortality. A pilot study, the Cardiac Arrhythmia Pilot Study (CAPS) (4), was conducted as a feasibility trial and was followed by the Cardiac Arrhythmia Suppression Trial (CAST) (5). CAST tested the hypothesis that suppression of premature ventricular contractions in post-myocardial infarction patients would result in a reduced risk of sudden cardiac death. The cardiology world was shocked in 1989 when CAST was terminated prematurely because the group randomized to the drug treatment arm had twice the mortality of the placebo group (5). A meta-analysis of studies with sodium channel blocking antiarrhythmic drugs confirmed the consistency of the data (6) and the practice of medicine responded; these drugs are now generally reserved for patients with symptomatic or life-threatening arrhythmias. However, drug developers concluded that the correct target was instead the potassium channel and began a search for drugs that would prolong repolarization and refractoriness. This may have been based on the supposition that this was the major action of amiodarone, a drug that was gaining favor in the United States in spite of its high risk of organ toxicity. Again, a clinical trial, Survival With ORal D-Sotalol (SWORD), markedly influenced the development of an entirely new class of drugs when it found that the d-isomer of sotalol failed to decrease mortality and in fact increased the overall mortality. The development of most of the drugs in this class was halted, with only ibutilide and dofetilide remaining to be developed for supraventricular arrhythmias.

The dramatic efficacy of amiodarone in a broad spectrum of arrhythmias led to its wide prescription and the need for controlled trials to determine its true value. Surprisingly, it was found to be no better than placebo in the Congestive Heart Failure–Survival Trial of Antiarrhythmic Therapy (CHF–STAT) (7). A meta-analysis of several trials concluded that amiodarone had a modest ability to improve mortality (8). Interestingly, although it is one of the most toxic drugs to organs of the body, compared to other antiarrhythmic drugs that clearly increase mortality, it is considered one of the safest (9).

With the advent of improved antiarrhythmic devices and their wider usage, it became apparent that a clinical trial was needed. Because of the severity of the arrhythmias, a comparison of the devices to active therapy was the only ethical approach. The Antiarrhythmic Versus Implantable Defibrillator (AVID) trial compared these devices to amiodarone and again changed the way cardiologists approached arrhythmia patients (10). AVID found that the devices were more effective than amiodarone. Subsequently, the Coronary Artery Bypass Graft Patch Trial (CABG Patch) found that the devices provided no added mortality benefit to bypass surgery alone (11).

These and other important trials have shaped the evolution of the practice of physicians caring for patients with arrhythmias. However, the scientific basis for these trials, the intricacies of their design, and the complexity of their outcomes have challenged physicians and called attention to the need for a readily available single source of information on these trials. The purpose of this book is to provide such a source in a novel framework. We invited clinician scientists intimately involved in the design and conduct of these trials to write a chapter summarizing the important aspects of the trial. We also invited leading authorities not intimately involved in the trial to provide an objective summary of the strengths and weaknesses of each trial and a discussion of issues that were either unresolved or created by the trial. The trials are discussed in the chronological order of their completion so that the reader can follow the sequence of events and conclusions as they evolved. A final chapter summarizes the trials that are currently underway and gives the reader a glimpse of the future.

We thank the many contributors who helped us prepare this review of the past 20 years of clinical trials in cardiac arrhythmias.

Raymond L. Woosley
Steven N. Singh

REFERENCES

1. Bigger JT, Jr, Weld FM, Rolnitzky LM. Prevalence, characteristics, and significance of ventricular tachycardia (three or more complexes) detected with ambulatory electrocardiographic recording in the late hospital phase of acute myocardial infarction. Am J Cardiol 1981;48:815–823.
2. ESVEM Investigators. The ESVEM Trial. Electrophysiologic Study Versus Electrocardiographic Monitoring for Selection of Antiarrhythmic Therapy of Ventricular Tachyarrhythmias. Circulation 1989;79(6):1354–1360.
3. Morganroth J, Bigger JT, Jr, Anderson JL. Treatment of ventricular arrhythmias by United States cardiologists: a survey before the Cardiac Arrhythmia Suppression Trial results were available. Am J Cardiol 1990;65:40–48.
4. CAPS Investigators. The effect of encainide, flecainide, imipramine and moricizine on ventricular arrhythmias during the year after myocardial infarction. Am J Cardiol 1988;61:501–509.
5. CAST Investigators. Preliminary report: Effect of encainide and flecainide on mortality in a randomized trial of arrhythmia suppression after myocardial infarction. N Engl J Med 1989;321:406–412.
6. Hine LK, Laird NM, Hewitt P, Chalmers TC. Meta-analysis of empirical long-term antiarrhythmic therapy after myocardial infarction. JAMA 1989;262(21):3037–3040.
7. Singh, SN, Fletcher RD, Fisher SG, Lewis HD, Deedwania PC, Massie BM, Colling C, Lazzeri D, and The Survival Trial of Antiarrhythmic Therapy in Congestive Heart Failure Investigaors. Amiodarone in patients with congestive heart failure and asymptomatic ventricular arrhythmia. N Engl J Med 1995;333:77–82.
8. Amiodarone Trials Meta-Analysis Investigators. Effect of prophylactic amiodarone on mortality after acute myocardial infarction and in congestive heart failure: meta-analysis of individual data from 6500 patients in randomised trials. Lancet 1997;350:1417–1424.
9. Vorperian VR, Havighurst TC, Miller S, January CT. Adverse effects of low dose amiodarone: a meta-analysis. J Am Coll Cardiol 1997;30:791–798.
10. The Antiarrhythmics Versus Implantable Defibrillators (AVID) Investigators. A comparison of antiarrhythmic-drug therapy with implantable defibrillators in patients resuscitated from near-fatal ventricular arrhythmias. N Engl J Med 1997;337:1576–1585.
11. Bigger JT and Coronary Artery Bypass Graft (CABG) Patch Trial Investigators. Prophylactic use of implanted cardiac defibrillators in patients at high risk for ventricular arrhythmias after coronary-artery bypass graft surgery. N Engl J Med 1997;337:1569–1575.

Contents

Contributors

Masood Akhtar, M.D. Clinical Professor of Medicine, University of Wisconsin Medical School–Milwaukee Clinical Campus; Director, Arrhythmia Service, Milwaukee Heart Institute, Sinai Samaritan Medical Center; and Director, Institute for Cardiac Rhythms, St. Luke's Medical Center, Milwaukee, Wisconsin

Jeffrey L. Anderson, M.D. Adjunct Professor, Department of International Medicine, University of Utah School of Medicine, Salt Lake City, Utah

Gust H. Bardy, M.D. Professor of Medicine, Division of Cardiology, Department of Medicine, University of Washington, Seattle, Washington

J. Thomas Bigger, Jr., M.D. Professor of Medicine and Pharmacology, Columbia University; Director, Arrhythmia Service, Columbia–Presbyterian Medical Center, New York, New York

Daniel M. Bloomfield, M.D. Assistant Professor of Medicine, Columbia University; Director, Syncope Center, Columbia–Presbyterian Medical Center, New York, New York

Alfred E. Buxton, M.D. Professor of Medicine and Director, Arrhythmia Services, Brown University School of Medicine and Rhode Island Hospital, Providence, Rhode Island

John A. Cairns, M.D., F.R.C.P.C. Dean, Faculty of Medicine, University of British Columbia, Vancouver, British Columbia, Canada

A. John Camm, M.D., F.R.C.P. Professor of Clinical Cardiology, Department of Cardiological Sciences, St. George's Hospital Medical School, London, England

Ronald W. F. Campbell, M.D.[†]   Department of Cardiology, Freeman Hospital, Newcastle Upon Tyne, England

John P. DiMarco M.D., Ph.D.   Professor of Medicine, Director of Cardiovascular Medicine, University of Virginia Health Sciences Center, Charlottesville, Virginia

Michael J. Domanski, M.D.   Head, Clinical Trials Group, National Heart, Lung and Blood Institute, National Institutes of Health, Bethesda, Maryland

Hernán C. Doval, M.D.   Heart Institute, Italian Hospital, Buenos Aires, Argentina

Andrew E. Epstein, M.D.   Professor of Medicine, Division of Cardiovascular Disease, Department of Medicine, The University of Alabama at Birmingham, Birmingham, Alabama

Derek V. Exner, M.D., M.P.H., F.R.C.P.   Clinical Trials Research, National Heart, Lung and Blood Institute, National Institutes of Health, Bethesda, Maryland

Susan G. Fisher, Ph.D.   Veterans Affairs Cooperative Studies Program, Hines, Illinois

Ross D. Fletcher   Georgetown University and Veterans Affairs Medical Centers, Washington, D.C.

Gary S. Francis, M.D.   Director, Coronary Intensive Care Unit, Department of Cardiology, The Cleveland Clinic Foundation, Cleveland, Ohio

Lawrence M. Friedman   National Heart, Lung and Blood Institute, National Institutes of Health, Bethesda, Maryland

H. Leon Greene, M.D.   Clinical Professor, Department of Medicine, University of Washington, Seattle, Washington

Mark E. Josephson, M.D.   Director, Harvard Thorndike Electrophysiology Institute, Beth Israel Deaconess Medical Center, Boston, Massachusetts

---

[†] Deceased.

Kerry L. Lee, Ph.D.   Associate Professor of Biostatistics, Duke Clinical Research Institute, Durham, North Carolina

Bradley Marchant, M.D.   Pfizer Limited, Kent, England

Jay W. Mason, M.D.   Professor and Chairman, Department of Medicine, University of Kentucky College of Medicine, Lexington, Kentucky

Arthur J. Moss, M.D.   Professor, Department of Medicine, University of Rochester Medical Center, Rochester, New York

Craig M. Pratt, M.D.   Professor, Section of Cardiology, Department of Medicine, Baylor College of Medicine, Houston, Texas

Eric N. Prystowsky, M.D.   Director, Clinical Electrophysiology Laboratory, Northside Cardiology, P.C., and St. Vincent Hospital, Indianapolis, Indiana

James A. Reiffel, M.D.   Professor of Clinical Medicine, Division of Cardiology, Department of Medicine, Columbia University, New York, New York

Dan M. Roden, M.D.   Director, Division of Clinical Pharmacology, Vanderbilt University Medical Center, Nashville, Tennessee

Jeremy N. Ruskin, M.D.   Director, Cardiac Arrhythmia Service, Massachusetts General Hospital, Boston, Massachusetts

Eleanor B. Schron, M.S., R.N., F.A.A.N.   Captain, U.S.P.H.S. Commissioned Corps, Division of Epidemiology and Clinical Applications, National Heart, Lung and Blood Institute, National Institutes of Health, Bethesda, Maryland

Bramah N. Singh, M.D., D.Phil.   Professor of Medicine, UCLA School of Medicine, and Department of Cardiology, West Los Angeles Veterans Affairs Medical Center, Los Angeles, California

Steven N. Singh, M.D., F.A.C.C.   Professor of Medicine and Pharmacology, Georgetown University and Veterans Affairs Medical Centers, Washington, D.C.

Lynne Warner Stevenson, M.D.   Director, Heart Failure and Cardiomyopathy Program, Brigham and Women's Hospital, Harvard Medical School, Boston, Massachusetts

William G. Stevenson, M.D.   Director, Cardiac Arrhythmia Service and Clinical Electrophysiology Laboratory, Brigham and Women's Hospital, Harvard Medical School, Boston, Massachusetts

Albert L. Waldo, M.D.   The Walter H. Pritchard Professor of Cardiology, Professor of Medicine, and Professor of Biomedical Engineering, Division of Cardiology, Department of Medicine, Case Western Reserve University, Cleveland, Ohio

David J. Wilber, M.D.   Professor of Medicine and Director, Clinical Electrophysiology, University of Chicago, Chicago, Illinois

Raymond L. Woosley, M.D., Ph.D.   Professor of Pharmacology and Medicine, Georgetown University Medical Center, Washington, D.C.

D. George Wyse, M.D., Ph.D.   Professor, Division of Cardiology, Department of Medicine, The University of Calgary, Calgary, Alberta, Canada

Yee Guan Yap, M.B.B.S., M.R.C.P.   British Heart Foundation Research Fellow in Cardiology, Department of Cardiological Sciences, St. George's Hospital Medical School, London, England

Peter J. Zimetbaum   Beth Israel Deaconess Medical Center, Boston, Massachusetts

Douglas P. Zipes, M.D.   Distinguished Professor of Medicine, Pharmacology, and Toxicology, Department of Medicine, and Director, Krannert Institute of Cardiology and the Division of Cardiology, Indiana University School of Medicine, Indianapolis, Indiana

Arrhythmia Treatment and Therapy

1

The International Mexiletine and Placebo Antiarrhythmic Coronary Trial (IMPACT) and the Chamberlain Trial

RONALD W. F. CAMPBELL[†]

Freeman Hospital, Newcastle Upon Tyne, England

INTRODUCTION

IMPACT (1) was published in 1984. It had been preceded by a very similar study, the Chamberlain study, published in 1980 (2). Both examined the role of prophylactic oral mexiletine in survivors of acute myocardial infarction. These were important studies of their time but, by present-day standards, they were statistically underpowered for the purpose of examining mortality. In their defense, both defined the effects of mexiletine against ventricular arrhythmias as the primary endpoint. In the era of the IMPACT and Chamberlain trials, there were relatively few antiarrhythmic agents available. Quinidine, procainamide, disopyramide, lidocaine, and the beta-blockers were, depending upon country-specific licensing, the agents available for managing ventricular arrhythmias. At that time, lidocaine was widely used in coronary care units (3). Numerous studies, albeit usually not placebo-controlled, had shown the efficacy of lidocaine to control ventricular ectopic beats and it was widely believed then that lidocaine, given prophylactically, could prevent primary ventricular fibrillation (4). Lidocaine had proved remarkably well tolerated in patients with depressed left ventricular function and proarrhythmia either did not occur or had not been recognized. It was natural, then, for mexiletine, an orally active analogue of lidocaine, to be investigated.

---

† Deceased.

By the early 1980s, coronary care units had focused attention not just on the acute phase of myocardial infarction but on the subsequent fate of those who survived and left the hospital. It was apparent that there was considerable first-year mortality (5,6) and that some risk factors might identify those with a particularly poor prognosis (7,8). The role of ventricular ectopic beats was under active investigation with reasonable evidence that high-frequency ventricular ectopic beats were indeed a risk factor (9,10) and perhaps were independent of indices of left ventricular function (7). A role for ventricular ectopic beats in late mortality was also seductively plausible. Ventricular fibrillation appears commonly to be initiated by an ectopic beat and, in that pre-CAST (11) era, it was easy to imagine why attention focused on post-MI interventions that might suppress ventricular ectopic beats with the expectation of improving prognosis.

Twenty years ago there was sufficient evidence to recognize that ventricular ectopic beats on their own were relatively poor positive predictive features for late death and that improved risk prediction could be provided by defining patients with multiple risk factors, including indices of left ventricular dysfunction, size of infarction, and continuing ischemia. At that time and even now there was little attempt to develop risk prediction for specific types of demise. In the two studies (1,2) that examined prophylactic mexiletine post-MI, it was not anticipated that mexiletine would have any action beyond an effect on ventricular arrhythmias. Whether mexiletine was imagined to bring benefit by suppressing triggers for ventricular fibrillation or whether it had a direct effect against ventricular fibrillation did not matter, but it was certainly not considered that mexiletine would prevent other mechanisms of post-MI mortality. Despite this, the risk predictors used to select patients in these studies related to total mortality rather than specifically to sudden, presumptively arrhythmic mortality.

THE CHAMBERLAIN STUDY

The Chamberlain study was published in 1980 (2). At the time it was innovative and, by the standards of the day, it was large. Its sample size had been based on crude statistical calculations which, with hindsight, were optimistic. Mexiletine was a well-regarded antiarrhythmic agent that had been shown to be capable of controlling ventricular arrhythmias associated with infarction (12), with little impact on LV function (13) and almost devoid of cardiovascular toxicity (14). That it was an analogue of lidocaine provided a further scientific basis for its evaluation in high-risk postinfarct patients. It was a multicenter trial, with three of the four UK trial centers adopting an identical protocol. The fourth center examined a second arrhythmic agent, aprindine. The trial design, however, allowed for this and in the evaluation of mexiletine versus placebo, data from the fourth center were amalgamated with that of the other three.

Patients

The patients included in the study had sustained a definite myocardial infarction within a time window of 6 to 14 days previously (Fig. 1). The criteria for infarction were standard and comprised history, ECG, and enzyme changes. An important element in the study was the selection of high-risk patients. These were identified as patients with persisting ST segment elevation (more than 2 mm for inferior infarcts or 3 mm for anterior infarcts) on either the second or third day after the infarct, pulmonary edema on a chest x-ray taken in the first 48 h, sinus tachycardia (>100 bpm) persisting for 24 h during the first 48 h, and left bundle branch block. In this study, ventricular ectopic beats were not a criteria for identifying high-risk patients but it had been assumed that in patients having at least one of the previously declared high-risk criteria, high-frequency ventricular ectopic beats were to be expected. Patients were excluded on the basis of overt hepatic or renal disease, right bundle branch block with left axis deviation, any degree of AV block during the enrollment window, the need for cardioactive drugs other than digitalis, nitrates, or diuretics, and Parkinsonism (this was because tremor was a recognized feature of high plasma concentrations of mexiletine and there was concern that in Parkinsonian patients the inability to track this important feature might place them at a disadvantage).

Study Design

Treatment allocation to mexiletine or placebo was on a double-blind basis with numbered, sequential treatment packs as the basis for randomization. As already

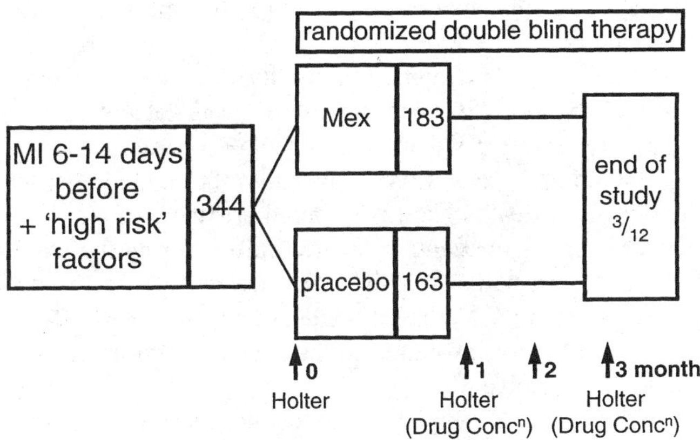

Figure 1　Schematic of the Chamberlain study.

mentioned, a second arrhythmic drug was examined in one center. This had the effect of reducing the placebo group size by a half, but it was considered unlikely to have any important statistical impact. Two different dosing regimens of mexiletine were permitted and were based on body weight. To maintain blinding, there was a similar "two-dose" matching placebo.

As it had been recognized that post-MI mortality declined in an exponential fashion, the study duration was for only 3 months, with patients being reviewed at monthly intervals. Twenty-four-hour ECG recordings were obtained on three occasions: prior to inclusion, at 1 month, and at 3 months. Blood samples were taken at 1 month and at 3 months, with standard hematological and clinical chemistry tests to monitor safety and to provide plasma concentrations of mexiletine.

In the event that unwanted effects occurred that were thought to be drug-related, the dose of mexiletine or placebo was reduced. Only if the problem persisted to an unacceptable level was the patient withdrawn from the study, although follow-up was continued. Withdrawal was also permitted when study medication had been omitted for several days after the development of arrhythmias that required active therapy, after reinfarction, and at the discretion of the physician. An attempt was made to analyze arrhythmic death, this being defined as an unexpected death that had been sudden and was not preceded by new symptoms. Determination of this mode of death was by group discussion and consensus.

Results

Three-hundred-forty-four patients were entered into the trial, of whom 181 received mexiletine and 163 placebo. The difference is due to the protocol difference at one of the centers, which resulted in reduction in size of the placebo cohort. The two groups were well-matched with respect to all important demographic features and risk factors.

On an intention-to-treat basis, mexiletine mortality was 13.2% versus 11.6% for the placebo group. The mortality increase of 1.6% was not statistically significant. This paper was a relatively early one to define 95% confidence limits for the mortality results which, in this case, were -5.4% to $+8.6\%$. On the criteria previously mentioned, 77% of deaths were considered arrhythmic.

Twenty-two of the 163 placebo patients were withdrawn during the study versus 15 of the mexiletine-treated patients. This difference is statistically significant. The imbalance was due to an increased incidence of unwanted effects in the mexiletine-treated patients with insomnia, tremor, nausea, vomiting, and constipation being statistically significantly.

As had been expected, there was a high prevalence of ventricular arrhythmias in the pretherapy tapes: 93% of patients showed ventricular ectopic beats;

25% showing couplets and 11% showing more than three consecutive ventricular ectopic beats. Multiform ventricular ectopic beats were found in 41% of patients. By contrast, runs of 10 or more ventricular ectopic beats and R-on-T beats were relatively rare. Based on crude incidence figures, there was no important change in these figures at 1 and 3 months, although the number of patients with couplets and with multiform ectopic beats was significantly reduced by mexiletine at 1 month. There was thus little evidence of mexiletine's ability to abolish any category of ventricular arrhythmia in these patients. By contrast, comparisons of the total number of ventricular ectopic complexes showed mexiletine to have a powerful effect with statistically significant reductions at 1 and 3 months.

The plasma concentrations of mexiletine showed that at 1 month and at 3 months 29% and 41%, respectively, of samples were below the minimum recommended plasma concentration of 0.75 µg/mL.

Implications

The mortality result was clearly disappointing, but probably not unexpected. The authors cited three other papers (15–17) that had failed to confirm a benefit of prophylactic antiarrhythmic drugs—phenytoin (15), procainamide (16), and aprindine (17). This was in contrast to early evidence of a mortality benefit of beta blockers (18,19). The authors noted that the mortality rate of 11.6% in the placebo group was less than the 20% expected by the entry criteria. In discussing why mortality was not reduced, one possibility suggested was that type 2 error may have concealed potential benefit given that the number of endpoints was low. Inadequate mexiletine dosing was another possibility, but the level of mexiletine-related unwanted events did not suggest that higher doses of mexiletine would have been tolerated.

Mortality was not the primary endpoint of the trial and the main thrust of the authors' discussion centered on the analysis of the 24-h tapes. The study claimed to be the most ambitious of its time, having analyzed almost 30,000 h of ECG. A reduction in ventricular ectopic beat numbers was expected and was found. The authors noted that ventricular arrhythmia suppression was not necessarily the same thing as ventricular fibrillation protection, but, perhaps most importantly, they recognized that selection criteria based principally on extensive acute myocardial damage might not have identified patients whose death would be modifiable by antiarrhythmic therapy. The authors' final sentence proved prophetic. *"This investigation emphasizes that the adverse prognostic significance of cardiovascular ventricular dysfunction cannot readily be influenced whether or not the late hospital course is complicated by complex ventricular arrhythmias."*

IMPACT

IMPACT was published in two papers (1,20). The first was a surprisingly long and detailed paper in the *Journal of the American College of Cardiology* in 1984. The other, almost 2 years later, was in the *European Heart Journal* (20).

Design

IMPACT bore many similarities to the Chamberlain trial (2) (Table 1), but there were important differences. The drug investigated was mexiletine but in a slow-release formulation; follow-up was up to 1 year; and inclusion demanded no more than a documented infarct in males aged 30 to 74 and women aged 45 to 74. Such patients were described at "moderate risk" rather than the high-risk patients that had been examined in the Chamberlain study. The exclusion list was more detailed than that of the Chamberlain study, but was similar in all important respects.

IMPACT was, as indicated in the title, an international, multicenter study, conducted in Europe and North America. This was an early study to reveal the detailed statistical basis for sample size calculation. The study was designed with a power of 0.89 to detect a reduction at 4 months from 30% to 18% in the rate of complex cardiac arrhythmias by mexiletine treatment. The authors recognized that based on such a primary endpoint, their study had a power of only 0.17 to detect a 25% reduction in 1-year mortality if the placebo mortality rate was 10%.

Patients

Six-hundred-thirty patients were enrolled, of whom 317 received mexiletine and 313 placebo (Fig. 2). The first published paper provides remarkably full details of baseline characteristics and contains interesting insights on medical practice of 15 years ago. Thirty-five percent of patients had received antiarrhythmic drugs in the time between the qualifying infarction and entry to the study. Seventeen percent were on beta-blockers and up to 16% on digitalis. Seventy percent of patients were receiving anticoagulants, but only 24% were taking antithrombotic agents. As in the Chamberlain study, the baseline Holter monitor showed that more than 90% of included patients had ventricular ectopic beats. Despite the fact that the patients in IMPACT were at lower risk than those enrolled in the Chamberlain study, the incidence of complex forms of ventricular ectopic beats was very similar.

Table 1　Chamberlain and IMPACT Studies

	Chamberlain Study	IMPACT
Primary endpoint	Mexiletine effect on ventricular arrhythmias first 3 mos. post-MI	Mexiletine effect on ventricular arrhythmias (frequent/complex) at 4 mos. and 1-year post-MI
Secondary endpoints	Mortality Unwanted effects	Mortality Unwanted effects
Patients		
n	344	630
time post-MI	6–14 days	4–24 days II
age		Men 30–74 years
gender		Women 45–74 years
risk factors	ST ↑ pulmonary edema; sinus tachycardia; left bundle branch block	
Follow-up duration	3 months	1 year
Holters	preinclusion, 1 month, 3 months	Baseline, 1 month, 4 months, 12 months
Mexiletine vs. placebo mortality	13% vs. 12% (p = ns)	7.6% vs. 4.8% (p = ns)
Mexiletine dose	250 mg @ 8 h patients ≥ 70 kg 250 mg @ 8 h patients < 70 kg	360 mg b.i.d. slow release
Mexiletine vs. placebo VE couplets at 1/12, 3/12, 4/12, 1 year	48% vs. 34% (p < 0.05) 46% vs. 36%	37% vs. 58% (p < 0.05) 42% vs. 60% (p < 0.05) 43% vs. 54% (p = ns)
Overall unwanted effect mexiletine vs. placebo	87% vs. 78% (p = ns)	88% vs. 85% (p = ns)
Unwanted effects—withdrawal mexiletine vs. placebo	17% vs. 4% (p < 0.001)	37% vs. 28% (p < 0.05)

Results

The primary endpoint of IMPACT concerned mexiletine's effect on recorded ventricular arrhythmias. Significant reductions in ventricular arrhythmias were detected at 1 and at 4 months into the study. At 12 months, a difference was still apparent but was no longer statistically significant. Corresponding antiarrhythmic effects were also seen in more complex forms of ventricular arrhythmias.

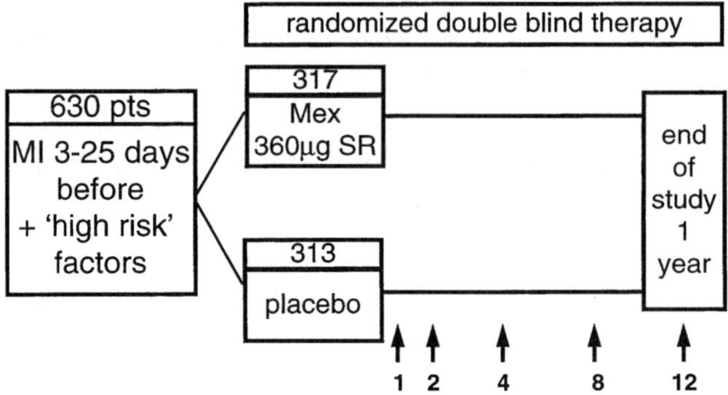

Figure 2   Schematic of the IMPACT trial.

Mortality analysis showed a rate of 7.6% in mexiletine-treated patients versus 4.8% in placebo-managed patients. Corresponding sudden death rates were 2.2% versus 1.3%. These differences were not statistically significant. One hundred sixty-nine baseline variables were examined with respect to subsequent mortality. Twelve were statistically significant based on absolute Z values. This was only slightly higher than expected by chance given the number of analyses.

In a relatively sophisticated further analysis of mortality, the interaction of treatment with each of 141 baseline variables was conducted. No statistically significant interactions were detected.

Adverse effects were sought by direct inquiry. Symptoms were described in 85% of placebo-treated patients and 88% in mexiletine-treated patients (not statistically significant). Tremor, loss of consciousness, nausea, and constipation, however, were significantly more frequent in mexiletine than placebo-treated patients but the differences were not large. Reduction of dose or discontinuation of therapy for unwanted effects was required in 28% of placebo-treated patients and 37% of mexiletine-treated patients. This difference was statistically significant and was principally because of intolerable tremor, insomnia, epigastric pain, and nausea. Interestingly, the main reason for reducing dose or stopping medication in the placebo group was the need to initiate antiarrhythmic therapy; the difference, however, of 5.4% placebo versus 3.5% mexiletine was not statistically significant.

Plasma Concentrations

As in the Chamberlain study, plasma concentrations of mexiletine were low. At the recommended dosage level, only 25% of mexiletine-treated patients achieved serum mexiletine levels of 0.7 µg or greater for at least three-quarters of their visit. Interestingly, mexiletine was detected in some placebo patients. A revealing anecdote disclosed that as part of an external quality control program, two aliquots of the same specimen were sent at different times for analysis to a central laboratory. For one pair, at one time the test was positive but in the other aliquot of the same specimen submitted at a later time, it was not.

The authors attempted to correlate antiarrhythmic activity with adherence to study medication. They found a relationship, although the differences were not impressive; frequent or complex cardiac arrhythmias (the primary endpoint) were present in 58% of poor adherers versus 45% of good adherers.

Implications

In discussion, the authors suggested that *mexiletine was quite effective in reducing the risk of arrhythmia during the first 4 months after discharge from the hospital.* They noted that the differences were primarily due to a large increase in ventricular ectopic activity compared with baseline in the placebo-treated patients at 1 and 4 months. This phenomenon was markedly blunted in the mexiletine-treated patients.

Holter Analysis: The Second Publication

In the second publication of IMPACT (20), the reporting emphasis was on 24-h electrocardiograms. There is a considerable repetition in this paper of the data in the first paper, but there are interesting new insights on methodology and new analyses. The Holter recordings from the study were all analyzed in a central laboratory running an analysis program developed at Washington University in St. Louis, Missouri. It ran on a DEC PDP–11/34 minicomputer. It is less than 15 years since this research was published, but already such a computer seems obsolete. The Holter instruments used were the Oxford Medilog System and it is a testimony to them and to the technicians applying them that only 4.6% of the 2292 tapes were unanalyzable. Two-thirds of the tapes were of good quality, defined as containing less than 2% in duration of noise.

The details of quality control in the Holter analysis were also revealed. One-hundred-ninety tapes were resubmitted and blinded for a rereading. There was 96% agreement of the two readings for the primary endpoint of the presence or absence of frequent or complex cardiac arrhythmias. There was 99% agreement for the presence or absence of runs of three or more premature ventricular complexes. Perhaps even more impressively, there was remarkably good correlation between the first and second readings on the total number of premature ventricular ectopic beats for 24 h.

In this second paper, the authors highlighted the importance of taking fatal events into account when examining nonfatal ones. They presented a new analysis whereby missing electrocardiograms occasioned by death were categorized as if frequent or complex cardiac arrhythmias had been present. This analysis slightly reduced the mexiletine/placebo differences, but the basic findings of the study were unchanged.

As had been noted in the original analysis, there were significantly fewer ventricular ectopic beats in the mexiletine-treated patients compared to those on placebo. These differences were very striking at 1 month and 4 months, but had diminished to a nonstatistically significant effect at 12 months. The authors noted the considerable change in ventricular ectopic activity that was observed in the placebo group as they remobilized and took up normal everyday activities. An analysis of that increase showed that the median change in total premature ventricular ectopic beats over 24 from baseline to the first month was equivalent to one ventricular ectopic beat per 24 h in the mexiletine group versus 40 for the placebo group. This difference was highly statistically significant.

COMPARISON AND DISCUSSION

The Chamberlain (21) and IMPACT (22,23) studies were ahead of their time in many respects. Both enrolled a tightly defined cohort of patients who had survived myocardial infarction. Both used statistical modeling to define the size of patient cohort to be enrolled. Both established efficacy of mexiletine against ventricular arrhythmias as the primary endpoint. Both recognized that mortality endpoints were unlikely to be accessible by virtue of the sample size. The Chamberlain study attempted, with partial success, to define high-risk survivors of myocardial infarction. Selection was based on features reflecting total mortality rather than presumptively arrhythmic mortality, which might have been more modifiable by an antiarrhythmic agent. The Chamberlain study permitted and indeed encouraged dose variation depending on body weight and an effort was made to maintain blinding by providing two-dose placebos. In the IMPACT study, lessons were learned from the Chamberlain results with respect to mexiletine tolerability. A slow-release version of mexiletine was adopted for the trial as it was anticipated that the more stable plasma concentrations would provide better tolerability. Adoption of this plan, however, precluded dose variation and, in the end, there was little evidence that mexiletine slow release was better tolerated than the conventional preparation.

The Good

Both studies provided remarkable data from ambulatory ECGs. These studies demonstrated that mobilizing and convalescent infarct patients could wear Holter monitors, and that these early systems were robust. Both studies recorded commendably high success rates for obtaining good-quality traces. In the discussion of both studies, there was a clear recognition that abolition of ventricular ectopic beats was a difficult goal. Mexiletine offered reduced numbers of ectopic beats but rarely achieved a 24-h recording free of ventricular ectopic activity. Finally, both studies made spirited attempts to correlate plasma concentrations of mexiletine or mexiletine compliance with subsequent efficacy.

The Bad

There were no truly bad features of either the Chamberlain or the IMPACT study. Both represented state-of-the-art clinical research methodology and thinking at the time of their publication.

Despite recognizing the importance of left ventricular function in determining prognosis, formal measurements were not undertaken. The protocol modification at one of the four participant centers of the Chamberlain study was a nuisance rather than a problem. The protocol had been designed to cope with the situation. The Chamberlain study was of a remarkably short duration. The reasons for this were established in the published paper and concerned the mortality patterns postinfarction. An exponential fall in mortality rates had been observed. The study was designed to address the highest risk early and thus economize on resources. This is unfortunate, as most other investigations have provided follow-up for 1 year. It makes cross-correlation of the Chamberlain study with others difficult.

Both studies were conducted at a time when management of post-MI patients was fundamentally different from that of the present day. These studies were prethrombolysis. ACE inhibitors were not in regular use, and the uptake of beta-blockers was relatively modest despite early supportive evidence. Aspirin did not feature and few, if any, patients were taking lipid-lowering therapies. Even in the U.S.-based IMPACT study, interventional rates in these infarct survivors were probably very low by comparison with current-day practice.

Impact of These Studies

Whilst the primary endpoint of both the Chamberlain and IMPACT studies was the antiarrhythmic effect of mexiletine, both publications reveal disappointment with a lack of effect on mortality. In both studies, there was a small, statistically insignificant mortality excess in mexiletine-treated patients. Although the studies were small and there was considerable scope for type 2 error, these were not propitious results for antiarrhythmic strategies postmyocardial infarction. At the very least, they should have signaled considerable caution in examining other antiarrhythmic interventions. To be fair, in the subsequent research involving the class 1c drugs flecainide and encainide (24), the concept that total abolition of ventricular ectopic beats should have been more achievable with the 1c agents rather than mexiletine is suggested. Nonetheless, the Chamberlain and IMPACT studies might have begun to raise fears of harm with antiarrhythmic interventions.

These studies were important for the design of subsequent investigations. They showed that it was possible, using relatively simple criteria, to define high-risk survivors of infarction. At least on relatively crude categorization, an important proportion of that mortality appeared sudden and presumptively arrhythmic. The difficulty of discussing the results when left ventricular function had not been well characterized provided a good reason to incorporate such assessments in other studies. Finally, these studies identified the dramatic importance of compliance and the difficulties of achieving stable plasma concentrations in infarct survivors. This issue has been a feature of all subsequent trials including the EMIAT (25) and CAMIAT (26) investigations of amiodarone, in which over 30% of patients either withdrew or stopped taking therapy.

A new attempt was made to correlate electrocardiographic findings of arrhythmias with the serum mexiletine levels at 1 month. Perhaps surprisingly, there were no striking differences although, on balance, those patients achieving higher mexiletine plasma serum concentrations had fewer arrhythmias. The effect was seen principally in the more complex forms of arrhythmias. This led the authors to suggest that mexiletine was more effective in preventing frequent or complex cardiac arrhythmias than infrequent single premature ventricular ectopic beats. This analysis of the study also showed that complete suppression of ventricular ectopic beats was rarely achieved, leading the authors to note that *premature ventricular complexes will be found when they are meticulously sought.*

In this analysis, the authors were interested in whether mexiletine prevented the appearance of ventricular ectopic beats as much as they were interested in the suppression of baseline ectopic beats. The results gave evidence that both effects were operating, perhaps not surprisingly. The study analyzed again underscored the remarkable lack of unwanted cardiac electrophysiological effects of mexiletine. There were no problems of bradyarrhythmias or AV conduction defects.

ACKNOWLEDGMENT

Academic Cardiology is supported by the British Heart Foundation.

REFERENCES

1. IMPACT Research Group. International mexiletine and placebo antiarrhythmic coronary trial: 1. Report on arrhythmia and other findings. J Am Coll Cardiol 1984; 4(6):1148–63.
2. Chamberlain DA, Jewitt DE, Julian DG, Campbell RW, Boyle DM, Shanks RG.

Oral mexiletine in high-risk patients after myocardial infarction. Lancet 1980; 2: 1324–1327.

3. Wyman MG, Hammersmith L. Comprehensive treatment plan for the prevention of primary ventricular fibrillation in acute myocardial infarction. Am J Cardiol 1974; 33:661–667.

4. Mogensen L. Ventricular tachyarrhythmias and lignocaine prophylaxis in acute myocardial infarction. Acta Med Scand 1970; suppl 513:1–580.

5. Lown B, Klein MD, Hershberg PI. Coronary and pre-coronary care. Am J Med 1969; 46:705.

6. Lown B, Vasaux C, Hood Jr WB, Fakhro AM, Kaplinsky E, Roberge G. Unresolved problems in coronary care. Am J Cardiol 1967; 20(4): 494–508.

7. Bigger JT, Fleiss JL, Kleiger R, Miller JP, Rolnitzky LM. The relationships among ventricular arrhythmias, left ventricular dysfunction, and mortality in the two years after myocardial infarction. Circulation 1984; 69:250–258.

8. Moss AJ, DeCamilla J, Davis H. Cardiac death in the first 6 months after myocardial infarction: potential for mortality reduction in the early posthospital period. Am J Cardiol 1977; 39(6):816–820.

9. Rehnqvist N. Ventricular arrhythmias after an acute myocardial infarction. Eur J Cardiol 1978; 7:169–187.

10. Kotler MN, Tabatznik B, Mower MM, Tominaga S. Prognostic significance of ventricular ectopic beats with respect to sudden death in the late postinfarction period. Circulation 1973; 47:959–966.

11. CAST. The Cardiac Arrhythmia Suppression Trial Investigators. Preliminary report: effect of encainide and flecainide on mortality in a randomised trial of arrhythmia suppression after myocardial infarction. N Engl J Med 1989; 321:406–412.

12. Campbell RWF, Dolder MA, Prescott LF, Talbot RG, Murray A, Julian DG. Comparison of procainamide and mexiletine in prevention of ventricular arrhythmias after acute myocardial infarction. Lancet 1975; 1(7919):1257–1260.

13. Renard M, de Hemptinne J, Gillet JM, Bernard R. Hemodynamic effects of parenteral and oral mexiletine. Acta Cardiol 1980; 25:75–80.

14. Achuff SC, Pottage A, Prescott L, Campbell RW, Murray A, Julian DG. Mexiletine in the prevention of ventricular arrhythmias in acute myocardial infarction. Postgrad Med J 1977; 53(suppl 1):163–165.

15. Peter T, Ross D, Duffield A, Luxton M, Harper R, Hunt D, Sloman G. Effect on survival after myocardial infarction of long-term treatment with phenytoin. Br Heart J 1978; 40(12):1356–1360.

16. Kosowsky BD, Taylor J, Lown B, Ritchie RF. Long-term use of procainamide following acute myocardial infarction. Circulation 1973; 47(6):1204–1210.

17. Hugenholtz PG, Hagemeijer F, Lubsen J, Glazer B, Durme JPV, Bogaert MG. One-year follow-up in patients with persistent ventricular dysrhythmias after myocardial infarction treated with aprindine and placebo. In: Sandoe E, Julian DG, Bell J, ed. Management of ventricular tachycardia—role of mexiletine. Amsterdam: Excerpta Medica, 1978: 572–578.

18. A Multicentre International Study. Improvement in prognosis of myocardial infarction by long term adrenoreceptor blockade using practolol. Br Med J 1975; 3: 735–740.

19. Wilhelmsson C, Vedin JA, Wilhelmsen L, Tibblin G, Werko L. Reduction of sudden deaths after myocardial infarction by treatment with Alprenalol. Lancet 1974; 2: 1157–1159.
20. IMPACT Research Group. International mexilitene and placebo antiarrhythmic coronary trial:II. Results from 24-hour electrocardiograms. Eur Heart J 1986; 7:749–759.
21. Chamberlain DA, Jewitt DE, Julian DG, Campbell RW, Boyle DM, Shanks RG. Oral mexiletine in high-risk patients after myocardial infarction. Lancet 1980; 2: 1324–1327.
22. IMPACT Research Group. International mexiletine and placebo antiarrhythmic coronary trial: 1. Report on arrhythmia and other findings. J Am Coll Cardiol 1984; 4(6):1148–1163.
23. IMPACT Research Group. International mexilitene and placebo antiarrhythmic coronary trial:II. Results from 24-hour electrocardiograms. Eur Heart J 1986; 7:749–759.
24. CAST. The Cardiac Arrhythmia Suppression Trial Investigators. Preliminary report: effect of encainide and flecainide on mortality in a randomised trial of arrhythmia suppression after myocardial infarction. N Engl J Med 1989; 321:406–412.
25. Camm AJ, Julian D, Janse G, Munoz A, Schwartz P, Simon P, Frangin G. The European Myocardial Infarct Amiodarone Trial (EMIAT). EMIAT Investigators. Am J Cardiol 1993; 72(16):95F–98F.
26. Cairns JA, Connolly SJ, Roberts R, Gent M. for the Canadian Amiodarone Myocardial Infarction Arrhythmia Trial Investigators. Randomised trial of outcome after myocardial infarction in patients with frequent or repetitive ventricular premature depolarisations: CAMIAT. Lancet 1997; 349(9053):675–682.

DAN M. RODEN

Vanderbilt University Medical Center, Nashville, Tennessee

IMPACT (International Mexiletine and Placebo Antiarrhythmic Coronary Trial) (1) was designed in the early 1980s, when what we knew about sudden cardiac death was that it was very common in the post-MI patient (2), was likely due to ventricular fibrillation (VF) in most patients, and that the risk increased as a function of the extent of LV damage and of frequency of PVCs (3). It was recognized that the mechanisms underlying ectopic activity and those underlying VF could be different, although we did not know much about the mechanisms of each. PVCs, we thought (and perhaps still do), acted in some way as a trigger to VF, so reducing the frequency of PVCs might help the problem of sudden death at least indirectly. The possibility that drugs might directly modify the risk of VF, independent of any such beneficial effect on the trigger, had been raised in animal experiments (4), but this concept did not achieve wide currency until the results of CAST, which so definitively showed that it was possible to nearly abolish PVCs and yet increase risk of sudden death.

Mexiletine, a close structural analog of lidocaine, was developed in the 1970s (5) when the benefits of lidocaine therapy for ventricular arrhythmias were near-unquestioned. Thus, there was an intense desire on the part of the cardiovascular community to be able to confer the perceived benefits of such therapy by chronic oral treatment with an analog that would produce the same electrophysiological effects but would not be subject to the extensive first-pass metabolism that prevents the oral use of lidocaine.

One of the first large trials with mexiletine, or indeed any oral antiarrhythmic, was conducted before IMPACT, in 344 patients judged within 1 to 3 days following an acute myocardial infarction to be at high risk for sudden death (6). Criteria applied were persistent ST segment elevation, pulmonary edema on chest x-ray, sinus tachycardia or left bundle branch block, all of which probably indicate more extensive infarction. In this study, the presence of ventricular arrhythmias was not an entry criterion, demonstrating that the dissociation between ventricular ectopy and sudden death was recognized. Patients did undergo Holter monitoring 6 to 10 days following the infarct. The trial was double-blind and randomized and a fixed dosage, based on weight, was used, although the dosage could be reduced in subjects who developed side effects. The trial lasted only 3 months, and there were monthly follow-up visits, with Holters at 1 and 3 months. Unexpected deaths were attributed to arrhythmia.

There was an imbalance in the number of patients assigned to the two arms: 181 to mexiletine and 163 to placebo. Nevertheless, the two groups were described as similar with respect to baseline characteristics. There was no significant difference in mortality in the two arms: 24/181 (13.2%) in patients randomized to mexiletine and 19/163 (11.6%) in those randomized to placebo. Although plasma concentrations below the therapeutic range were documented in a substantial proportion of patients (e.g., 29% at 1 month), there was also a relatively high incidence of side effects in drug-treated patients. Thus, it is unlikely that fixed higher dosages of mexiletine could have been used, although titration to a target concentration (as in BHAT) or to PVC suppression (as in CAST) were other formal possibilities. As in other trials, the frequency of ventricular arrhythmias rose in the 3 months following infarction in placebo-treated patients, but this trend was blunted in the drug-treated patients. Most (>90%) of patients had some ventricular ectopy at baseline, but very frequent ectopics or runs were seen in a minority.

One conclusion drawn by the investigators was that severe ventricular arrhythmias were a serious prognostic factor in this group. However, the power of the trial appears insufficient to make any definitive comment in this regard. More generally, the major result—that mexiletine did not reduce mortality in a predefined high-risk group—probably holds, despite the small size of the trial. The trial did not have the power to formally test the possibility that mexiletine exerted a beneficial effect in patients with baseline arrhythmia (the PVC hypothesis). Nevertheless, the subgroup analysis did not suggest this result. Moreover, if the drug exerted a benefit in such a subgroup, it would have had to exert substantial harm in the complementary subgroup in order to have produced the overall mortality effect observed.

The IMPACT investigators viewed this result as showing that mexiletine should not be further assessed in very high-risk patients. The problem with this approach is that very large numbers of patients would therefore be required to provide sufficient power to detect a mortality-sparing effect of drug in a lower risk group. Therefore, IMPACT was essentially designed as a pilot study and its primary endpoint was reduction in ectopic beat frequency, not mortality. Patients with recent myocardial infarction were again recruited, but the high-risk criteria used in the previous trial were not applied. Again, arrhythmia at entry was not a criterion, and Holter monitors were obtained at baseline (3–25 days postinfarct) and at 1, 4, and 12 months. The power calculation when the trial began assumed a 40% reduction in ectopic beats by drug (an anticipated 30% prevalence in the placebo group vs. 18% in the drug-treated group) and 600 patients. This number gave a power of 89% of detecting such a reduction in ectopic beat frequency, but only 17% for detecting a 20 to 25% reduction in mortality if placebo mortality in the first year was assumed to be 10%. As in the previous trial, only a minority of patients in IMPACT had baseline arrhythmia, and mexiletine appeared to exert a very modest antiarrhythmic effect over time. For example, 92 out of 300 drug-treated patients had "frequent or complex arrhythmia" (the predefined endpoint) at baseline versus 112/298 placebo-treated patients (30.7% vs. 37.6%). More importantly, the mortality rates were smaller than expected on placebo (4.8%) and were substantially (but, because of the power considerations above, not statistically significantly) higher on drug (7.6%). The Holter recordings were subject to considerable quality control (7), an important step later adopted in CAST. At 1 and 4 (but not 12) months, the incidence was significantly higher in placebo-treated patients (e.g., 41.7% vs. 59.9% at 4 months). Interestingly, the mindset of the investigators was so focused on PVC suppression that the 12-month result was termed "a favorable trend in antiarrhythmic efficacy" of the drug (7). Another important trial design aspect was the implementation of a system of computer-linked coordinating centers, an approach that presaged current international drug trial efforts (8).

Issues of whether the dosage was sufficient to reduce arrhythmias or mortality were considered (especially as the plasma concentrations were, in this trial as in the previous one, frequently "subtherapeutic); however, as in the previous trial, the incidence of side effects and of arrhythmia suppression suggested that use of fixed higher dosages was unlikely to give a substantially different result. A later trial targeting "therapeutic concentrations" of procainamide, quinidine, or mexiletine in a high-risk group (inducible arrhythmias 1 to 4 weeks following myocardial infarction) showed no effect (or trend) on mortality, but the study was very small (9).

With the benefit of hindsight, it is easy to criticize the design, conduct, and interpretation of trials such as IMPACT. The trial was powered to detect a change in what we now think of as a marginally relevant endpoint; it used fixed doses of antiarrhythmic; and a "low-risk" group was recruited. However, we should be very careful not to adopt a sort of intellectual arrogance with respect to what we think we now understand about mechanisms of drug action, and sources of variability in patient response to drugs. IMPACT was one of the first large trials to actually address the possibility that chronic antiarrhythmic drug therapy might save lives. One important outcome of IMPACT was that it was possible to conduct a large multicenter trial to address this issue; another was that mexiletine was probably not the right drug—or at least probably not in the population studied in IMPACT—with which to test this hypothesis. Nevertheless, the feasibility aspects of the trial did provide important, and unfortunately often overlooked, lessons as the larger and definitive trials of antiarrhythmic therapy the late 1980s and 1990s (i.e., CAST, AVID, etc.) unfolded. The molecular lessons of the long QT syndromes (where mexiletine may play a role, although this is far from proven), and the striking success of the mechanism-based nonpharmacological therapy of ablation (as well as ICDs) are eloquent testimony to how far we have come in management of arrhythmias since the design of IMPACT.

ACKNOWLEDGMENTS

Supported in part by grants from the United States Public Health Service (HL49989, HL46681). Dr. Roden is the holder of the William Stokes Chair in Experimental Therapeutics, a gift from the Daiichi Corporation.

REFERENCES

1. IMPACT Research Group. International mexiletine and placebo antiarrhythmic coronary trial: I. Report on arrhythmia and other findings. J Am Coll Cardiol 1984; 4: 1148–1163.
2. Lown B, Wolf M. Approaches to sudden death from coronary heart disease. Circulation 1971; 44:130–140.
3. Schulze RAJ, Strauss HW, Pitt B. Sudden death in the year following myocardial infarction. Relation to ventricular premature contractions in the late hospitals phase and left ventricular ejection fraction. Am J Med 1977; 62:192–199.
4. Nattel S, Pedersen DH, Zipes DP. Alterations in regional myocardial distribution and arrhythmogenic effects of aprindine produced by coronary artery occlusion in the dog. Cardiovasc Res 1981; 15:80–85.
5. Campbell NPS, Chaturvedi NC, Shanks RG, Kelly JG, Strong JE, Adgey AAJ. The development of mexiletine in the management of ventricular dysrhythmias. Postgrad Med 1977; 53 (suppl I):114–119.
6. Chamberlain DA, Jewitt DE, Julian DG, Campbell RWF, Boyle DMC, Shanks RG. Oral mexiletine in high-risk patients after myocardial infarction. Lancet 1980; 2: 1324–1327.
7. IMPACT Research Group. International Mexiletine and Placebo Antiarrhythmic Coronary Trial (IMPACT): II. Results from 24-hour electrocardiograms. Eur Heart J 1986; 7:749–759.
8. Alamercery Y, Wilkins P, Karrison T. Functional equality of coordinating centers in a multicenter clinical trial. Experience of the International Mexiletine and Placebo Antiarrhythmic Coronary Trial (IMPACT). Controlled Clin Trials 1986; 7:38–52.
9. Denniss AR, Ross DL, Cody DV, Russell PA, Young AA, Richards DA, Uther JB. Randomized controlled trial of prophylactic antiarrhythmic therapy in patients with inducible ventricular tachyarrhythmias after recent myocardial infarction. Eur Heart J 1988; 9:746–757.

2

The Cardiac Arrhythmia Suppression Trials (CAST): A Retrospective Perspective

D. GEORGE WYSE
The University of Calgary, Calgary, Alberta, Canada

OVERVIEW OF BACKGROUND FOR STUDY DESIGN

It is now over 10 years since the beginning of the planning phase for the Cardiac Arrhythmia Suppression Trials (CAST). Accordingly, it may be instructive to review briefly the state of knowledge upon which the trial was based in the context of that time period.

At that point in time the implantable cardioverter defibrillator was only in its early developmental stage. The primary treatment modality for cardiac arrhythmias was pharmacological. Several promising new agents seemed poised to launch a new era of pharmacological arrhythmia management. Furthermore, contemporary evidence indicated that ambulatory electrocardiographic (AECG) recordings effectively identified a subgroup of patients with recent myocardial infarction who had increased risk of death (1), presumably at least partly on the basis of fatal arrhythmia.

The confluence of contemporary evidence seemed ideal for the launch of a study to evaluate critically the hypothesis that selective pharmacological arrhythmia treatment after myocardial infarction had salutary benefit. Studies of antiarrhythmics after myocardial infarction to that point in time had not selected high-risk patients and the available antiarrhythmic agents were poorly tolerated by patients (2). Furthermore, recent studies had demonstrated the benefit of beta-adrenoceptor blocking agents in patients who had had a recent myocardial infarction. There was considerable optimism that pharmacological manipulation of arrhythmic death and other risk following myocardial infarction was a concept whose time had come. Sadly, antiarrhythmic drug therapy would prove to be undeserving of this optimistic viewpoint and contrasts sharply with other preventative drug therapies such as angiotensin-converting enzyme inhibitors and statin cholesterol lowering agents when they were subsequently evaluated in this same setting.

The initial study plan for CAST outlined in the Request for Proposals (RFP) of the National Heart, Lung and Blood Institute (NHLBI) was based on a research plan proven successful for beta-adrenoceptor blocking agents, in particular propranolol. That is, pharmacological agents would be evaluated in a double-blind, placebo-controlled design among patients who had had a recent myocardial infarction. The one refinement that was added to the RFP in comparison to earlier antiarrhythmic drug studies was that patients would be selected as those having higher risk for arrhythmic death on the basis of reduced left ventricular function and frequent and/or complex ventricular ectopy on a 24-h AECG.

Given this broad outline, respondents to the RFP were asked to describe the protocol they would use to evaluate the hypothesis that use of antiarrhythmic drugs in a selected population of postmyocardial infarction patients would reduce the risk of arrhythmic death. Approximately 25 responding centers selected to undertake the study began to meet as the Steering/Planning Committee. It was at this time that the investigators made the fateful decision to follow a protocol that would evaluate the ''suppression hypothesis.'' Simply stated, the ''suppression hypothesis'' stated that if the risk of arrhythmic death was conferred by frequent and complex ventricular ectopy acting as ''triggers'' for fatal ventricular tachycardia/fibrillation (VT/VF), then the proposed benefit of antiarrhythmic drugs would be most clearly seen in those subjects whose ventricular ectopy was suppressed by the antiarrhythmic drugs. Accordingly, it was agreed that only patients whose arrhythmia was suppressed by drugs would be included in the randomized, placebo-controlled portion of the study. Fortunately, it was also agreed that patients whose arrhythmia could not be suppressed by open-label drug titration would be followed, but not randomized. Part of the rationale for this approach was that if arrhythmia suppression could be causally linked to reduced arrhythmic death, then in subsequent trials arrhythmia suppression could be studied as a validated surrogate endpoint. These decisions in the planning phase had important consequences with respect to the ultimate results of CAST.

PROTOCOL FOR CAST

The first inclusion criterion was a history of proven myocardial infarction 6 days to 2 years prior to the qualifying AECG (3). There was considerable debate among the Planning/Steering Committee about the most appropriate time window within which the qualifying myocardial infarction should have occurred. During the planning phase, the investigators had access to unpublished databases that suggested the rate of occurrence of arrhythmic death following myocardial infarction was linear over at least 4 years. Accordingly, it was decided that the qualifying infarction could have occurred up to 2 years prior to enrollment. The second inclusion criterion was reduced left ventricular function. This criterion was used differentially, depending on the recency of myocardial infarction, in order to enroll a higher risk study group. When the onset of myocardial infarction was <90 days from qualifying AECG, the left ventricular ejection fraction (LVEF) was ≤0.55, and when it was ≥90 days, LVEF was ≤0.40. The third and final inclusion criterion was a 24-h AECG, with at least 18 analyzable hours, showing an average ≥6 ventricular premature depolarizations (VPDs) per hour. There were a number of exclusion criteria (3), which mainly dealt with perceived requirement for antiarrhythmic drug therapy, medical contraindications, potential administrative problems, and lack of consent.

The study began with an open-label titration phase. A lower dose of the first drug to be evaluated was randomly assigned from the three drugs available (see below). After allowing an appropriate period of time to achieve steady state, the degree of arrhythmia suppression was measured by a repeat 24-h AECG. The doses of antiarrhythmic drug and the time to steady state were based on data from the pilot study, Cardiac Arrhythmia Pilot Study (CAPS) (4). The protocol allowed for a higher dosage of the first drug to be used when suppression was not achieved. Furthermore, up to two doses each of a second, and sometime third, drug could be evaluated in the open-label titration phase when suppression was not achieved or intolerable adverse effects were noted. Flecainide use was not permitted when LVEF was <0.30. Therefore, the potential number of drug/dose trials before categorization of a patient as "nonsuppressed" was 6 for those with LVEF ≥0.30 and 4 for those with LVEF <0.30. It was required that drug titration be completed within 90 days of enrollment. Suppression of arrhythmia was defined as ≥ 80% reduction in the total number of VPDs, plus ≥90% suppression of runs of VPDs. When suppression was proven using a well-tolerated drug and dose, the patient was randomized into the main study with equal probability to drug or matching placebo administered in a double-blind fashion. Partially suppressed patients were similarly randomized in a separate stratum in a substudy. Those patients whose VPDs were nonsuppressed (i.e., same or increased frequency) were not randomized but were followed without any specific antiarrhythmic therapy using the same schedule as the main study.

Figure 1 presents an overview of the CAST protocol showing the three general groups of patients enrolled: those who entered drug titration but who were not randomized for a variety of reasons (19%); those whose arrhythmia was suppressed during drug titration and who were randomized to active drug or placebo (main study, 75%); and those whose arrhythmia was partially suppressed and who were randomized to the best active drug or placebo (6%).

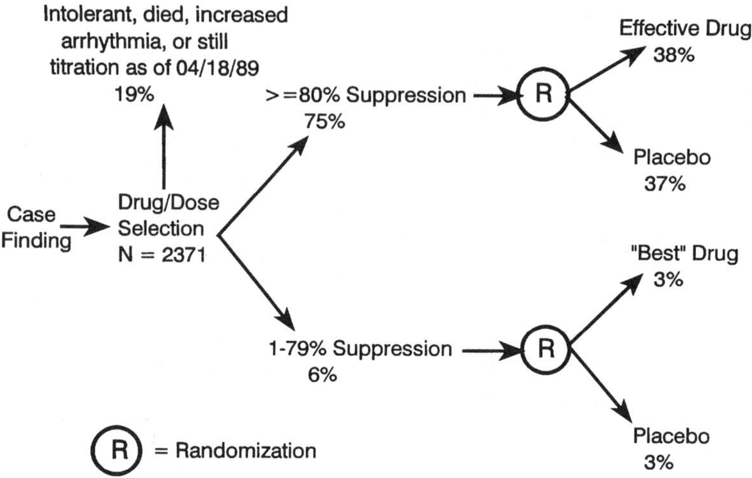

Figure 1   Overview of the CAST protocol illustrating the three general groups of patients (see text).

DRUG SELECTION FOR CAST

Clearly one of the most fateful decisions in the planning of CAST was the selection of the three antiarrhythmic drugs—encainide, flecainide, and moricizine. As with many decisions made in the planning phase, the preliminary literature search and deliberation leading to a recommendation to the Planning/Steering Committee was undertaken by a subcommittee of the investigators. The investigators responding to the RFP included some who had participated in CAPS but even more who had not participated in that study. Accordingly, the variety of drugs proposed included virtually all approved and investigational drugs available at that time. In considering these suggestions, the drug selection subcommittee first set criteria for levels of evidence needed to properly evaluate the available drugs. For some older agents, such as quinidine, it was felt that there was already ample evidence that these drugs were poorly tolerated and had low efficacy. Indeed, in CAPS, the drug imipramine was included as a ''surrogate'' for the class 1a agents, and it was shown that this drug had poor efficacy and was not well tolerated (5). Amiodarone was considered by the subcommittee but it was felt that the many adverse effects of this agent would lead to an unacceptably high dropout rate. Several other suggestions, such as combination therapy with a class 1a and 1b antiarrhythmic agents, were rejected because there were too few data upon which to base a decision. CAPS was the most robust data upon which to base a decision concerning newer drugs available at that time (4). The CAPS data clearly showed that encainide and flecainide were very effective for suppression of VPDs in this patient population and they were tolerated as well as or better than placebo (5). Moricizine was not quite as effective as the other two agents but was also well tolerated. Importantly, moricizine's efficacy did not seem to be reduced after encainide or flecainide had failed to adequately suppress VPDs. On the basis of the recommendation of the drug selection subcommittee, the Planning/Steering Committee accepted that encainide, flecainide, and moricizine be the three drugs used in the trial. The investigators were again at least partly motivated by the notion that they wished to evaluate the suppression hypothesis. In testing the suppression hypothesis, it seemed less important whether a particular drug or group of drugs was selected and more important that the strategy produced effective VPD suppression as quickly as possible, with the fewest adverse effects in order to minimize dropouts. Accordingly, the study adopted the randomly selected sequences for drug titration of flecainide–moricizine–encainide or encainide–moricizine–flecainide for those patients with LVEF $\geq$0.30 and encainide–moricizine or moricizine–encainide for those with LVEF $<$0.30.

RESULTS OF CAST

The results of CAST are now well know to most and are illustrated in Figures 2 and 3. CAST enrollment was prematurely terminated on April 18, 1989, on

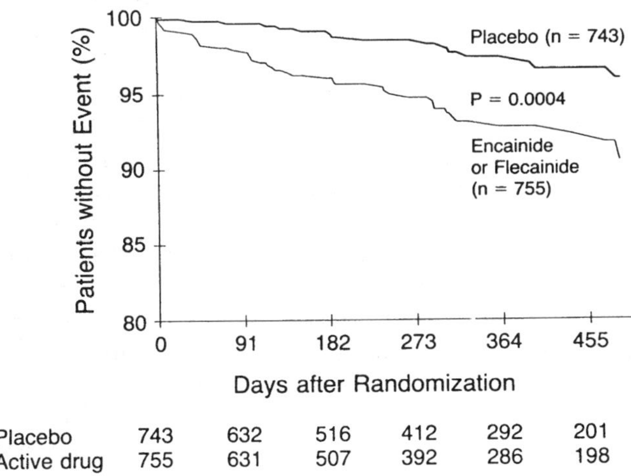

Placebo	743	632	516	412	292	201
Active drug	755	631	507	392	286	198

Figure 2 Effect of encainide and flecainide on arrhythmic death in CAST. (Reproduced with permission from Ref. 3.)

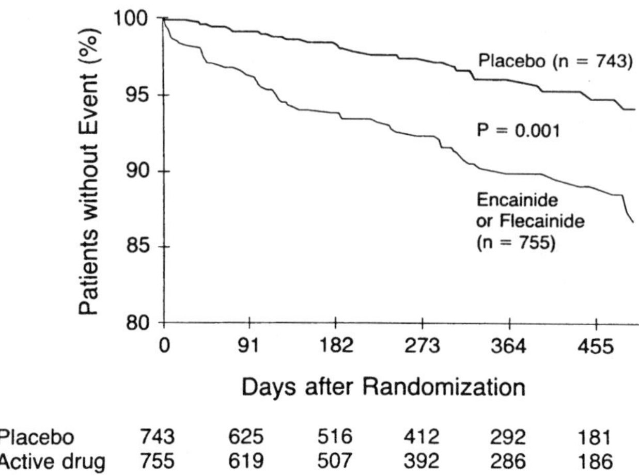

| Placebo | 743 | 625 | 516 | 412 | 292 | 181 |
| Active drug | 755 | 619 | 507 | 392 | 286 | 186 |

Figure 3 Effect of encainide and flecainide on total mortality in CAST. (Reproduced with permission from Ref. 3.)

recommendation of the Data and Safety Monitoring Board (DSMB) when it became clear that there was excess mortality in those subjects treated with antiarrhythmic drugs. The primary endpoint of CAST was arrhythmic death or resuscitated cardiac arrest (Fig. 2), but the harmful effects of the drugs were consistent whether the primary endpoint or total mortality (Fig. 3) was examined. Further subgroup analysis suggested that the harmful effect was confined to those treated with encainide and flecainide. The actual recommendation of the DSMB was that randomization to encainide and flecainide be discontinued. The Executive Committee immediately stopped enrollment when informed of these results and began to discontinue treatment with encainide and flecainide as quickly as possible. Although the investigators were unaware of it, it became apparent later that there was actually a trend for benefit in those patients randomized to moricizine (Fig. 4). Even without the benefit of that particular knowledge, the Steering Committee met quickly and prepared to disseminate the trial results as soon as possible for safety reasons. At that time, both flecainide and encainide were already being prescribed outside the trial. The result of that effort was the ''preliminary report'' (6), followed later by a more detailed report when the data analysis was complete (3). The Steering Committee also made a decision to continue with randomization to moricizine or its placebo, and based on the preliminary results, some changes were made in the protocol.

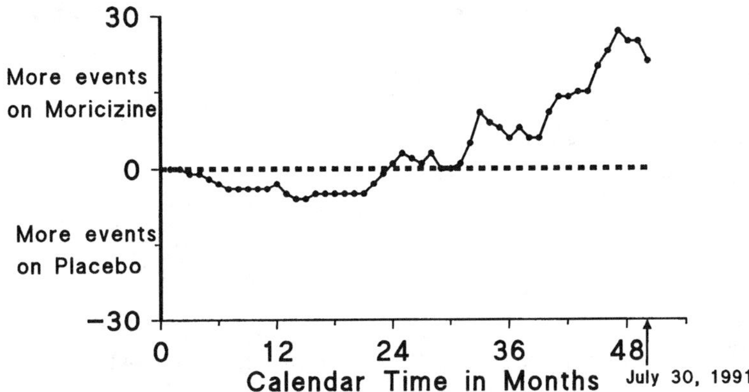

Figure 4 Temporal trends for death or nonfatal cardiac arrest in the long-term phase of CAST-II. The vertical axis is the number of events in patients receiving moricizine minus the number of events in patients receiving placebo.

MODIFICATION OF PROTOCOL FOR CAST-II

Although at the end of CAST the Steering Committee did not know there was a favorable trend with moricizine, it was widely speculated to be the case. The investigators wished to maximize their opportunity to detect such a beneficial effect. To do so, several changes were made in the protocol before randomization restarted (7). First, however, it was decided to continue all randomized patients in CAST who had already been randomized to moricizine or its placebo. It was apparent from the preliminary CAST data that the rate of endpoints in the subset of patients enrolled more than 90 days after their qualifying myocardial infarction who had well-preserved ventricular function was very low. Accordingly, it was determined that only those with a qualifying myocardial infarction 4 days to 90 days prior to the qualifying AECG and left ventricular ejection fraction ≤0.40 would be included. Those surviving and consenting CAST patients who were previously randomized to encainide, flecainide, or their placebos or who were in the titration phase at the time CAST was ended were also allowed to continue if they still met the AECG criteria after their original treatment was discontinued. A third (higher) dose of moricizine was also permitted in CAST-II. These patients were retitrated in the new protocol and randomized with equal probability to moricizine or placebo when suppression or partial suppression was observed. The flow of patients between CAST and CAST-II is illustrated in Figure 5. Of the 1374 patients randomized in CAST-II, 360 had been previously randomized to

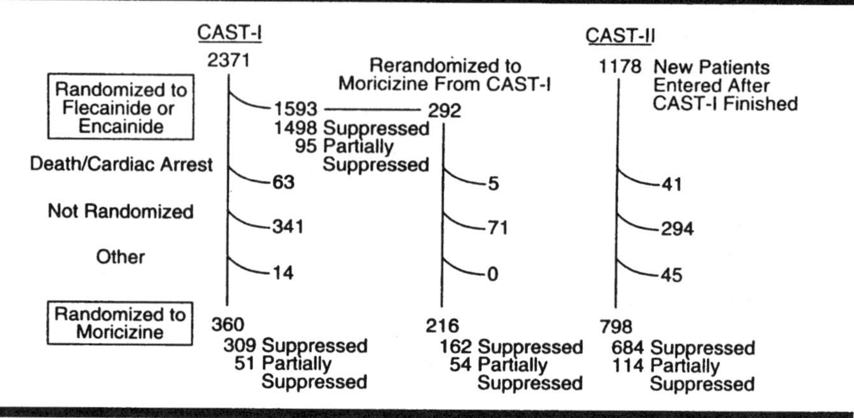

Figure 5 Flow diagram of patients who entered CAST and CAST-II. (Reproduced with permission from Ref. 8.)

moricizine or placebo in CAST, 216 were formerly on flecainide, encainide, or their placebo, and 798 were new patients who qualified under the CAST-II protocol.

One other major change in the protocol was made. In CAST, the titration phase had been open-labeled. Clearly, open-label titration left the possibility that there were a significant number of events attributable to drug effects occurring during the open-label phase. Thus it was decided that the first 14 days of titration in CAST-II would be double-blinded to evaluate the frequency of events in the titration phase. With approval of these changes, enrollment and randomization were restarted. An overview of the CAST-II protocol is presented in Figure 6.

RESULTS OF CAST-II

As can be seen in Figure 4, the favorable trend with moricizine did not persist. Enrollment in CAST-II was terminated on July 30, 1991, on the recommendation of the DSMB because of a preset futility criterion. That is, it was determined at a specially scheduled review of the data that there was virtually no likelihood of showing a benefit from moricizine, even if the study was continued to its planned termination. Indeed, if the study had been continued, it was more likely that results similar to those seen in CAST with encainide and flecainide would have been observed (Fig. 4). In the randomized, long-term portion of CAST-II, there was no difference between active drug and placebo with respect to the primary endpoint of arrhythmic death or resuscitated cardiac arrest (Fig. 7). In comparing

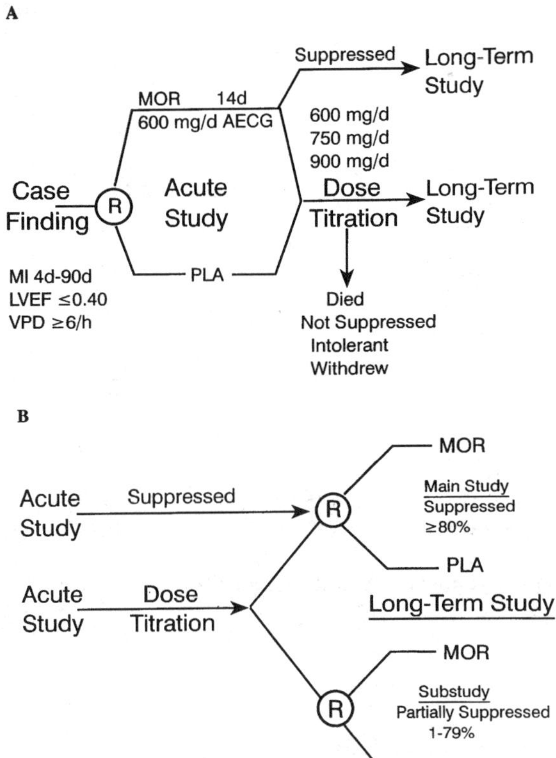

Figure 6 Overview of the CAST-II protocol. Panel A represents the placebo-controlled initial 2 weeks of therapy (acute study). Panel B represents the placebo-controlled treatment after assessment of arrhythmia suppression (long-term study).

Figures 4 and 7, it should be noted that Figure 4 illustrates total mortality and Figure 7 illustrates arrhythmic mortality. Furthermore, in the first 14 days of the titration phase, moricizine actually increased total mortality (Fig. 8). With the publication of these results, the main findings of CAST and CAST-II were complete. A number of subsequent analyses of the database provided some further insight into various aspects of arrhythmia management in this postmyocardial infarction group.

ANALYSIS OF CAST/CAST-II BY ORIGINAL DESIGN

As was outlined at the beginning of this chapter, part of the philosophy behind the initial planning of CAST/CAST-II was that the particular drug used was less

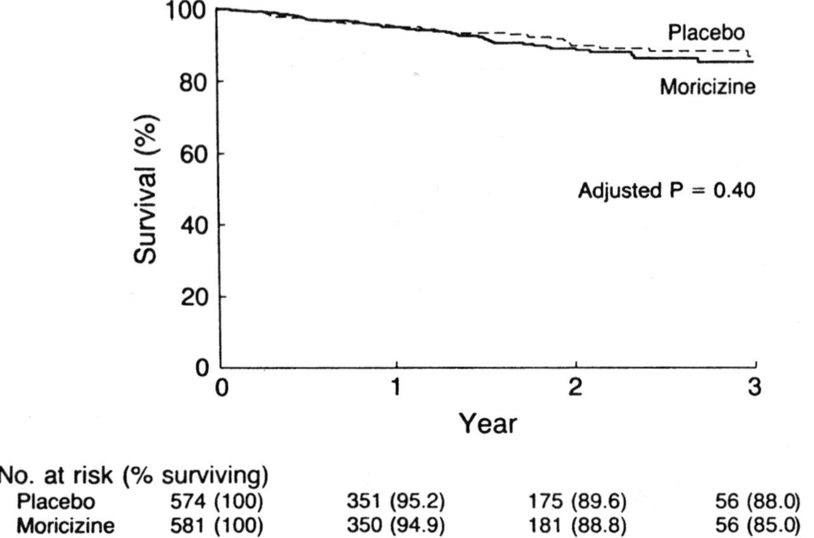

No. at risk (% surviving)

Placebo	574 (100)	351 (95.2)	175 (89.6)	56 (88.0)
Moricizine	581 (100)	350 (94.9)	181 (88.8)	56 (85.0)

Figure 7 Effect of moricizine on arrhythmic death in the long-term phase of CAST-II. (Reproduced with permission from Ref. 7.)

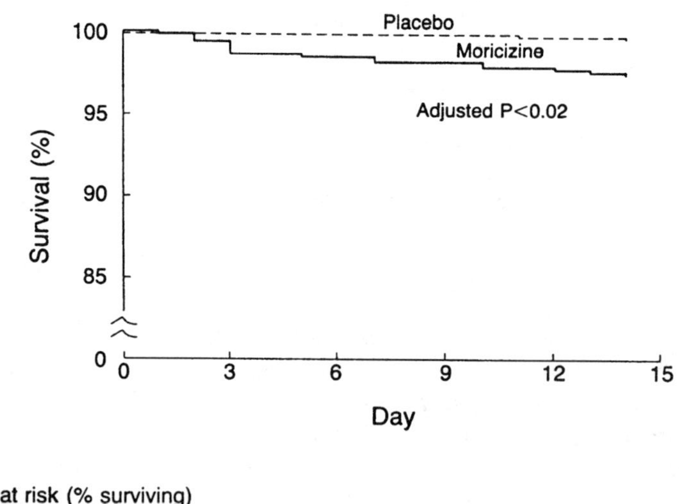

No. at risk (% surviving)

Placebo	660 (100)	659 (99.9)	658 (99.7)
Moricizine	665 (100)	655 (98.5)	608 (97.7)

Figure 8 Effect of moricizine on total mortality or nonfatal cardiac arrest during the first 14 days of treatment in CAST-II. (Reproduced with permission from Ref. 7.)

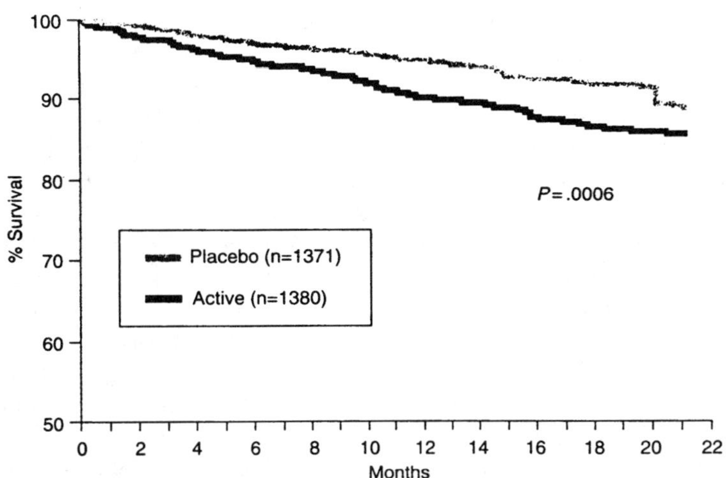

Figure 9   Effect of encainide, flecainide, and moricizine on total mortality in CAST and CAST-II by the original trial design. (Reproduced with permission from Ref. 8.)

important than the actual suppression of arrhythmia. These two studies clearly showed that arrhythmia suppression and survival benefit could be separated from one another. Thus it seems likely that arrhythmia suppression is a by-product rather than the primary effect of drugs that prevent arrhythmic death. The exact interplay between these factors is incompletely understood even at this time. Nevertheless, an analysis of the data according to the original design has been published (8). The results of this analysis (Fig. 9) reinforce the conclusion that arrhythmia suppression in itself is not sufficient to ensure a survival benefit in these patients.

IMPORTANT CAST/CAST-II SUBANALYSES

There have indeed been several subanalyses of the CAST/CAST-II databases. Some of these are particularly instructive with respect to the problem of arrhythmia management in the postmyocardial infarction population.

One of the more instructive analysis was evaluation and follow up of the 318 patients in CAST who were not randomized because their arrhythmia was not suppressed, they had adverse drug effects, or they withdrew consent. These 318 patients were compared to 942 randomized patients who were treated with placebo (9). The mortality in the nonrandomized patients was greater than that of the randomized placebo patients but they were also different in several other

respects. When compared to randomized placebo patients with similar characteristics (e.g., age, left ventricular ejection fraction), the difference in mortality between the two groups disappeared. However, inability of these sicker patients to
progress from drug titration to randomization at least partly explains the lower
than expected mortality in the randomized placebo group in CAST. Perhaps the
most interesting finding in the nonrandomized group, however, was that transient
ECG changes (mostly proarrhythmia) during drug titration markedly and independently increased the hazard ratio for arrhythmic death or resuscitated cardiac
arrest (relative risk 7.0; $p < 0.005$) (9), even when antiarrhythmic therapy was
not given. A subsequent analysis also demonstrated that the converse was also
true, that ease of arrhythmia suppression was an independent favorable prognostic
factor (10). Thus, ease of VPD suppression by drugs in this population in itself
identifies lower risk patients and conversely increased VPDs caused by drugs in
itself identifies higher risk patients.

Other important insights emerged from additional analyses. Certainly, the
concept that proarrhythmia from antiarrhythmic drugs was a problem only at the
onset of therapy was no longer tenable. Proarrhythmic mortality continued to
occur for the duration of CAST. Other observations relevant to proarrhythmia
were made using the CAST and CAPS databases. For example, fatal proarrhythmia occurred in spite of the fact that there was little evidence of measured arrhythmia increase (11). Furthermore, increased arrhythmia on AECG categorized as

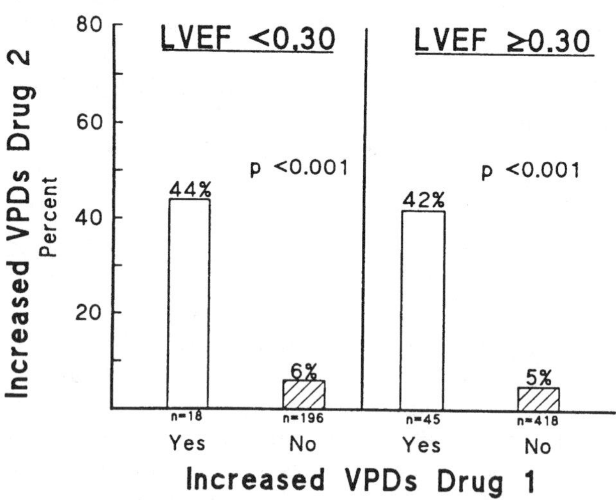

Figure 10   Proarrhythmia on the second antiarrhythmic drug in relation to its occurrence
on the first antiarrhythmic drug during drug titration in CAPS, CAST, and CAST-II. (Reproduced with permission from Ref. 11.)

proarrhythmia is frequently spontaneous variability, particularly when the baseline VPD count is low. Finally, when proarrhythmic increases in VPD frequency occur with one drug, they are much more likely to be seen with a second drug (Fig. 10). The deadly combination of poor left ventricular function, heart failure, and antiarrhythmic drugs was strongly noted in CAST (12,13). One consequence of this deadly combination can be seen in Figure 4, where the early favorable trend of treatment with moricizine began to disappear as more patients with poorer ventricular function were enrolled and treated with moricizine in CAST-II. The important salutary benefit of beta-blockers was also seen in CAST/CAST-II as it has been in virtually every study that has looked at the postmyocardial infarction population (14). In particular, beta-blocker therapy was shown to reduce the risk of arrhythmic death as well as total mortality. In those with a history of heart failure, beta-blocker therapy delayed the recurrence of heart failure (14). Finally, the CAST/CAST-II data underline the deficiencies in our methods of selecting an appropriate subset of high-risk patients who are most likely to benefit from antiarrhythmic therapy. Simply setting an upper limit on left ventricular ejection fraction and the detection of frequent VPDs on an AECG seems, in retrospect, to be inadequate.

CONCLUSION

CAST/CAST-II were important studies from which there are many lessons to be learned. In many ways, their results have changed forever the way we think about arrhythmia, antiarrhythmic drugs, and management of the postmyocardial infarction patient.

REFERENCES

1. Bigger JT, Jr, Fleiss JL, Kleiger R, Miller JP, Rolnitzky LM. The relationships among ventricular arrhythmias, left ventricular dysfunction, and mortality in the 2 years after myocardial infarction. Circulation 1984; 69:250–258.
2. Furberg CD. Effect of antiarrhythmic drugs on mortality after myocardial infarction. Am J Cardiol 1983; 52:32C–36C.
3. Echt DS, Liebson PR, Mitchell LB, Peters RW, Obias-Manno D, Barker AH, Arensberg D, Baker A, Friedman L, Greene HL, Huther ML, Richardson DW, and the CAST Investigators. N Engl J Med 1991; 324:781–788.
4. The CAPS Investigators. The Cardiac Arrhythmia Pilot Study. Am J Cardiol 1986; 54:91–95.
5. The Cardiac Arrhythmia Pilot Study (CAPS) Investigators. Effects of encainide, flecainide, imipramine and moricizine on ventricular arrhythmias during the year after acute myocardial infarction: the CAPS. Am J Cardiol 1988; 61:501–509.

6. The Cardiac Arrhythmia Suppression Trial (CAST) Investigators. Preliminary report: effect of encainide and flecainide on mortality in a randomized trial of arrhythmia suppression after myocardial infarction. N Engl J Med 1989; 321:406–412.

7. The Cardiac Arrhythmia Suppression Trial II Investigators. Effect of the antiarrhythmic agent moricizine on survival after myocardial infarction. N Engl J Med 1992; 327:227–233.

8. Epstein AE, Hallstrom AP, Rogers WJ, Liebson PR, Seals AA, Anderson JL, Cohen JD, Capone RJ, Wyse DG, for the CAST Investigators. Mortality following ventricular arrhythmia suppression by encainide, flecainide, and moricizine after myocardial infarction. The original design concept of the Cardiac Arrhythmia Suppression Trial (CAST). JAMA 1993; 270:2451–2455.

9. Wyse DG, Hallstrom A, McBride R, Cohen JD, Steinberg JS, Mahmarian J, and the CAST Investigators. Events in the Cardiac Arrhythmia Suppression Trial (CAST): mortality in patients surviving open label titration but not randomized to double-blind therapy. J Am Coll Cardiol 1991; 18:20–28.

10. Goldstein S, Brooks MM, Ledingham R, Kennedy HL, Epstein AE, Pawitan Y, Bigger JT. Association between ease of suppression of ventricular arrhythmia and survival. Circulation 1995; 91:79–83.

11. Wyse DG, Morganroth J, Ledingham R, Denes P, Hallstrom A, Mitchell LB, Epstein AE, Woosley RL, Capone R, for the CAST and CAPS Investigators. New insights into the definition and meaning of proarrhythmia during initiation of antiarrhythmic drug therapy from the Cardiac Arrhythmia Suppression Trial and its pilot study. J Am Coll Cardiol 1994; 23:1130–1140.

12. Hallstrom A, Pratt CM, Greene HL, Huther M, Gottlieb S, DeMaria A, Young JB, for the Cardiac Suppression Trial Investigators. Relations between heart failure, ejection fraction, arrhythmia suppression and mortality: Analysis of the Cardiac Arrhythmia Suppression Trial. J Am Coll Cardiol 1995; 25:1250–1257.

13. Josephson RA, Chahine RA, Morganroth J, Anderson J, Waldo A, Hallstrom A, for the CAST Investigators: Prediction of cardiac death in patients with very low ejection fraction after myocardial infarction: a Cardiac Arrhythmia Suppression Trial (CAST) study. Am Heart J 1995; 130:685–691.

14. Kennedy HL, Brooks MM, Barker AH, Bergstrand R, Huther ML, Beanlands DS, Bigger JT, Goldstein S, for the CAST Investigators. Beta-blocker therapy in the Cardiac Arrhythmia Suppression Trial. Am J Cardiol 1994; 74:674–680.

CAST: Critique

JEREMY N. RUSKIN

Massachusetts General Hospital, Boston, Massachusetts

The Cardiac Arrhythmia Suppression Trial (CAST) is among the most important clinical trials in the history of cardiac arrhythmia research. The trial was designed to examine the hypothesis that suppressing asymptomatic or mildly symptomatic ventricular ectopic activity after myocardial infarction would reduce the rate of sudden death. This study, which was preceded by a well-designed feasibility study, the Cardiac Arrhythmia Pilot Study, is the first long-term, multicenter, multidrug, placebo-controlled trial of the safety and efficacy of antiarrhythmic drug therapy in reducing the risk of sudden death (1). The results surprised most observers and challenged commonly held beliefs about antiarrhythmic drugs and their role in the treatment of asymptomatic ventricular arrhythmias. The results of CAST-I, which was terminated prematurely in 1989, demonstrated beyond question that the use of encainide and flecainide, two class IC antiarrhythmic agents, to treat asymptomatic or minimally symptomatic ventricular arrhythmias in patients after myocardial infarction was associated with a substantial increase in all-cause mortality and sudden death (2,3). Furthermore, this risk was highly consistent across all patient subgroups and persisted despite the effective suppression of spontaneous ventricular premature beats by these agents. Observations on the efficacy of ethmozine in a similar, but higher-risk, subpopulation (CAST-II), revealed an excess mortality rate with ethmozine during the first 2 weeks of exposure to the drug and no realistic possibility of demonstrating a long-term survival benefit, resulting in premature termination of the trial in 1991 (4).

Although the basis for the excess mortality rate in CAST-I is not clearly defined, this unexpected outcome is best explained by the induction of lethal ventricular arrhythmias (i.e., a proarrhythmic effect) by encainide and flecainide. Other causes of sudden cardiac death, such as asystole, atrioventricular block, and electromechanical dissociation, may also have occurred. While a large majority of excess deaths appeared to be the result of an increase in arrhythmic events, deaths due to acute myocardial infarction with shock or congestive heart failure also occurred more commonly on encainide and flecainide than on placebo, confirming the negative inotropic potential of class IC agents in the setting of acute ischemic injury (3). The fact that nonfatal ischemic endpoints such as myocardial infarction and angina pectoris were significantly more common on placebo to a degree that virtually balanced the excess mortality rate on active drug suggests that encainide and flecainide may have converted nonfatal ischemic events to fatal events by both arrhythmic and nonarrhythmic (mechanical) mechanisms. This effect may result from an interaction between encainide and flecainide and an acutely ischemic substrate. This hypothesis is further supported by the observation that the relative risk for death on encainide or flecainide over placebo was higher in patients with a history of non-Q-wave myocardial infarction than patients with Q-wave MI. In the placebo group, non-Q-MI patients had a significantly lower rate of death and cardiac arrest than Q-wave MI patients (1.0% vs. 4.6%, respectively; $p = 0.04$) (5). Encainide and flecainide were associated with a significantly increased rate of death and cardiac arrest compared with placebo in both non-Q-wave MI patients (8.7%; $p < 0.01$) and Q-wave MI patients (7.8%; $p = 0.04$) (5). However, the relative risk for death on encainide or flecainide over placebo in the non-Q-wave MI patients was 8.7, significantly higher than the 1.7 observed for the Q-wave MI patients ($p = 0.03$) (5). These rather striking observations suggest that the non-Q-wave MI substrate, which likely represents an incomplete infarct that may be vulnerable to chronic residual or recurrent ischemia, exposed patients to a significantly heightened relative risk of death due to an interaction with the proarrhythmic and, possibly, the negative inotropic effects of the IC drugs. Of additional interest is the fact that nonfatal arrhythmic events were equally distributed between active drug and placebo, confirming that the adverse cardiac events on class IC agents were usually fatal.

The mechanisms by which encainide and flecainide increase the risk of sudden death in this population have not been fully defined. Both drugs significantly depress conduction velocity, and this may facilitate reentry under some conditions (6,7). Like other class IC agents, encainide and flecainide appear to exert proarrhythmic effects in patients with sustained ventricular arrhythmias more frequently than other classes of antiarrhythmic drugs. Both encainide and flecainide are associated with inefficient suppression of the sustained ventricular arrhythmias induced by programmed electrical stimulation (8). In addition, encainide and other sodium-channel blockers have been shown to raise the energy requirements for ventricular defibrillation in experimental models (9). More recently, experimental studies examining the modulation of flecainide binding by adrenergic influences have shown reversal of flecainide effects in normal tissue but a paradoxical amplification of flecainide-induced conduction slowing in depolarized tissue in response to adrenergic stimulation (10). These disparate effects in normal and depressed cardiac tissues result in significant dispersion of both conduction and recovery and would, thereby, be expected to enhance susceptibility to reentrant arrhythmias. Which of these mechanisms, if any, contribute to the occurrence of sudden death in patients treated with encainide and flecainide after myocardial infarction is unknown. The interaction of acute ischemia superimposed on healed myocardial infarction in enhancing vulnerability to ventricular fibrillation is well established in experimental models (11). How these interactions might increase susceptibility to drug-induced ventricular proarrhythmia is unknown. These gaps in our knowledge emphasize the need for more basic physiological research on the mechanisms and proarrhythmic effects of antiarrhythmic drugs in clinically relevant experimental models.

The adverse effects of encainide and flecainide on mortality in CAST were highlighted by an extremely low incidence of sudden death (1.2%) and total mortality (3.0%) in the placebo group (2,3). The unexpectedly low mortality placebo group may have been due in part to the unique design of CAST, in which patients with drug-responsive arrhythmias were identified and selected for the randomized, placebo-controlled trial in an open-label titration phase. Deaths during the open-label titration phase and the exclusion of patients with drug-resistant arrhythmias may have contributed to the selection of a low-risk population for the randomized trial (12). The incidence of increased ventricular premature depolarizations (VPD) during therapy was low and equivalent for encainide, flecainide, and moricizine (3% to 5%) and indistinguishable from that seen with placebo (13). When an increase in VPD frequency occurred with the first drug, it was also much more likely to be present with the second drug (13). Furthermore, a marked increase in VPD frequency during initiation of drug therapy independently predicted an increased risk of subsequent arrhythmic death (independent RR 2.34; $p = 0.005$) in the absence of continued antiarrhythmic drug therapy (13). These observations support the contention that patients selected for the main trial were at particularly low risk because those who were at highest risk (i.e., patients whose arrhythmias were exacerbated or not suppressed by drug therapy) were excluded from the study. Of the nonrandomized patients, approximately 70% were not randomized because of lack of suppression of ventricular premature depolarizations or adverse events, or both (14). Despite these limitations, the risk associated with the use of encainide and flecainide in this patient population is clear and inescapable.

The occurrence of a proarrhythmic effect of the magnitude observed in CAST is both striking and unexpected. Previous uncontrolled studies suggested that patients with no history of sustained arrhythmias, like those entered in CAST, were at extremely low risk for class IC drug-induced ventricular proarrhythmia (15). The results of CAST dispelled this view. Despite the fact that the pharmaceutical database experience with encainide and flecainide prior to CAST exceeded 3000 patients, there was no indication of a serious proarrhythmic effect (15,16). In contrast, the high proarrhythmic event rate in the CAST population receiving encainide and flecainide was evident after only 10 months of follow-up in a randomized subset of only 725 patients treated with these agents (2,3,16). The reasons for this discrepancy are complex and include the fact that patients with recent myocardial infarction were generally excluded from the pharmaceutical experience with these drugs (16). In addition, in the flecainide database, as in other uncontrolled observational studies on antiarrhythmic drugs, arrhythmic events that occurred more than 14 days after the initiation of drug therapy were generally attributed to the natural history of the underlying heart disease and not to a drug-induced proarrhythmic mechanism. Survival analyses in CAST have demonstrated that an excess rate of sudden death persisted throughout the entire 10-month follow-up period among patients treated with encainide and flecainide (2,3). This effect would not have been detectable in the absence of a parallel placebo control group. This critical observation challenged traditional concepts of proarrhythmia and disproved the long-held belief that patients are susceptible to drug-induced arrhythmias only in the early period of drug exposure (16,17). The results of CAST, therefore, underscore the power and importance of randomized, placebo-controlled clinical trials in evaluating new therapies and in the detection of unsuspected benefits or liabilities thereof (16).

Despite the limitations of CAST, some practical conclusions can be drawn from the trial (12). First, encainide, flecainide, and other class IC antiarrhythmic drugs should not be used to treat patients with ischemic heart disease. Whether patients with recent myocardial infarction would benefit from other forms of antiarrhythmic therapy directed at the prevention of sudden cardiac death remains to be determined, but studies to date with dofetilide and amiodarone have failed to demonstrate a beneficial effect on all-cause mortality in this population (19). A recent trial with d-sotalol showed an adverse effect on mortality similar to that observed in CAST (20). At the present time, therefore, there is no indication for the use of antiarrhythmic drugs either to suppress ventricular ectopic activity or as routine prophylaxis in patients post myocardial infarction. Beta-adrenergic blocking agents should be administered after infarction to all patients who tolerate them, since they remain the only class of antiarrhythmic drug of established benefit in reducing the risk of sudden cardiac death in this patient population (21). The use of flecainide to treat patients with symptomatic sustained ventricular arrhythmias remains an approved indication if efficacy is established with the use of objective endpoints. In patients with ischemic heart disease and probably with other forms of advanced structural heart disease, it is generally accepted that the use of class IC agents should be avoided whenever possible. As a result of CAST, these agents are currently used largely in patients with symptomatic atrial fibrillation or sustained ventricular arrhythmias occurring in the absence of underlying structural heart disease.

CAST, despite its limitations and in part because of its unexpected outcome, is one of the most important milestones in contemporary cardiology. In addition to serving as the most definitive study of asymptomatic ventricular arrhythmias, CAST challenged old preconceptions and set new standards for research in the field of cardiac arrhythmias (12). The trial has resulted in enormous public health benefit by virtually eliminating the common pre-CAST practice of using potentially dangerous antiarrhythmic agents in patients with asymptomatic ventricular arrhythmias following acute myocardial infarction. The study also established beyond a doubt the fact that it is possible to achieve marked suppression of spontaneous ventricular ectopy in patients with heart disease while at the same time increasing risk for arrhythmic death, and thereby eliminated VPB suppression as an acceptable therapeutic endpoint. CAST has also changed our concepts of drug-induced proarrhythmia and emphasized the inability to detect and quantify this phenomenon objectively in the absence of placebo-controlled trials. These findings have exerted a profound impact on the current labeling and future development of antiarrhythmic drugs. The unexpected findings of CAST have provided the impetus and ethical justification for additional placebo-controlled mortality trials of different classes of antiarrhythmic agents in patients at high risk for sudden death. The generally accepted requirement for placebo-controlled mortality trials as part of the development of new antiarrhythmic agents can also be attributed directly to the results of CAST. Such studies are particularly important to assess objectively both the efficacy and safety of new agents in patients with structural heart disease. The study has also catalyzed renewed interest in the mechanisms of action and proarrhythmic effects of antiarrhythmic drugs and in the electrophysiology of sudden cardiac death (12).

REFERENCES

1. Cardiac Arrhythmia Pilot Study (CAPS) Investigators. Effect of encainide, flecainide, imipramine and moricizine on ventricular arrhythmia during the year after acute myocardial infarction: the CAPS. Am J Cardiol 1988; 61:501–509.
2. The Cardiac Arrhythmia Suppression Trial (CAST) Investigators. Preliminary report: effect of encainide and flecainide on mortality in a randomized trial of arrhythmia suppression after myocardial infarction. N Engl J Med 1989; 321:406–412.
3. Echt DS, Liebson PR, Mitchell LB, Peters RW, Obias-Manno D, Barker AH, Arensberg D, Baker A, Friedman L, Greene HL, et al. Mortality and morbidity in patients receiving encainide, flecainide, or placebo. The Cardiac Arrhythmia Suppression Trial. N Engl J Med 1991; 324(12):781–788.
4. The Cardiac Arrhythmia Suppression Trial II Investigators. Effect of the antiarrhythmic agent moricizine on survival after myocardial infarction. N Engl J Med 1992; 327(4):227–233.
5. Akiyama T, Pawitan Y, Greenberg H, Kuo CS, Reynolds-Haertle RA for the CAST Investigators. Increased risk of death and cardiac arrest from encainide and flecainide in patients after non-Q-wave acute myocardial infarction in the Cardiac Arrhythmia Suppression Trial. Am J Cardiol 1991; 68(17):1551–1555.
6. Winkle RA, Mason JW, Friggin IC, Ross D. Malignant ventricular tachyarrhythmias associated with the use of encainide. Am Heart J 1981; 102:857–864.

9. Echt DS, Black IN, Barbey IT, Cone DR, Cab E. Evaluation of antiarrhythmic drugs on defibrillation energy requirements in dogs: sodium channel block and action potential prolongation. Circulation 1989; 79:1106–1117.

10. Packer DL, Munger TM, Johnson SB, Cragun KT. Mechanism of lethal proarrhythmia observed in the Cardiac Arrhythmia Suppression Trial: role of adrenergic modulation of drug binding. Pacing Clin Electrophysiol 1997; 20:455–467.

11. Garan H, McComb JM, Ruskin JN. Spontaneous and electrically induced ventricular arrhythmias during acute ischemia superimposed on 2 week old canine myocardial infarction. J Am Coll Cardiol 1988; 11(3):603–611.

12. Ruskin, J. The Cardiac Arrhythmia Suppression Trial. Editorial. New Engl J Med 1989; 321:386–388.

13. Wyse DG, Morganroth J, Ledingham R, Denes P, Hallstrom A, Mitchell LB, Epstein AE, Woosley RL, Capone R for the CAST and CAPS Investigators. New insights into the definition and meaning of proarrhythmia during initiation of antiarrhythmic drug therapy from the Cardiac Arrhythmia Suppression Trial and its pilot study. J Am Coll Cardiol 1994; 23:1130–1140.

14. Wyse DG, Hallstrom A, McBride R, Cohen JD, Steinberg JS, Mahmarian J. Events in the Cardiac Arrhythmia Suppression Trial (CAST). Mortality in patients surviving open label titration but not randomized to double-blind therapy. J Am Coll Cardiol 1991; 18 (1):20–28.

15. Morganroth I, Anderson IL, Gentzkow GD. Classification by type of ventricular arrhythmia predicts frequency of adverse cardiac events from flecainide. J Am Coll Cardiol 1986; 8:607–615.

16. Pratt CM, Moye LA. The Cardiac Arrhythmia Suppression Trial. Background, interim results and implications. Am J Cardiol 1990; 65 (4):20B–29B.

16. Rinckenherger RL, Prystowsky EN, Jackman WM, Naccarelli GV, Heger W, Zipes DP. Drug conversion of nonsustained ventricular tachycardia to sustained ventricular tachycardia during serial electrophysiologic studies: identification of drugs that exacerbate tachycardia and potential mechanisms. Am Heart J 1982; 103:177–184.

17. Herre IM, Titus C, Franz MR. Inefficacy and proarrhythmia of flecainide and encainide in patients with sustained ventricular tachycardia. Circulation 1988; 78 (suppl 11):11–61.

18. Minardo ID, Heger II. Miles WM, Zipes DP. Prystowsky EN. Clinical characteristics of patients with ventricular fibrillation during antiarrhythmic drug therapy. N Engl J Med 1988; 319:257–262.

19. Julian DG, Camm AJ, Frangin G, Janse MJ, Munoz A, Schwartz PJ, Simon P. Randomised trial of effect of amiodarone on mortality in patients with left-ventricular dysfunction after recent myocardial infarction: EMIAT. European Myocardial Infarct Amiodarone Trial Investigators. Lancet 1997; 349 (9053):667–674.

20. Waldo AL, Camm AJ, de Ruyter H, Friedman PL, MacNeil DJ, Pauls JF, Pitt B, Pratt CM, Schwartz PJ, Veltri EP. Effect of d-sotalol on mortality in patients with left ventricular dysfunction after recent and remote myocardial infarction. The SWORD Investigators. Lancet 1996; 348 (9019):7–12.

21. The Norwegian Multicenter Study Group. Timolol-induced reduction in mortality and reinfarction in patients surviving acute myocardial infarction. N Engl J Med 1981; 304:801–807.

3

The Cardiac Arrest in Seattle: Conventional versus Amiodarone Drug Evaluation (CASCADE) Study

H. LEON GREENE*

University of Washington, Seattle, Washington

INTRODUCTION

Resuscitation from an episode of out-of-hospital ventricular fibrillation (VF) carries with it the risk of recurrent VF in the ensuing years (1–8). The risk of recurrent cardiac arrest is high in most patients, although lower in patients who have a new Q-wave myocardial infarction associated with the episode of VF. Therefore, high-risk patients can be identified who need aggressive therapy for their arrhythmias. Low-risk patients do not warrant aggressive therapy.

In the 1980s, antiarrhythmic drug therapy was enthusiastically promoted in this patient population (9–11). Few studies compared various drug treatments in such a high-risk population, in part because resuscitation rates in most cities were low. In Seattle, with its advanced Medic system, survival from out-of-hospital VF was common. The success of resuscitation in Seattle has been attributed to early bystander cardiopulmonary resuscitation (CPR), the rapid response time

*****The CASCADE Investigators:** H. Leon Greene, MD (Principal Investigator). Gust H. Bardy, MD, Jeanne E. Poole, MD, Peter J. Kudenchuk, MD, G. Lee Dolack, MD, Leonard A. Cobb, MD, Ellen L. Graham-Renfroe, RN, Judy L. Powell, RN, Amy C. Galloway, RN, and Joanne Kellie, RN, *Harborview Medical Center/University of Washington Medical Center, University of Washington, Seattle, Washington.* Christopher L. Fellows, MD, Carolyn L. Main, RN, and Mary McMahon-Busch, RN, *Virginia Mason Medical Center, Seattle, Washington*; David R. Broudy, MD, John Sanders, RN, and Judy E. Garni, RN, *Providence Medical Center, Seattle, Washington*; Charles Maynard, PhD, Alfred P. Hallstrom, PhD, and Ruth McBride, *Coordinating Center, Seattle, Washington.*

39

of the Medics, and early defibrillation attempts (1–5). This setting provided the ideal environment for comparison of different antiarrhythmic drug therapies. Furthermore, widespread use of the implantable cardioverter defibrillator (ICD) did not appear until the late 1980s and early 1990s (12,13).

Amiodarone was thought to be an excellent antiarrhythmic drug for the treatment of high-risk patients (14,15). However, it was unclear whether electrophysiological testing and/or Holter ambulatory electrocardiographic recording was useful in this patient population, although electrophysiological studies had gained widespread acceptance for the guidance of therapy with other conventional antiarrhythmic drugs (11). The adverse drug effects of the various antiarrhythmic agents were known (16–18), but it was unclear how often these complications of therapy resulted in discontinuation of treatment.

The Cardiac Arrest in Seattle: Conventional vs. Amiodarone Drug Evaluation (CASCADE) study was designed to compare empiric treatment with amiodarone to treatment with conventional antiarrhythmic drugs guided by electrophysiological testing and/or Holter recording in these high-risk survivors of out-of-hospital VF (19).

METHODS

Because there are clinical and electrophysiological differences between patients with recurrent sustained ventricular tachycardia (VT) and patients with out-of-hospital VF (20,21), the CASCADE study limited enrollment to patients with out-of-hospital VF (Fig. 1). Patients were considered to be candidates for the

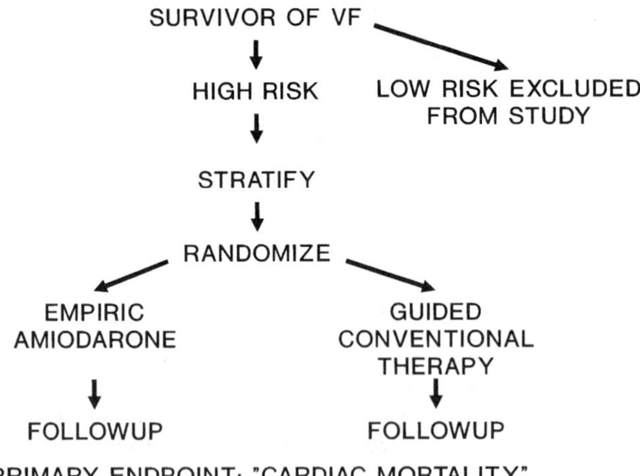

Figure 1 Protocol for the CASCADE study.

CASCADE study if the episode of VF did not occur with a new Q-wave myocardial infarction. This selection process included high-risk patients who were more likely to have had a previous myocardial infarction, low ejection fraction, history of congestive heart failure, and to be male gender. In general, patients included in the CASCADE study had a risk of recurrent VF approaching 20% at 1 year (4). These patients were also likely to be inducible at electrophysiological study, to have frequent and/or complex arrhythmias on Holter ambulatory electrocardiographic recording, and to be older.

After patients were stabilized from resuscitation from their episode of VF, and as soon as they had recovered neurologically to be able to give informed consent, they were approached regarding enrollment in the study. In some cases, patients were referred from hospitals outside the Seattle area, but no patients were enrolled beyond 6 months following their episode of spontaneous out-of-hospital VF. Low-risk patients were excluded from the study. All patients had left ventricular ejection fraction measured, usually by radionuclide ventriculography. High-risk patients underwent a baseline, drug-free ambulatory Holter electrocardiographic recording and catheter-based electrophysiological study with programmed electrical stimulation. In order for inclusion in the CASCADE study, patients had to have either: (1) inducible sustained VT or VF at electrophysiological study or (2) frequent ($\geq$ 10 ventricular premature depolarizations per hour) complex arrhythmias on Holter monitoring, or both. Following stratification (based upon cardiac disease, ejection fraction, and prior drug failure), patients had therapy randomized either to empiric amiodarone or conventional antiarrhythmic drug therapy guided by invasive electrophysiological testing and/or Holter monitoring. Randomization occurred following surgery in those patients who were deemed to require cardiac surgery, primarily coronary artery bypass graft surgery.

Patients randomly assigned to amiodarone received a loading dose of 1200 mg/day for up to 10 days and then 600 mg/day (range 200–800 mg/day) for 1 to 2 months. Amiodarone doses were then subsequently tapered to 100 to 400 mg/day, based upon symptomatic adverse effects. Though the maintenance dose of amiodarone was aggressively reduced to avoid symptomatic adverse effects, the dose was increased if VT was seen on routine Holter monitoring, performed at 1 month, 3 months, 6 months, and at 12 months and yearly thereafter. Serum levels of amiodarone were not used. Thyroid function tests and pulmonary function tests were measured at least at 6-month intervals.

Patients randomized to conventional therapy had their treatment guided by suppression of inducible sustained VT or VF and/or suppression of spontaneous ambient ventricular ectopy on Holter recording. The sequence of drug therapy was usually procainamide (administered intravenously at electrophysiological study), quinidine, disopyramide, tocainide, mexiletine, encainide, flecainide, propafenone, or combination therapy. Serum levels of conventional antiarrhythmic drugs were measured as indicated clinically. Drugs that had previously been ineffective or discontinued because of adverse effects were not repeated. Successful treatment was considered to be suppression of inducible sustained VT or VF. If a drug therapy could not be found which completely suppressed inducible sustained arrhythmias, the best antiarrhythmic drug was chosen based upon slowing of the induced VT cycle length or the aggressiveness of the protocol required to induce VT or VF (22). For patients who were noninducible at baseline electrophysiological study, Holter recording alone was used to determine drug therapy. Successful suppression of ectopy was considered to be ≥70% suppression of ventricular premature depolarizations, and >90% suppression of runs of VT. Patients who had neither a positive electrophysiological study nor adequate ectopy on Holter recording were excluded from the study prior to randomization because of the absence of a marker for adjustment of conventional antiarrhythmic drug therapy.

During the course of the study, the results of the Cardiac Arrhythmia Suppression Trial (CAST) were published, suggesting that encainide, flecainide, and moricizine were potentially ineffective drugs, although the CAST population was decidedly different than the CASCADE patients (23–25). Therefore, use of the class I antiarrhythmic drugs tested in CAST was restricted toward the end of the CASCADE study. Furthermore, as evidence accumulated that the mortality rate was still quite high in the patients initially treated in the CASCADE study and that the ICD was a successful treatment (26–27), all patients were offered the ICD toward the latter half of the CASCADE study, unless there were clinical reasons not to attempt implantation of this device [which at this time required thoracotomy (28)].

The primary endpoint of this study was the composite of total cardiac mortality (encompassing sudden arrhythmic cardiac death and nonarrhythmic cardiac death), documented resuscitated out-of-hospital VF, and syncope followed by a shock from the ICD in those patients in whom such a device had been deployed (29–32). If a patient had experienced a death due to amiodarone pulmonary toxicity, it would have been counted as a primary endpoint because it was a direct result of antiarrhythmic drug treatment. Amiodarone pulmonary toxicity was defined by a constellation of clinical parameters that included dyspnea on exertion, dyspnea at rest, cough, pulmonary rales, interstitial fibrosis on chest x-ray, and a reduction in the pulmonary diffusion capacity (in the absence of congestive heart failure or pulmonary infection). Secondary endpoints were arrhythmic mortality, total mortality, arrhythmia recurrence (sustained VT), ventricular ectopic activity and VT on Holter recording, adverse drug effects, recurrent hospitalization, compliance, and crossover.

Because the ICD was relatively new at the inception of CASCADE, a strict definition was used for the endpoints determined by the ICD. Complete syncope followed by a shock from the ICD was required to qualify as an endpoint. Dizziness, dyspnea, palpitations, or near-syncope followed by a shock from the ICD was not counted in this analysis. This definition included only those shocks that could reasonably be considered to be equivalent to an episode of VF. As such, it probably undercounted the number of ICD events, if one assumes that it could convert a serious ventricular tachyarrhythmia prior to complete loss of consciousness.

The null hypothesis stated that there would be no difference in mortality between patients treated with amiodarone and patients treated with conventional antiarrhythmic drugs. We estimated that the expected mortality would be approximately 40% at 2.5 years, 29% as arrhythmic events, and 11% as nonarrhythmic events. The alternative to the null hypothesis was that amiodarone would decrease arrhythmic mortality from 29% to 10% without affecting nonarrhythmic mortality. The power to detect this difference was estimated to be 0.91. Data were analyzed using t-tests, chi-square tests, the Kaplan-Meier method by standard technique. Patients were analyzed by intention-to-treat. Other statistical and monitoring techniques have been reported (33–36). Noncardiac deaths were censored in the survival analysis.

RESULTS

Two hundred twenty-eight patients had therapy randomized, 113 to amiodarone and 115 to conventional antiarrhythmic therapy (Table 1) (37–40). Both randomization groups had similar clinical characteristics. The average age was 62. Most patients (82%) had coronary artery disease, and of patients with coronary artery disease, 81% had experienced a prior myocardial infarction. Nearly one-half of the patients had a history of congestive heart failure, and the baseline ejection fraction was 0.35. Spontaneous ectopy was common, and over half of the patients had inducible sustained VT or VF. The mean time from index cardiac arrest to randomization was 3 weeks. Discharge medications, exclusive of antiarrhythmic agents, were similar. Approximately one-half of patients had an ICD implanted.

The mean maintenance dose of amiodarone was 183 mg/day at 12 months, 158 mg/day at 24 months, and 185 mg/day at 36 months in the patients who continued to take the drug. In the conventional antiarrhythmic drug group, type 1 agents were used most commonly: quinidine—33 patients; procainamide—26; disopyramide—3; tocainide—4; mexiletine—8; moricizine—1; flecainide—12; propafenone—1; combinations—17; beta-blocker only—1; amiodarone crossover—4; and none—5. The maximum number of drug trials was 7 with a mean of 1.5 ± 1.5 (±S.D.). Inducibility was successfully suppressed in 35 of 57 patients, and an additional 10 patients had inducible VT rendered slow and hemodynamically stable. Twelve of 57 patients continued to have inducible VT that was not adequately slowed, and they were given the drug that slowed the induced arrhythmia most. In this relatively small patient population, there was no differ-

Table 1 Baseline Characteristics of the 228 CASCADE Patients

Characteristics	Total (%) ($n = 228$)	Amiodarone therapy (%) ($n = 113$)	Conventional therapy (%) ($n = 115$)
Male gender	202 (89)	103 (91)	99 (86)
Age (years)	62 ± 10	63 ± 10	62 ± 10
Coronary artery disease	188 (82)	96 (85)	92 (80)
Prior myocardial infarction	153 (81)	80 (83)	72 (78)
Congestive heart failure	102 (45)	54 (48)	48 (42)
Drug failure before randomization[a]	103 (45)	51 (45)	52 (45)
Drug therapy at VF	50 (22)	29 (26)	21 (18)
After VF, before randomization	53 (23)	22 (19)	31 (27)
Cardiac surgery	158 (69)	84 (74)	74 (64)
Before VF	57 (25)	27 (24)	30 (26)
After VF and before or within 30 days after randomization	101 (44)	57 (50)	44 (38)
Left ventricular ejection fraction	0.35 ± 0.10	0.35 ± 0.15	0.35 ± 0.14
Baseline Holter recording			
Ventricular premature complexes/hour	167 ± 240	129 ± 170[b]	208 ± 292[b]
Complex ventricular ectopy	174/194 (90)	89/99 (90)	85/95 (89)
VT	109/194 (56)	56/99 (57)	53/95 (56)
Sustained VT or VF inducible at baseline electrophysiological study	110/183 (60)	53/90 (59)	57/93 (61)
Time from index VF to randomization (days)	21 ± 23	22 ± 24	20 ± 22
Drugs at initial hospital discharge			
Digitalis	84 (37)	35 (31)	49 (43)
Diuretics	109 (48)	52 (46)	57 (50)
β-blockers	13 (6)	7 (6)	6 (5)
Nitrates	42 (18)	20 (18)	22 (19)
Antihypertensives	61 (27)	29 (26)	32 (28)
Calcium antagonists	42 (18)	22 (19)	20 (17)
Automatic implanted cardioverter/defibrillator[c]	105 (46)	53 (47)	52 (45)

[a] Either (1) spontaneous sustained arrhythmias with adequate dose and serum level of drug before or after index ventricular fibrillation event or (2) inducible sustained arrhythmia with adequate dose and serum level of drug at electrophysiological testing after index ventricular fibrillation event.
[b] $p = 0.02$; all other comparisons $p > 0.05$.
[c] Automatic implanted cardioverter/defibrillator.
VF = ventricular fibrillation; VT = ventricular tachycardia.
Source: Ref. 37.

ence in survival in patients whose inducible arrhythmias were suppressed compared to those whose arrhythmias were not suppressed. Holter-guided therapy was successful in suppressing spontaneous arrhythmias in 25 of 45 patients (56%). Patients treated with amiodarone had an excellent suppression of spontaneous ventricular ectopy, with only 15 patients having VT on Holter monitoring between discharge and 6 months.

Consistent with other studies, ejection fraction was a powerful predictor of outcome. Patients with low ejection fraction were more likely to suffer cardiac death, cardiac arrest, or have a syncopal episode followed by a shock from the ICD. Survival was similar in patients with coronary artery disease and in patients with noncoronary etiologies.

Table 2 summarizes the events in follow-up. The conventional group had 55 events, compared with 38 in the amiodarone group. Most of these events were cardiac, with only 6 noncardiac deaths throughout the entire study.

Table 3 lists the actuarial event rates for the two groups. The composite endpoint of total cardiac mortality, resuscitated cardiac arrest, plus syncopal ICD shocks was the main endpoint of the study. Amiodarone patients had a better survival than patients treated with conventional agents. A strict definition of cardiac death, excluding patients successfully resuscitated from recurrent VF and excluding patients who had a syncopal shock from an ICD, was 15% at 2 years for amiodarone-treated patients and 22% for patients treated with conventional drugs ($p = 0.07$).

Patients were treated with the ICD primarily during the last half of the CASCADE study. All patients who were candidates for the rather extensive surgical procedure required were offered the device during the last half of the study;

Table 2 Events

	Amiodarone ($n = 113$)	Conventional ($n = 115$)
Total events	38	55
Noncardiac death	4	2
Cardiac death/VF	34	53
Sudden arrhythmic cardiac (not resuscitated)	13	19
Sudden arrhythmic cardiac (resuscitated/survived)	11	21
Resuscitated by medics	6	9
Syncope, shock from implanted cardioverter/ defibrillator	5	12
Nonarrhythmic cardiac death	10	13

VF = ventricular fibrillation.
Source: Ref. 37.

Table 3 Actuarial Event Rates

	Total cardiac mortality, resuscitated CA, plus syncopal ICD shocks		Total cardiac mortality, resuscitated CA, syncopal ICD shocks, plus sustained VT		All ICD shocks[a]		Syncopal ICD shocks[a]	
Year	Amio	Conv	Amio	Conv	Amio	Conv	Amio	Conv
1	9%	23%	15%	34%	20%	43%	2%	19%
2	18%	31%	22%	48%	23%	58%	2%	19%
3	24%	44%	34%	55%	31%	58%	2%	19%
4	34%	48%	48%	64%				
5	37%	54%	53%	71%				

[a] Analysis limited to patients with coronary artery disease only.
CA = cardiac arrest; amio = amiodarone; conv = conventional drugs; VT = ventricular tachycardia.
Source: Refs. 37–39.

therefore, this therapy was not randomized. Whether the ICD shock analysis was limited to patients with coronary artery disease only or extended to all patients, survival free of syncopal episodes followed by a shock from the ICD was better for the patients treated with amiodarone. Furthermore, the total number of shocks was decreased by the use of amiodarone. Predictors of shocks from the ICD were low ejection fraction ($p = 0.002$), female gender ($p = 0.007$), and conventional drug therapy ($p = 0.015$). The only predictor of syncopal shocks was conventional drug therapy ($p = 0.035$).

Though the dose of amiodarone was lower than reported in other studies, adverse effects of amiodarone were common. Twenty-nine percent of patients discontinued amiodarone for 6 months or longer, and 11% stopped amiodarone and crossed over to conventional therapy. Though pulmonary toxicity is difficult to diagnose, it was suspected in nine patients. The actuarial incidence was 6% at 1 year, 10% at 2 years, 10% at 3 years, 12% at 4 years, and 12% at 5 years. No patient died from amiodarone pulmonary toxicity. The mean diffusion capacity decreased from a baseline of 69% of the predicted value to 62% during the course of the study ($p = 0.003$). Thyroid function abnormalities were also common. Seven patients developed hyperthyroidism, and 18 patients developed hypothyroidism or abnormalities of thyroid function requiring hormone replacement. With the relatively low doses of amiodarone used in this study, serious neurological effects were not seen, but corneal microdeposits and skin sensitivity to sunlight and discoloration were seen.

Table 4 Annual Rates of Rehospitalization

	Total ($n = 224$)	Amiodarone ($n = 112$)	Conventional ($n = 112$)
Average follow-up/patient (years)	2.88	3.12	2.64
Number hospitalized	168	88	80
Number of hospitalizations	512	259	253
Annual rate of rehospitalization	79/100	74/100	85/100

Source: Ref. 40.

The analysis of the rehospitalization rate was performed on 224 patients. Four patients were excluded because they died during the index hospitalization for study enrollment. Table 4 shows the annual rates of rehospitalization. The average patient follow-up was 2.88 years. The rate of rehospitalization was 79 admissions per 100 patients per year. Evaluation of baseline characteristics revealed that the only predictor of rehospitalization was left ventricular ejection fraction ≤ 0.30 ($p = 0.001$) and mean left ventricular ejection (0.33 $\pm$ 0.14 in patients rehospitalized versus 0.41 $\pm$ 0.15 in patients not rehospitalized; $p = 0.002$). No other factors predicted rehospitalization. Overall, the time to first rehospitalization was not different among patients treated with amiodarone compared with conventional drugs, although patients treated with conventional therapy were more often admitted for change of antiarrhythmic drugs. The presence of an ICD was associated with a shorter length of stay.

DISCUSSION

The CASCADE study demonstrated that amiodarone therapy administered empirically is superior to conventional antiarrhythmic drug therapy guided by electrophysiological testing and/or Holter monitoring. Furthermore, the CASCADE study shows that amiodarone reduces the number of shock from the ICD.

The CASCADE study was begun in an era prior to the recognition of the adverse effects of the class IC drugs demonstrated by the CAST study. Fortunately, the Ic drugs were used infrequently in the CASCADE study. Furthermore, the ICD was not extensively used in the mid and late 1980s. The main results of the CASCADE study were published in 1993, well before the AVID study showed that the ICD is superior to antiarrhythmic drugs, primarily amiodarone (41,42). Relatively low-dose amiodarone in CASCADE appeared to be safe, although the incidence of suspected pulmonary toxicity was higher in CASCADE than reported in other studies.

A composite endpoint was used for the main outcome of the CASCADE study and had been defined before the study had begun. Difficulty in classification of cardiac events made total cardiac mortality a more relevant measure of drug effectiveness than purported arrhythmic death.

Application of the lessons of the CASCADE study is dependent upon identification of high-risk survivors of out-of-hospital VF. Whereas many studies evaluate primarily patients with recurrent sustained VT, the CASCADE study population was limited to patients who had been resuscitated from an episode of out-of-hospital cardiac arrest with documented VF. Similar studies have shown the relatively good outcome of patients who have had VF in the setting of an acute Q-wave myocardial infarction. It is unclear how accurately one can make a diagnosis of VF due to other transient or reversible causes of arrhythmias, and the prognostic value of these other transient/reversible causes is not clear.

With the recent publication of the AVID study showing the superiority of the ICD for treatment of these patients, the application of the CASCADE study is more limited. Empiric amiodarone therapy is simple and relatively inexpensive, but antiarrhythmic devices are more successful in prolonging survival. Nevertheless, amiodarone can be used successfully to suppress recurrent arrhythmias in patients receiving frequent ICD shocks.

LIMITATIONS

The CASCADE study did not have a placebo arm. Because of the seriousness of the qualifying arrhythmia, it was felt that no patient should be treated with a placebo. The CAST study suggested that, in fact, some antiarrhythmic drugs given to other patient populations may actually worsen the mortality. The CASCADE study only provides evidence that amiodarone is better than conventional antiarrhythmic agents. How patients treated in the CASCADE study compare with the natural history of patients treated with neither antiarrhythmic drug nor the ICD cannot be determined.

Patients treated with amiodarone did not have serial electrophysiological testing to guide therapy. There still remains considerable debate regarding the utility of electrophysiological testing with amiodarone, although some studies suggest even further improvement in survival if electrophysiological testing is used. The CASCADE study was designed to test a simple regimen that did not require repeated, expensive, and invasive procedures.

Because of the size of the CASCADE study, it is impossible to analyze subsets of the patient population to see which patients might have benefited the most from their therapy.

Evaluation of adverse effects from drugs was obviously subjective. The study was not blinded. Biopsies were not required to make a diagnosis of pulmonary toxicity, for example. Therefore, the reported incidence of suspected amiodarone pulmonary toxicity may be too high.

CONCLUSIONS

The CASCADE study demonstrated the superiority of amiodarone over conventional antiarrhythmic drugs in patients who had been resuscitated from an episode of out-of-hospital VF. Survival free of cardiac death, resuscitated VF, or syncopal shock from an ICD was better for the amiodarone patients (82% vs. 69% at 2 years; 66% vs. 52% at 4 years; and 53% vs. 40% at 6 years; $p = 0.007$). Patients requiring antiarrhythmic drug therapy following an episode of out-of-hospital VF should be offered amiodarone.

ACKNOWLEDGMENTS

Supported in part by grants from the Medic I Foundation of Seattle, Washington, Wyeth-Ayerst Laboratories of Philadelphia, Pennsylvania, grant R01 HL31472 and contract N01 HC25117 from the National Heart, Lung, and Blood Institute, Bethesda, Maryland.

REFERENCES

1. Schaffer WA, Cobb LA. Recurrent ventricular fibrillation and modes of death in survivors of out-of-hospital ventricular fibrillation. N Engl J Med 1975; 393:260–262.
2. Cobb LA, Baum RS, Alvarez H III, Schaffer WA. Resuscitation from out-of-hospital ventricular fibrillation: 4 years follow-up. Circulation 1975; 52 (suppl 3):III-223–III-235.
3. Cobb LA, Werner JA, Trobaugh GB. Sudden cardiac death: II. Outcome of resuscitation, management, and future directions. Mod Concepts Cardiovasc Dis 1980; 49:37–42.
4. Hallstrom AP, Cobb LA. Predicting risk of recurrence in sudden cardiac death syndrome. Emerg Health Serv Rev 1984; 2:49–62.
5. Cobb LA, Hallstrom AP, Weaver WD, Trobaugh GB, Greene HL. Considerations in the long-term management of survivors of cardiac arrest. Ann NY Acad Sci 1984; 432:247–257.
6. Goldstein S, Landis JR, Leighton R, Ritter G, Vasu CM, Wolfe RA, Acheson A, VanderBrug-Mendendorp S. Predictive survival models for resuscitated victims of

out-of-hospital cardiac arrest with coronary heart disease. Circulation 1985; 71:873–880.

7. Weaver WD, Cobb LA, Hallstrom AP, Copass MK, Ray R, Emery M, Fahrenbruch C. Considerations for improving survival from out-of-hospital cardiac arrest. Ann Emerg Med 1986; 15:1181–1186.

8. Weaver WD, Copass MK, Bufi D, Ray R, Hallstrom AP, Cobb LA. Improved neurologic recovery and survival after early defibrillation. Circulation 1984; 69:943–954.

9. Moosvi AR, Goldstein S, Medendorp SV, Landis JR, Wolfe RA, Leighton R, Ritter G, Vasu CM, Acheson A. Effect of empiric antiarrhythmic therapy in resuscitated out-of-hospital cardiac arrest victims with coronary artery disease. Am J Cardiol 1990; 65:1192–1197.

10. Grayboys TB, Lown B, Podrid PJ, DeSilva R. Long-term survival of patients with ventricular arrhythmia treated with antiarrhythmic drugs. Am J Cardiol 1982; 50:437–443.

11. Mason JW, Winkle RA. Accuracy of the ventricular tachycardia-induction study for predicting long-term efficacy and inefficacy of antiarrhythmic drugs. N Engl J Med 1980; 303:1073–1077.

12. Winkle RA, Mead RH, Ruder MA, Gaudiani VA, Smith NA, Buch WS, Schmidt P, Shipman T. Long-term outcome with the automatic implantable cardioverter-defibrillator. J Am Coll Cardiol 1989; 13:1353–1361.

13. Maloney J, Masterson M, Khoury D, Trohman R, Wilkoff B, Simmons T, Morant V, Castle L. Clinical performance of the implantable cardioverter defibrillator: electrocardiographic documentation of 101 spontaneous discharges. Pacing Clin Electrophysiol 1991; 14:280–285.

14. Heger JJ, Prystowsky EN, Jackman WM. Amiodarone—clinical efficacy during long-term therapy for recurrent ventricular tachycardia or ventricular fibrillation. N Engl J Med 1981; 305:539–545.

15. Herre JM, Sauve MJ, Malone P, Griffin JC, Helmy I, Langberg JJ, Goldberg H, Scheinman MM. Long-term results of amiodarone therapy in patients with recurrent sustained ventricular tachycardia or ventricular fibrillation. J Am Coll Cardiol 1989; 13:442–449.

16. Greene HL, Graham EL, Werner JA, Sears GK, Gorham JR, Kudenchuk PJ, Trobaugh GB. Toxic and therapeutic effects of amiodarone in the treatment of cardiac arrhythmias. J Am Coll Cardiol 1983; 2:1114–1128.

17. Kudenchuk PJ, Pierson DJ, Greene HL. Prospective evaluation of amiodarone pulmonary toxicity. Chest 1984; 86:541–548.

18. Hallstrom AP, Cobb LA, Yu BH, Weaver WD, Fahrenbruch CE. An antiarrhythmic drug experience in 941 patients resuscitated from an initial cardiac arrest between 1970 and 1985. Am J Cardiol 1991; 68:1025–1031.

19. CASCADE Investigators. Cardiac Arrest in Seattle: Conventional versus Amiodarone Drug evaluation (the CASCADE Study). Am J Cardiol 1991; 67:578–584.

20. Adhar GC, Larson LW, Bardy GH, Greene HL. Sustained ventricular arrhythmias: differences between survivors of cardiac arrest and patients with recurrent sustained ventricular tachycardia. J Am Coll Cardiol 1988; 12:159–165.

21. Denniss AR, Ross DL, Richards DA, Holley LK, Cooper MJ, Johnson DC, Uther JB. Differences between patients with ventricular tachycardia and ventricular fibril-

lation as assessed by signal-averaged electrocardiogram, radionuclide ventriculography and cardiac mapping. J Am Coll Cardiol 1988; 11:276–283.

22. Waller TJ, Kay HR, Spielman SR, Kutalek SP, Greenspan AM, Horowitz LN. Reduction in sudden death and total mortality by antiarrhythmic therapy evaluated by electrophysiologic drug testing: criteria of efficacy in patients with sustained ventricular tachyarrhythmia. J Am Coll Cardiol 1987; 10:83–89.

23. The Cardiac Arrhythmia Suppression Trial (CAST) Investigators. Preliminary report: effect of encainide and flecainide on mortality in a randomized trial of arrhythmia suppression after myocardial infarction. N Engl J Med 1989; 321:406–412.

24. Echt DS, Liebson PR, Mitchell LB, Peters RW, Obias-Manno D, Barker AH, Arensberg D, Baker A, Friedman L, Greene HL, Huther ML, Richardson DW, and the CAST Investigators. Mortality and morbidity in patients receiving encainide, flecainide, or placebo. The Cardiac Arrhythmia Suppression Trial. N Engl J Med 1991; 324:781–788.

25. The Cardiac Arrhythmia Suppression Trial II Investigators. Effect of the antiarrhythmic agent moricizine on survival after myocardial infarction. N Engl J Med 1992; 327:227–233.

26. Lehmann MH, Steinman RT, Schuger CD, Jackson K. The automatic implantable cardioverter defibrillator as antiarrhythmic treatment modality of choice for survivors of cardiac arrest unrelated to acute myocardial infarction. Am J Cardiol 1988; 62:803–805.

27. Newman D, Sauve MJ, Herre J, Langberg JJ, Lee MA, Titus C, Franklin J, Scheinman MM, Griffin JC. Survival after implantation of the cardioverter defibrillator. Am J Cardiol 1992; 69:899–903.

28. Zipes DP, Roberts D. Results of the international study of the implantable pacemaker cardioverter-defibrillator: a comparison of epicardial and endocardial lead systems. Circulation 1995; 92:59–65.

29. Greene HL, Richardson DW, Barker AH, Roden DM, Capone RJ, Echt DS, Friedman LM, Gillespie MJ, Hallstrom A, Verter J. Classification of deaths after myocardial infarction as arrhythmic or nonarrhythmic (the Cardiac Arrhythmia Pilot Study). Am J Cardiol 1989; 63:1–6.

30. Epstein AE, Carlson MD, Fogoros RN, Higgins SL, Venditti FJ Jr. Classification of death in antiarrhythmia trials. J Am Coll Cardiol 1996; 27:433–42.

31. Kim SG, Fogoros RN, Furman S, Connolly SJ, Kuck KH, Moss AJ. Standardized reporting of ICD patient outcome: the report of a North American Society of Pacing and Electrophysiology Policy Conference, February 9–10, 1993. Pacing Clin Electrophysiol 1993; 16:1–5.

32. Pratt CM, Greenway PS, Schoenfeld MH, Hibben ML, Reiffel JA. Exploration of the precision of classifying sudden cardiac death. Implications for the interpretation of clinical trials. Circulation 1996; 93:519–24.

33. Friedman LM, Furberg CD, DeMets DL. Monitoring response variables. In: Fundamentals of Clinical Trials, 2nd ed. Littleton, MA: PSG Publishing, 1985:213–239.

34. Halperin M, Lan KKG, Ware JH, Johnson NJ, DeMets DL. An aid to data monitoring in long-term clinical trials. Controlled Clin Trials 1982; 3:311–323.

35. Lan KKG, DeMets DL. Discrete sequential boundaries for clinical trials. Biometrika 1983; 70:659–663.

36. Fleming TR, Harrington DP, O'Brien PC. Designs for group sequential tests. Controlled Clin Trials 1984; 5:348–361.
37. The CASCADE Investigators. Randomized antiarrhythmic drug therapy in survivors of cardiac arrest (the CASCADE Study). Am J Cardiol 1993; 72:280–287.
38. Greene HL, for the CASCADE Investigators. The CASCADE Study: Randomized antiarrhythmic drug therapy in survivors of cardiac arrest in Seattle. Am J Cardiol 1993; 72:70F–74F.
39. Dolack GL, for the CASCADE Investigators. Clinical predictors of implantable cardioverter-defibrillator shocks (results of the CASCADE trial). Am J Cardiol 1994; 73:237–241.
40. Maynard C, for the CASCADE Investigators. Rehospitalization in surviving patients of out-of-hospital ventricular fibrillation (the CASCADE study). Am J Cardiol 1993; 72:1295–1300.
41. The AVID Investigators. Antiarrhythmics Versus Implantable Defibrillators (AVID)—rationale, design, and methods. Am J Cardiol 1995; 75:470–475.
42. The Antiarrhythmics Versus Implantable Defibrillators (AVID) Investigators. A comparison of antiarrhythmic drug therapy with implantable defibrillators in patients resuscitated from near-fatal ventricular arrhythmias. N Engl J Med 1997; 337:1576–1583.

JAMES A. REIFFEL
Columbia University, New York, New York

The CASCADE trial (1) is a landmark study in our progress toward successful secondary prevention of ventricular fibrillation (VF) by pharmacotherapy. CASCADE was designed to test prospectively two of the dominant approaches to preventive therapy in use at the time the trial was conceived: guided therapy with class I antiarrhythmics (termed ''conventional therapy'' by the investigators), versus empiric treatment with amiodarone. Subjects were survivors of VF who were felt to be at high risk for recurrence, and whose VF was not due to an acute reversible cause and/or did not take place during the acute phase of a transmural myocardial infarction. The exclusion of low-risk subjects prevented dilution of the results. The primary endpoint measure was cardiac survival, a useful composite of freedom from cardiac mortality, recurrent resuscitated cardiac arrest, or a syncopal ICD shock (the latter two presumed to have represented fatal events in the absence of the therapy applied). In CASCADE, amiodarone was associated with better survival, fewer recurrences, and fewer ICD shocks following syncope than was class I drug therapy. The class I therapy was primarily guided by serial electrophysiological testing in patients inducible at baseline, and by serial Holter monitor testing in noninducible subjects. Details of the CASCADE trial are available in the original report (1) as well as in Chapter 3 of this book.

On first glance, CASCADE appears to be a demonstration of the superiority of amiodarone over class I antiarrhythmics. Cardiac survival at years 1 through 6 for the two therapies, respectively, was 91 vs. 77%; 82 vs. 69%; 76 vs. 56%; 66 vs. 52%; 63 vs. 46%; and 53 vs. 40%, for example. The confirmation of previous beliefs that the rate of recurrence is greatest in the first few years, and then slower later on, and that survival declines as left ventricular ejection fraction falls were also important observations in CASCADE. The results of CASCADE, coupled with other studies such as ESVEM (2), which suggested that class I agents are inferior to sotalol, has led to a dramatic reduction in the use of sodium channel blocking agents as first-line therapy for ventricular tachyarrhythmias.

Unfortunately, several serious design and clinical care flaws existed in CASCADE. These flaws, when carefully considered, provide for alternative interpretations, raise several new questions, and/or leave several important old questions unanswered. A full understanding of and application of CASCADE requires an understanding of what was not demonstrated as well as what was. These issues may be considered as follows.

WEAKNESSES

1. Because of the high recurrence rate observed during the first 3 years of CASCADE, implantation of defibrillators (ICD) concomitant with the assigned antiarrhythmic drug administered was utilized routinely during the second half of the trial. Although the distribution of ICD implantation was equivalent in the two drug therapy arms of CASCADE, it is not certain whether the effects of the ICD were equal in the two arms. Drug–device interactions vary from drug to drug. Amiodarone is likely to slow ventricular tachycardia, which often precedes VF, more than the class I drugs used most frequently in CASCADE, thus reducing the likelihood of syncope prior to ICD discharge, which was part of the composite cardiac survival endpoint. This would reduce the apparent true arrhythmic event rate in the amiodarone arm. Defibrillation thresholds (DFT) may be raised by antiarrhythmics. Since an increase in DFT may decrease shock efficacy, thus increasing the length of the tachycardia and the possibility of syncope, unequal effects on DFTs could have affected the reported results. Additionally, since the ICD may have truly prevented fatal events, as it is designed to, whether from drug inefficacy or proarrhythmia, the ICD must certainly have altered the actual event rate in some, though in an undetermined manner. Because in all likelihood the class I drugs are indeed less efficacious and more proarrhythmic than amiodarone, it is likely that this effect led to a reduced event rate in the conventional drug arm. This effect would separate the survival curves in a manner discordant from the drug–device interaction effects noted above. Accordingly, it would have been interesting to see the survival data presented separately for the patients with and without implanted ICDs to better assess their effects on the results, but these data were not reported.

2. Additional weaknesses involved the drug selection and dosing protocols. Empiric use of amiodarone was tested in CASCADE, as it was being widely used in this manner. However, it was already recognized that arrhythmia recurrence rates in patients rendered noninducible by amiodarone were particularly low. These data have been borne out over time (3). In this light, CASCADE would have been a more useful trial if a guided amiodarone arm had also been

employed. This issue is of particular importance when one considers the AVID trial (4). In AVID, outcome on amiodarone in sustained ventricular tachyarrhythmia patients was not as good, in terms of survival, as in patients treated with an ICD. Yet, in part the AVID trial design was influenced by the amiodarone survival data in CASCADE, although it was already clear in CASCADE that survival with empiric amiodarone was still too low to be acceptable. Remember, this caused the addition of ICD implantation. Accordingly, one could question the need for AVID since CASCADE had already shown less than an ideal benefit from empiric amiodarone, though in a smaller study. A better comparison for AVID might have been the ICD versus guided amiodarone. This design would have had more support if CASCADE had included a guided amiodarone arm, which likely would have had better survival when noninducibility was achieved than did empiric therapy. Moreover, had the CASCADE investigators shown the comparative data for the presence and absence of the ICD as was suggested above, and had a benefit been shown in the ICD group, which is likely, the need for AVID as it was performed could have been questioned even further.

Of additional concern in CASCADE as regards drug administration and dosing was the inclusion in the conventional arm of nonresponders (in both EP study and Holter-guided patients), and the approach used to taper the amiodarone dosing over time. Among the 115 conventional therapy patients, 57 were inducible at baseline and were to have their drug guided by EP testing. Of these 57, 12 (over 20%) were neither suppressed nor slowed at repeat testing, yet they were left on an empiric sodium blocker. Similarly, about 20% of the Holter-guided patients failed to achieve adequate suppression of target ectopy, yet they continued on conventional therapy empirically. Inclusion of these patients may have contributed to the poorer survival data for the conventional drug limb. An analysis excluding these patients would have been of interest, but as with the ICD issue, it, too, was not provided. Conversely, the amiodarone in CASCADE was progressively decreased in dose over time until nonsustained ventricular tachycardia returned on follow-up monitoring. This resulted in average doses under 200 mg/day during long-term therapy. Such doses are lower than are typically used for VF therapy and may have contributed to the less than desirable results for survival with amiodarone in CASCADE. How these two curve-altering effects taken in combination might have changed the results cannot be retrospectively determined, although they are of importance to both clinical practice and future trial designs.

3. Most importantly, there is yet another and truly major weakness in CASCADE. This serious shortcoming is the lack of appropriate use of best medical care in the CASCADE patients. Of particular note is the dramatic underuse of beta blockade. In CASCADE, 82% of the patients had coronary artery disease, 81% had a prior myocardial infarction, the mean left ventricular ejection fraction was 35%, and all had suffered VF. Yet, only 6% were receiving beta-blockers.

By the time CASCADE was developed, the benefits of beta-blockers in such patients was universally recognized. Beta-blockers reduce mortality, reduce VF, reduce ischemia, and reduce catecholamine reversal of antiarrhythmic drug effects among their many beneficial actions. Virtually certain is the [presumed] fact that had beta-blockers been used concomitantly with the conventional agents in CASCADE, as would have been appropriate, an entirely different survival curve would have been generated. Had this been the case, one can only wonder what the AVID protocol might have been. It is possible that in CASCADE the results with conventional therapy plus a beta-blocker would have been indistinguishable from those of amiodarone (which has some inherent antiadrenergic actions). In retrospect, from the recent EMIAT and CAMIAT trials (5,6), we now know that beta blockade is even important in terms of survival benefit in combination with amiodarone. This was not known, however, when CASCADE was performed, so the low beta-blocker use in the amiodarone arm, in contrast to the conventional therapy arm, cannot be viewed as a weakness of the study. Also, as regards best medical therapy, the trial report did not provide any data as to the use and distribution of ACE inhibitors, which, if unequal and/or inadequate, could have altered the trial results and made them difficult to extrapolate to the current treatment era.

UNANSWERED QUESTIONS

1. Several important but unanswered questions remain from CASCADE. Would guided amiodarone therapy have been associated with better cardiac survival than was empiric amiodarone? One can only speculate but the meta-analysis by Roberts (4) suggests this is likely. If so, would the AVID protocol have been different? Probably so. Would the addition of beta-blocker therapy have improved the survival results in the conventional therapy arm? It is hard to imagine that the answer would not be yes. If so, how would the conventional therapy arm have fared against amiodarone? It seems probable that the difference would have been smaller, perhaps significantly so. If one extrapolates from ESVEM, the addition of beta blockade to class I therapy would have reduced mortality substantially, and made it similar to that achieved with a class II/III agent (7). How were the results affected by the concomitant ICD use? Again, this cannot be retrospectively determined, although the answer has great potential impact.

2. Additional important but unanswered questions in CASCADE include: How would amiodarone have fared against sotalol? Sotalol was not used in CASCADE, though ESVEM suggests that it is a better agent than class I drugs, and hence a better comparison to study against amiodarone. In part, AVID was to have addressed this question. However, in AVID, extremely little sotalol was used—and again, beta-blockers were underutilized as well. This probably repre-

sents, at least in part, physicians' inappropriate reticence about using beta-blockers in patients with ventricular dysfunction. So AVID, like CASCADE, was essentially an empiric amiodarone comparison trial—this time against the ICD. Since AVID showed a survival benefit against amiodarone of only a few months, the importance of low beta-blocker use and nonguided amiodarone therapy in AVID, as well as in CASCADE, as a model, should not be underestimated! Also unanswered was how CASCADE would appear had an on-therapy analysis been performed. This is an important question to ask for most trials, since on-therapy data demonstrate actual treatment results, rather than the treatment strategy results which are demonstrated by intention-to-treat analyses. However, since in CASCADE the amiodarone arm had the higher discontinuation rate but the lower event rates, an on-therapy analysis probably would not have altered the outcome conclusions. Important, as regards the discontinuation rates in CASCADE, is one additional question. This relates to the pulmonary toxicity experience. In CASCADE, the incidence of pulmonary toxicity attributed to amiodarone was 10% by 4 years, despite a mean dose under 200 mg/day. Pulmonary toxicity was distinguished from heart failure in this prospectively performed study, and should be looked at seriously. If these rates are reliable, they have important implications for other low-dose circumstances with amiodarone (e.g., the treatment of atrial fibrillation). Unfortunately, the pulmonary data in CASCADE were not presented as events plotted against actual affected individuals doses, so that the questions "is there a threshold dose effect or a linear dose-related effect present" was not answered. Of note, since EMIAT and CAMIAT (5,6) suggested a pulmonary toxicity rate of perhaps 1.5% per year with approximately 200 mg/day dosing, the CASCADE data may be valid and important for clinicians to recall.

QUESTIONS RAISED

In addition to questions left unanswered, CASCADE also raised some additional questions.

1. Can the results of CASCADE be extrapolated to a broader population? In addition to the concerns addressed above, including changes in the medical care of VF patients with heart disease and the greater use of ICDs in recent years, there are concerns about the CASCADE population itself. Low-risk patients were excluded. Fewer prior drug failures (average 1.5) were seen in the CASCADE trial than in other concurrent VT/VF trials. Only 50% were inducible at baseline EPS, despite most having coronary disease. However, in light of the AVID data, it is likely that the CASCADE results are meaningful to a broader group than the AVID type population alone.

2. On a larger scale, should class I antiarrhythmics, even guided, ever be used any more for VF; should empiric amiodarone be used any more for VF; what is the optimal role for combined drug–device therapy, and how does one judge the beneficial contributions of each component; and what is the true pulmonary toxicity profile of low-dose amiodarone? CASCADE, taken together with ESVEM, probably does suggest that class I drugs should be relegated to choices further down the therapeutic line than first- or second-line therapy. When used, class I agents should be coupled with beta-blockers if possible. CASCADE also suggests that empiric amiodarone, in the absence of concomitant beta blockade, does not provide adequate protection from VF in high-risk subjects. Whether guided therapy with amiodarone or empiric therapy with amiodarone coupled with beta-blockers would fare better remains to be determined. The Roberts meta-analysis (3) and the EMIAT and CAMIAT data suggest that these approaches are likely to be different than that of empiric amiodarone and worth testing. As for the drug–device combination and pulmonary toxicity questions, only further prospective observations in the future will provide the answers we seek.

REFERENCES

1. The CASCADE Investigators. Randomized antiarrhythmic drug therapy in survivors of cardiac arrest (the CASCADE study). Am J Cardiol 1993; 72:280–287.
2. Mason JW, for the Electrophysiologic Study Versus Electrocardiographic Monitoring Investigators. A comparison of seven antiarrhythmic drugs in patients with ventricular tachyarrhythmias. N Engl J Med 1993; 329:452–458.
3. Roberts SA, Viana MA, Nazari J, Bauman JL. Invasive and noninvasive methods to predict the long-term efficacy of amiodarone: a compilation of clinical observations using meta-analysis. PACE 1994; 17:1590–1602.
4. The AVID Investigators. Antiarrhythmics Versus Implantable Defibrillators (AVID): rationale, design, and methods. Am J Cardiol 1995; 75:470–475.
5. Julian DG, Camm AJ, Frangin G, Janse MJ, Munoz A, Schwartz PJ, Simon P, for the European Myocardial Infarction Amiodarone Trial Investigators. Randomized trial of effect of amiodarone on mortality in patients with left ventricular dysfunction after recent myocardial infarction: EMIAT. Lancet 1997; 349:667–674.
6. Cairns JA, Connolly SJ, Roberts R, Gent M, for the Canadian Amiodarone Myocardial Infarction Arrhythmia Trial Investigators. Randomized trial of outcome after myocardial infarction in patients with frequent or repetitive ventricular premature depolarizations: CAMIAT. Lancet 1997; 349:675–682.
7. Reiffel JA, Hahn E, Hartz V, Reiter MJ, for the ESVEM Investigators. Sotalol for ventricular tachyarrhythmias: beta-blocking and class III contributions, and relative efficacy versus class I drugs after prior drug failure. Am J Cardiol 1997; 79:1048–53.

4

The Electrophysiological Study Versus Electrocardiographic Monitoring (ESVEM) Trial

JAY W. MASON

University of Kentucky College of Medicine, Lexington, Kentucky

The ESVEM (Electrophysiological Study Versus Electrocardiographic Monitoring) trial was an investigator-initiated clinical trial supported by the National Institutes of Health through the RO-1 mechanism (1–5). The trial is interesting beyond its clinical findings because of the controversy it caused and the changing clinical environments in which it was conceived, conducted, reported, and interpreted.

DESIGN OF THE ESVEM TRIAL

The ESVEM trial arose from discussions among members of the now defunct Southwest Cardiology Research Group (SOCREG). This group, formed by the Universities of Arizona, California at San Diego, Colorado, New Mexico, Oklahoma, and Utah, agreed in the fall of 1983 to pursue a comparison of outcomes of patients with ventricular tachyarrhythmias managed by electrophysiological study (EPS) or Holter monitoring (HM). Continued discussions in the winter and spring led to a grant application submitted to NIH on July 2, 1984. A site visit took place in Bethesda, Maryland, on November 28, 1984. The award started on July 1, 1985, and trial enrollment began on October 1, 1985. Five of the six SOCREG and two other University-based enrollment centers formed the initial group. The group was later doubled to 14 centers to expand enrollment. The

59

clinical coordinating center was at the University of Utah and the data coordinating center was at the University of Arizona. Both of these centers participated in enrollment along with the Baylor College of Medicine, the University of Colorado, Columbia University, the University of New Mexico, and the University of Oklahoma in the original group, and Newark Beth Israel Medical Center, Northwestern University, Oregon Health Sciences University, the University of British Columbia, the University of California at San Francisco, the University of Massachusetts, and the University of Pennsylvania in the expanded group. Due to low enrollment, Northwestern University and the University of British Columbia later dropped out of the trial.

The underlying hypothesis of the trial was that either electrophysiological study or Holter monitoring gave more accurate predictions of the ability of an antiarrhythmic drug to prevent recurrence of ventricular tachycardia or sudden death. A mortality endpoint was not appropriate for examination of this very specific hypothesis. We were comparing the accuracy of the prediction of prevention of VT and VF made by the two methods rather than survival per se. Our primary interest was not in whether the drug therapies, with their multiple effects (electrophysiological, autonomic, cardiovascular, and extracardiac), affected survival, but rather whether a prediction of prevention of ventricular tachyarrhythmia by electrophysiological study or Holter monitoring was more reliable.

Patients were screened for enrollment if they had documented, sustained VT, cardiac arrest due to VT or VF, or syncope without electrocardiographic documentation (Fig. 1). In the latter case, patients were also required to have reproducibly inducible, sustained, monomorphic ventricular tachycardia with a rate below 226 beats per minute. Patients without medical exclusions then underwent electrophysiological study and Holter monitoring. Those patients who met EPS and HM criteria and gave consent were then enrolled and randomized. The randomization process allocated one-half of the enrollees to the HM limb and the other half to the EPS limb. Patients in both limbs then underwent serial drug testing with efficacy determined by the method to which they were randomized. Drugs the patient was eligible to receive (basically, those drugs the patient had not received previously or for which there was no contraindication) were then administered in random order until one of them was predicted effective. In the HM limb, a drug was considered provisionally effective if it reduced ectopy sufficiently (Fig. 2) as judged by comparing an on-drug 24-h Holter to the initial off-drug 48-h Holter. A final efficacy prediction was made after the patient underwent treadmill exercise without VT. In the EPS limb, a drug efficacy prediction was made if arrhythmia induction was suppressed (Fig. 2). Exercise testing was also performed in this limb, but was not required for a prediction of efficacy. After drug efficacy was predicted or all drugs had been tested without efficacy, the patient was discharged for long-term follow-up, which included scheduled clinic visits, drug level measurements, and Holter monitor studies.

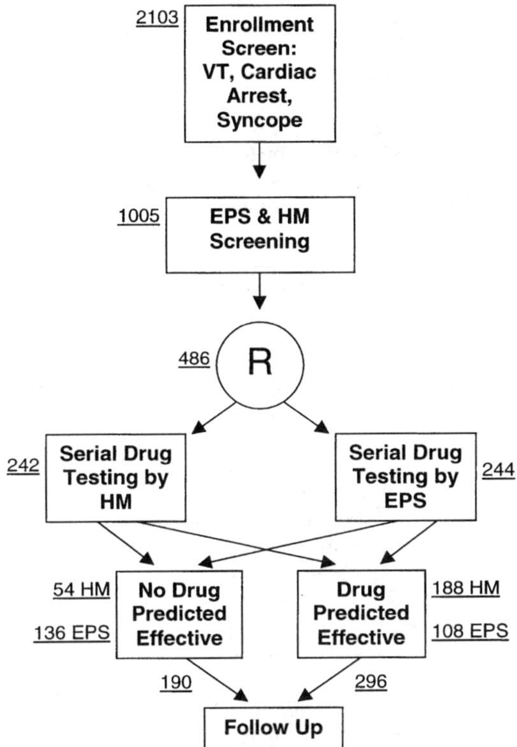

Figure 1 Enrollment and patient flow. The underlined figures outside the boxes indicate the number of patients entering each phase of the trial. R = 1:1 randomization of the 486 eligible, consenting patients; HM = Holter monitoring limb; EPS = electrophysiological study limb.

Comparative efficacy of the seven drugs used in the trial was a prespecified secondary analysis. We began the study with five drugs: quinidine, procainamide, sotalol, mexiletine, and imipramine. Imipramine performed poorly because our hemodynamically impaired ESVEM population could not tolerate its hypotensive and intense vagolytic effects. Thus, it was removed from the trial in accordance with protocol and was replaced by propafenone. Pirmenol was added as well in order to make two investigational agents available throughout the trial. Mexiletine had recently been approved, necessitating this addition. The investigational drugs (at that point, sotalol and pirmenol) were needed to help attract enrollees.

The original sample size estimate for this trial of 520 patients was based upon time-to-documented arrhythmia recurrence or sudden death. Using an expo-

<table>
<tr>
<td>

Holter Eligibility Criteria:

≥ 480 PVCs in 48 hours,
excluding PVCs in long VT runs

</td>
<td>

Holter Drug Efficacy Criteria:

Suppression of :
PVCs by 70%
PVC pairs by 80%
Unsustained VT by 90%
Sustained VT by 100%
VT > 5 beats on treadmill

</td>
</tr>
<tr>
<td>

EPS Eligibility Criteria:

Induction of sustained VT twice
in patients presenting with
sustained VT
Induction of sustained VT or VF
twice in patients presenting with
cardiac arrest
Induction of sustained VT with
rate ≤ 225 twice in patients
presenting with undiagnosed
syncope

</td>
<td>

EPS Drug Efficacy Criteria:

Induction of no more than 15
beats of VT using a minimum
of 2 extrastimuli at 3 ventricular
drive rates, with each
extrastimulus setting delivered
twice and decremented by
10ms from an initial CL of
400ms, and a maximum of up
to 3 extrastimuli at 2 pacing
sites depending on what was
required to induce VT or VF at
baseline.

</td>
</tr>
</table>

Figure 2 Holter and electrophysiology eligibility and drug efficacy criteria. The boxes on the left display the threshold Holter monitor and electrophysiological study criteria for randomization. The boxes on the right indicate the minimum degree of arrhythmia suppression required to declare drug efficacy in the two limbs.

nential survival model, we calculated that 290 patients with drug efficacy predictions would be needed. We wanted to be able to detect a difference in arrhythmia recurrence of 15% in the two groups with a power of 0.80 and a two-tailed significance level of 0.05. At about 2 years of enrollment, with approximately 56% of patients randomized achieving an efficacy prediction during the first few years of the trial, and the annual arrhythmia recurrence rate near the estimated 25%, the total enrollment requirement was recalculated to be 518 patients. Ultimately, fewer subjects were needed to supply 290 or more efficacy predictions.

RESULTS OF THE ESVEM TRIAL

Enrollment of 486 patients resulted in 296 patients (61%) with drug efficacy predictions (Fig. 1). Clinical characteristics of the patients are summarized in

Table 1 Clinical Characteristics of the Patients

	Randomized patients	Patients with efficacy predicted
n	486	296
Mean age (years)	65 ± 10	65 ± 10
Male	88%	87%
Previous MI	82%	80%
VT	73%	66%
Cardiac arrest	22%	23%
Syncope	8%	5%
Mean LVEF	0.32 ± 0.12	0.33 ± 0.12
Mean PVC count	320 ± 428	338 ± 417

Table 1. There were no significant differences among patients in the two randomization limbs. Those with efficacy predicted were clinically similar to those without, except that they had higher LVEF and were more likely to have been tested in the HM limb (2).

Drug efficacy was much more frequent in the HM limb (77%) in comparison to the EPS limb (45%) and the median time to achievement of an efficacy prediction was shorter in the HM limb (10 vs. 25 days).

There were 278 arrhythmia recurrences in the 486 randomized patients. One hundred fifty of the 296 patients with an efficacy prediction had a recurrence, while 128 events occurred in the 190 patients with no drug predicted to be effective (Fig. 3). There was a strikingly higher actuarial arrhythmia recurrence rate in the latter group, supporting the validity of drug efficacy testing in the ESVEM population. That is, serial drug testing either brought about a better outcome, or accurately identified patients that would experience fewer events independent of drug influences. This conclusion is further supported by the fact that the 190 patients without a drug efficacy prediction received more aggressive therapy. In fact, their therapy would be considered today to be superior to that received by the other 296 patients because the 190 patients without drug efficacy predicted were treated more frequently with implanted cardioverter-defibrillators (ICDs) (6,7) and amiodarone (8). Among the 190 patients without an efficacy prediction, 15% had an ICD implanted, 41% received amiodarone, and another 15% had both an ICD and amiodarone, while among the 296 with efficacy predicted one patient received and ICD and none received amiodarone while continuing on therapy predicted effective.

The primary analysis of the trial was the comparison of arrhythmia recurrence in the EPS and HM limbs among the 296 patients with a prediction of drug efficacy. There was no difference in this primary endpoint (Fig. 4). One must

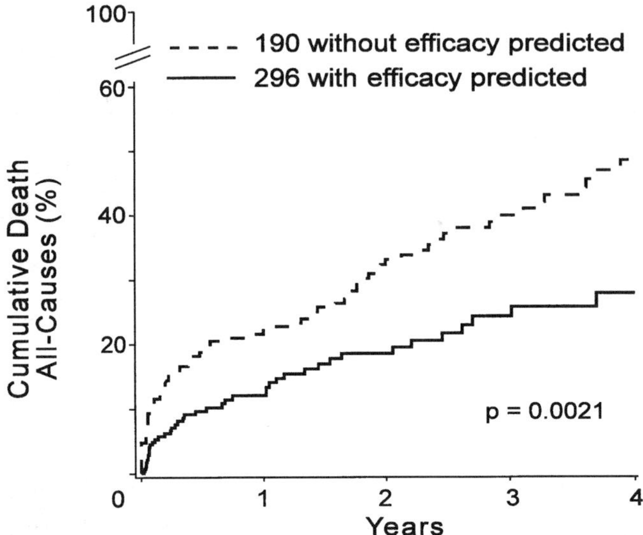

Figure 3 Comparison of actuarial mortality in patients with and without a drug efficacy prediction. The outcome of patients with a drug efficacy prediction was significantly better. Since patients were not randomly assigned to these groups, the difference in mortality might be related to differences in therapy, differences in patient characteristics, or both. (Reproduced with permission from Ref. 5.)

conclude that the two testing methods, as used in the ESVEM trial, are equally accurate in predicting efficacy of the antiarrhythmic drugs used in the trial. In addition, we found no significant differences in all-cause mortality, cardiac mortality, and arrhythmic mortality in the two limbs.

There was a significant difference in costs associated with the two techniques. Both the initial hospitalization and long-term care cost more in the EPS limb (9–11).

The comparative efficacy of the antiarrhythmic drugs used in the ESVEM trial was a prespecified analysis identified early in the design of the trial. Sotalol was compared to the other six drugs because more patients received it chronically than any other drug (Table 2), and because a class comparison (Vaughn-Williams Class I vs. Class III) was also prespecified. As shown in Table 2, sotalol was predicted to be effective more frequently than the other drugs. There were fewer arrhythmia recurrences in patients taking sotalol (Fig. 5), and the relative risks of death, cardiac death, and arrhythmic death for patients taking sotalol compared to those receiving any of the other drugs were 0.50 for each endpoint. Sotalol was also better tolerated and resulted in fewer therapy-ending side effects. As a

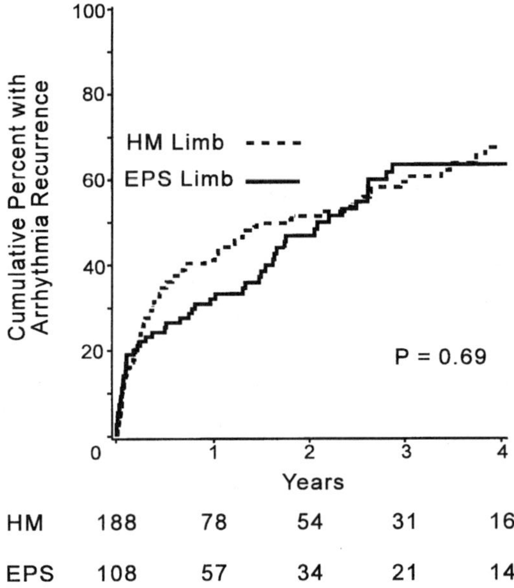

Figure 4 Comparison of actuarial recurrence of VT and cardiac arrest in the Holter monitoring and the electrophysiological study limbs in patients with a drug efficacy prediction. There was no significant difference in this primary endpoint, indicating equal accuracy of Holter monitoring and electrophysiological study in predicting antiarrhythmic drug efficacy in patients with previous VT or cardiac arrest. (Reproduced from Ref. 3.)

Table 2 Drug Usage and Efficacy in the ESVEM Trial

Drug	*n* Patients tested	% with efficacy predicted			*n* Patients treated	% with recurrence
		by HM	by EPS	Overall		
Sotalol	234	56	35	43	85	50
Mexiletine	226	67	12	36	58	61
Propafenone	220	48	14	28	45	61
Procainamide	158	50	26	34	39	71
Quinidine	157	59	16	33	38	62
Imipramine	129	45	10	21	15	73
Primenol	109	55	19	32	27	69

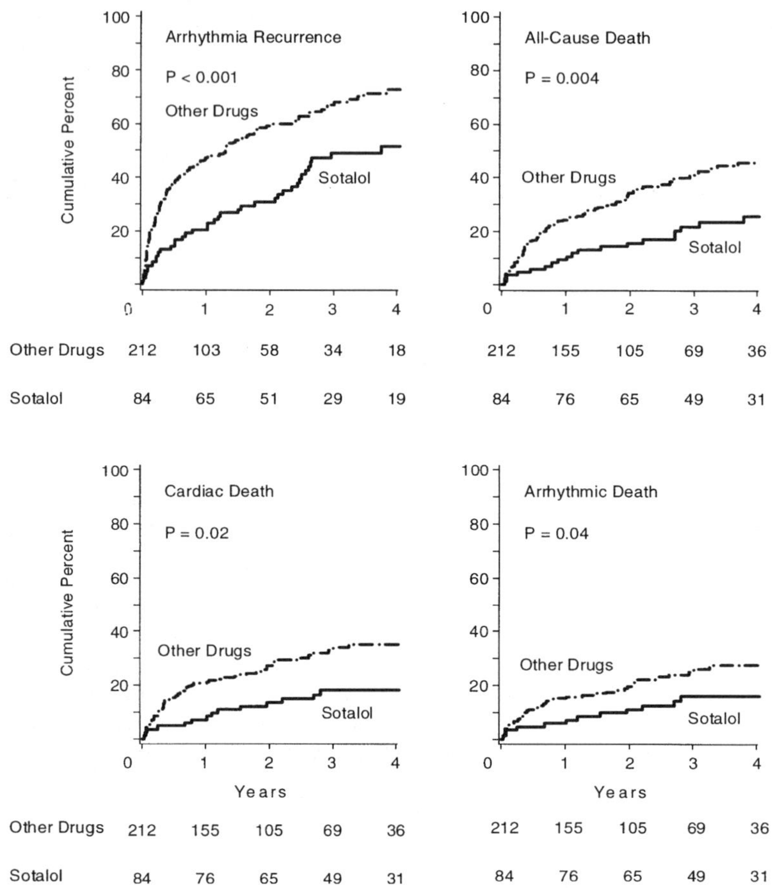

Figure 5 Comparison of actuarial arrhythmia recurrence and mortality in patients receiving sotalol and patients receiving other drugs. In this intention-to-treat analysis, sotalol therapy was associated with significantly better outcomes for all four endpoints. An analysis censoring patients if they stopped taking the drug predicted effective yielded similar results. (Reproduced from Ref. 4.)

result of all of these factors, patients initially exposed to sotalol were much more likely to still be receiving the drug during follow-up. For example, the actuarial probability that a patient given sotalol and tested by HM would have efficacy predicted and still be on the drug at 1 year was 33%, and if tested by EPS, 23%. The corresponding figures for the other six drugs combined were 17% and 5%.

Table 3 Ancillary Findings of the ESVEM Trial

Ref.[a]	Finding and significance
12	Sodium channel blockers prolong late potentials and slow VT
13	Heart period variability in patients with MI and VT/VF
14	Concordance of HM and EPS does not improve efficacy prediction
15	VT is usually not initiated by a distant ectopic beat
16	The fractal dimension of PVC occurrence predicts outcome
17	Cardiac arrest presentation is not more ominous than VT presentation
18	Arrhythmia suppression by both HM and EPS greatly limits the frequency of drug efficacy predictions without improving accuracy of the predictions
19	Patients with arrhythmia suppression on the first but not the second 24-h HM have outcomes similar to those with suppression on both
20	Easy reproducibility of VT/VF induction does not provide a better baseline for drug testing than less easily reproduced VT/VF at EPS
21	Significance of unsustained VT in patients with sustained VT
22	SAECG does not predict drug efficacy in patients with VT
23	Unsustained predicts sustained VT
24	Heart rate variability changes predict onset of ventricular tachyarrhythmias
25	HM criteria of drug efficacy: trade-off between sensitivity and specificity
26	Unexplained syncope has a poor prognosis
27	ESVEM patients with VT on HM have a higher prevalence of ischemic disease, but otherwise are clinically similar and have a similar outcome to those without
28	In- but not out-of-hospital deaths are usually classified as arrhythmic
29,30,31, *32,33*	HRV changes indicate a complex causal relationship between the ANS and VT
34,35	Repolarization changes precede onset of VT

[a] Italicized references are published as abstracts only at this time.

ANCILLARY FINDINGS OF THE ESVEM TRIAL

The ESVEM investigators proposed several ancillary studies (12–35). Those studies that have been published as full manuscripts or abstracts are listed in Table 3.

SIGNIFICANCE OF THE ESVEM TRIAL

The ESVEM trial provides a good illustration of how the clinical relevance and significance of a trial may change over time, and how interpretation of a trial's results may differ among experts. It is interesting to consider the significance of the ESVEM trial in four different time periods: during its design, at the time the results were reported, now, and in the future.

Period 1: During Design, 1983

The relative merits of EPS and HM for the assessment of antiarrhythmic drug efficacy in patients with ventricular arrhythmias was a matter of considerable controversy in 1983 when the ESVEM trial was being designed. Proponents of the two techniques had recently published large studies supporting their methods (36,37). The controversy had blossomed at national meetings and a clear line was drawn, with Bernard Lown's group and many practicing cardiologists and internists on one side, and the new, growing group of invasive electrophysiologists on the other, including the groups from Montefiore Hospital, Stanford University, University of Pennsylvania, and many others. The invasive approach was relatively new at that time, and many considered it to be excessively aggressive and overly unpleasant for the patient. Other now-popular alternatives, amiodarone and ICDs, were not available at that time. Thus, determination of the relative merits of the two techniques seemed an urgent matter and one that would have a strong influence upon clinical practice. The designers and investigators in the trial were nearly all invasive electrophysiologists, and most of them believed that EPS was the best approach, but recognized that it must be proven.

Period 2: Reporting of Results, 1992

Nine years passed between the initial design phase of the trial and preliminary announcement of its results at the April, 1992, American College of Cardiology Scientific Sessions in Dallas, Texas. The trial itself took 6 years, and the other 3 years were taken up by design and preparation prior to initiation of the trial, and by data verification and analysis after the trial. Passage of a decade from conception of a clinical trial to its reporting is not unusual, and it is also not unusual for the clinical relevance and significance of the original question scrutinized by the trial to change in that period of time. This was true of the ESVEM trial. Between 1983 and 1992 several changes in the management of patients with ventricular tachyarrhythmias had taken place. By 1992, the majority of patients with ventricular tachyarrhythmias who were to receive drug therapy were undergoing EPS for drug selection. A small, randomized trial had been published showing superiority of the invasive approach (38), and even the Lown group had begun to use EPS in some patients (39). In addition, amiodarone had been approved and was routinely used without EPS or HM guidance. Finally, use of ICDs was increasing and some experts considered them to be first-line therapy for ventricular tachyarrhythmias, eliminating the need for drug testing altogether.

Thus, use of HM for drug efficacy testing had become a secondary method, used primarily when VT/VF was not inducible at EPS or when EPS could not be used for drug selection for other reasons. And, reliance upon antiarrhythmic drugs and drug efficacy testing had diminished. These changes set the stage for an explosive response to the announcement of the ESVEM trial results.

Response to ESVEM Trial Results

At the time the results were announced, electrophysiologists had convinced their referring physicians of the value of EPS and of its perceived superiority over HM in management of ventricular tachyarrhythmias. These arrhythmia specialists' practices depended upon referrals of patients with ventricular arrhythmias for EPS. Their hospitals had invested considerably in equipment and space for performance of EPS. These referrals were also fueling an increase in ICD implantations. There was open concern over the possibility that knowledge of the equivalence of EPS and HM in the ESVEM trial would lead internists and general cardiologists to stop referring patients with ventricular tachyarrhythmias and manage them themselves by selecting antiarrhythmic drugs using HM, since, unlike EPS, HM was available universally and did not require interpretation by a specialist.

The clinical electrophysiology community aggressively attacked the ESVEM trial. ESVEM results were presented on the morning of Tuesday, April 14, 1992. By early afternoon a group of academic clinical cardiac electrophysiologists, including one of the ESVEM investigators, had come together and arranged a press conference to criticize the trial. The findings of the trial were covered on ABC's national evening news broadcast that night, and this group's opposition to the findings was included in the coverage. Subsequently several articles in the medical press and in non-peer-reviewed magazines (40) included a wide range of criticisms. When the results of the trial were published the next year, additional criticism followed (41–46). Many of these criticisms have been rebutted by ESVEM investigators and others (5,47–51). Based upon what were perceived to be excessive arrhythmia recurrence and mortality rates in the ESVEM trial (though, in fact, the rates were consonant with those of all prospective trials done in patients with ventricular tachyarrhythmias during that period of time) ESVEM's "take-home" message for many arrhythmia specialists was that the efficacy of drugs, selected by HM or EPS, was too poor to justify antiarrhythmic therapy alone; ICDs seemed preferable.

The ESVEM finding regarding sotalol's superior efficacy over the five class I drugs used in the trial was not as controversial as the other findings, though dissatisfaction with the main trial results carried over to this issue (41). Though comparison of drugs was a secondary objective of the trial, the efficacy of sotalol turned out to be the trial's most influential result. It not only increased the use of sotalol for ventricular tachyarrhythmias, but it helped generate interest in the potential efficacy of class III drugs and beta-blockade in patients with life-threatening ventricular arrhythmias.

Period 3: The Present, 1998

The clinical relevance of the ESVEM trial has changed considerably in the 6 years since the results of the trial were announced. The trend toward use of ICDs has continued, and two prospective randomized trials supported the ICD strategy instead of drug therapy for ventricular arrhythmias (6,7) The need to shorten hospital stays has also contributed to the now well-established preference to implant an ICD rather than laboriously evaluate drug efficacy with serial testing. At the present time, in the United States, choice of either HM or EPS to carry out drug efficacy assessment now rarely has to be made. Even when drugs are used in conjunction with ICDs, they are assessed by EPS because the ability of the ICD to detect and terminate VT or VF in the presence of the new drug cannot be evaluated by HM. In other countries in which ICDs are in short supply or unavailable, the original question explored by the ESVEM trial remains relevant.

Period 4: The Future

Renewed future relevance of the ESVEM trial seems unlikely but not out of the realm of possibility. ICD implantation is more costly than drug therapy in survivors of ventricular tachyarrhythmias, as demonstrated by the AVID trial (52). If the pressure to reduce health care costs was to result in unavailability of ICDs, drug efficacy assessment would become commonplace again. If much more effective antiarrhythmic drugs were to become available in the future, there might again be interest in drug efficacy assessment, if those new drugs were at least as effective as the ICD and could be evaluated by HM or EPS.

CONCLUSIONS

The ESVEM trial—its history and results, and the response of experts to its outcome—teach several lessons in clinical trial design and reporting. First, whenever possible, a clinical trial should investigate a fundamental biological or therapeutic question that has permanent relevance. The objective of the ESVEM trial, comparison of two testing methods (HM and EPS), had immediate relevance when the trial was designed, but no significance beyond the application of the two methods. During the decade that passed between the conception and the reporting of ESVEM trial findings, the clinical relevance of the comparison had diminished. The value of the trial would have been greater if it had also explored a more basic issue in clinical arrhythmology. That is not to say that purely practical therapeutic questions should not be explored in randomized clinical trials. Many such questions demand an answer. But, a risk of obsolescence awaits such trials.

Second, the duration of a clinical trial, from its conception to reporting of its results, should be as short as possible, preferably not greater than 5 years. Diagnostic and therapeutic advances are occurring so rapidly in present-day medicine that few therapeutic dilemmas persist more than 5 years.

Third, a controversial and potentially unpopular trial result should not be revealed suddenly. The academic community should be alerted to the findings to provide it time to understand their implications and to develop strategies for dealing with them.

REFERENCES

1. The ESVEM Investigators. The ESVEM trial. Electrophysiologic study versus electrocardiographic monitoring for selection of antiarrhythmic therapy of ventricular tachyarrhythmias. Circulation 1989; 79:1354–1360.
2. The ESVEM Investigators. Determinants of predicted efficacy of antiarrhythmic drugs in the electrophysiologic study versus electrocardiographic monitoring trial. Circulation 1993; 87:323–329.
3. Mason JW for the Electrophysiologic Study Versus Electrocardiographic Monitoring (ESVEM) Investigators. A Comparison of Electrophysiologic Testing with Holter Monitoring to Predict Antiarrhythmic-Drug Efficacy for Ventricular Tachyarrhythmias. N Engl J Med 1993; 329:445–451.
4. Mason JW for the Electrophysiologic Study Versus Electrocardiographic Monitoring (ESVEM) Investigators. A Comparison of Seven Antiarrhythmic Drugs in Patients with Ventricular Tachyarrhythmias. N Engl J Med 1993; 329:452–458.
5. Mason JW, Marcus FI, Bigger JT, Lazzara R, Reiffel JA, Reiter MJ, Mann D. A summary and assessment of the findings and conclusions of the ESVEM trial. Prog Cardiovasc Dis 1996; 38:347–358.
6. The Antiarrhythmics Versus Implantable Defibrillators (AVID) Investigators. A comparison of antiarrhythmic-drug therapy with implantable defibrillators in patients resuscitated from near-fatal ventricular arrhythmias. N Engl J Med 1997; 337:1576–1583.
7. Moss AJ, Hall WJ, Cannom DS, et al. Improved survival with an implanted defibrillator in patients with coronary disease at high risk for ventricular arrhythmia. Multicenter Automatic Defibrillator Implantation Trial Investigators. N Engl J Med 1996; 335:1933–1940.
8. The CASCADE Investigators. Randomized antiarrhythmic drug therapy in survivors of cardiac arrest (the CASCADE study). Am J Cardiol 1993; 72:280–287.
9. Omoigui NA, Marcus FI, Mason JW, Hahn EA, Hartz VL, Hlatky MA, for the ESVEM Investigators. Cost of initial therapy in the electrophysiologic study versus electrocardiographic monitoring trial (ESVEM). Circulation 1995; 91:1070–1076.

10. Hlatky MA. Cost and efficacy analysis in the ESVEM trial: implications for diagnosis and therapy for ventricular tachyarrhythmias. Prog Cardiovasc Dis 1996; 38(5): 371–376.

11. Hlatky MA, Boothroyd DB, Johnstone IM, Marcus FI, Hahn E, Hartz V, Mason JW, for the Investigators. Long-term cost-effectiveness of alternative management strategies for patients with life-threatening ventricular arrhythmias. J Clin Epidemiol 1997; 50:185–193.

12. Freedman RA, Steinberg JS, for the ESVEM Investigators. Selective prolongation of QRS late potentials by sodium channel blocking antiarrhythmic drugs: relation to slowing of ventricular tachycardia. J Am Coll Cardiol 1991; 17:1017–1025.

13. Bigger JT, Jr, Fleiss JL, Rolnitzky LM, Steinman RC, with data contributed by the CAPS and ESVEM Investigators. Stability over time of heart period variability in patients with previous myocardial infarction and ventricular arrhythmias. Am J Cardiol 1992; 69:718–723.

14. Reiter MJ, Mann DE, Reiffel JE, Hahn E, Hartz V, and the ESVEM Investigators. Significance and incidence of concordance of drug efficacy predictions by Holter monitoring and electrophysiologic study in the ESVEM trial. Circulation 1995; 91: 1988–1995.

15. Anderson KP, Walker R, Dustman T, Fuller M, Mori M, for the ESVEM Investigators. Spontaneous sustained ventricular tachycardia in the Electrophysiologic Study Versus Electrocardiographic Monitoring (ESVEM) trial. J Am Coll Cardiol 1995; 26:489–96.

16. Karagounis LA, Stein KM, Bair T, Albright D, Anderson JL for the ESVEM Investigators. Fractal dimension predicts arrhythmia recurrence in patients being treated for life-threatening ventricular arrhythmias. J Electrocardiol 1995; 28:71–73.

17. Caruso AC, Marcus FI, Hahn EA, Hartz VL, Mason JW, and the ESVEM Investigators. Predictors of arrhythmic death and cardiac arrest in the ESVEM trial. Circulation 1997; 96:1888–1892.

18. Reiter MJ, Mann DE, Reiffel JA, Hahn E, Hartz V, and the ESVEM Investigators. Significance and incidence of concordance of drug efficacy predictions by Holter monitoring and electrophysiological study in the ESVEM trial. Circulation 1995; 91:1988–1995.

19. Reiter JM, Karagounis LA, Mann DE, Reiffel JA, Hahn E, Hartz V and the ESVEM Investigators. Reproducibility of drug efficacy predictions by Holter monitoring in the Electrophysiologic Study Versus Electrocardiographic Monitoring (ESVEM) trial. Am J Cardiol 1997; 79:315–22.

20. Mann DE, Hartz V, Hahn EA, Reiter MJ and the ESVEM Investigators. Effect of reproducibility of baseline arrhythmia induction on drug efficacy predictions and outcome in the ESVEM trial. Am J Cardiol 1997; 80:1448–1452.

21. Anderson KP, Mori M, for the ESVEM Trial Investigators. The clinical significance of nonsustained ventricular tachycardia in patients with sustained ventricular tachyarrhythmias. Ann Noninvas Electrocardiol 1996; 1:33–43.

22. Steinberg JS, Freedman RA, for the ESVEM Investigators. The signal averaged ECG does not predict drug efficacy in sustained ventricular arrhythmias. Circulation 1987; 76:IV–344.

23. Mason JW and the ESVEM Investigators. Unsustained VT as a predictor of spontaneous sustained VT in the ESVEM study. Circulation 1991; 84 (suppl II):II–348.

24. Marks ML, Dustman TJ, Fuller MS, Ben-Haim S, Mori M, Johnston M, Anderson KP. Frequency domain characteristics of heart rate variability preceding recorded spontaneous sustained ventricular tachycardia. Circulation 1993; 88:1–116.

25. Reiffel J, Mann D, Reiter M, Freedman R, Huang SKS, Hahn E, Hartz V, and the ESVEM Investigators. A comparison of Holter suppression criteria for declaring drug efficacy in patients with sustained ventricular tachyarrhythmias in the ESVEM trial. J Am Coll Cardiol 1994; 279A.

26. Olshansky B, Hahn EA, Hartz VL, Prater SP, Mason JW. Clinical significance of syncope in the electrophysiologic study versus electrocardiographic monitoring (ESVEM) trial. The ESVEM Investigators. Am Heart 1994; 137:878–86.

27. Anderson KP, Mori M, Lyver S, Dustman T, Fuller MS, for the ESVEM Investigators. Clinical characteristics and outcome of patients with ventricular tachycardia on the baseline Holter recording in the electrophysiologic study versus electrocardiographic monitoring trial (ESVEM). Circulation 1994; 90(4):I–339.

28. Olshansky B, Hartz V, Hahn E, Mason JW and the ESVEM Investigators. Out-of-hospital versus in-hospital death I the ESVEM trial. J Am Coll Cardiol (Special Issue) 1995; 314A.

29. Li C, Shusterman V, Gottipaty V, Fahrig S, Anderson KP for the ESVEM Investigators. Changes in the energy distribution of heart rate variability in patients with chronic sympathetic predominance. PACE 1997; 20(II):1104.

30. Shusterman V, Aysin B, Gottipaty V, Fahrig S, Anderson KP for the ESVEM Investigators. Physiological saturation in the markers of sympathetic activity preceding spontaneous sustained ventricular tachycardia. PACE 1997; 20(II):1158.

31. Anderson KP, Shusterman V, Aysin B, Weiss R, Brode S, Gottipaty V. Distinctive RR dynamics preceding two modes of onset of spontaneous sustained ventricular tachycardia. (ESVEM) Investigators. Electrophysiologic Study Versus Electrocardiographic Monitoring. J Cardiovasc Electrophysiol 1999; 10:897–904.

32. Aysin B, Shusterman V, Grave I, Gottipaty V, Fahrig S, Anderson KP for the ESVEM Investigators. Differences in circadian variations of ventricular tachycardia and premature ventricular complexes. J Am Coll Cardiol 1997; 29:293A.

33. Shusterman V, Aysin B, Gottipaty V, Weiss R, Brode S, Schwantzman D, Anderson KP. Autonomic nervous system activity and the spontaneous initiation of ventricular tachycardia. ESVEM Investigators. Electrophysiologic Study Versus Electrocardiographic monitoring trial. J Am Coll Cardiol 1998; 32:1891–1899.

34. Konety S, Shusterman V, Shah SI, Gottipaty V, Fahrig S, Anderson KP for the ESVEM Investigators. Dissociation in QT-RR relationship preceding sustained ventricular tachycardia. PACE 1997; 20(II):1112.

35. Shusterman V, Konety S, Flanigan S, Shah SI, Fahrig S, Gottipaty V, Anderson KP. Short-term changes in RR and QT-intervals are related to the rate and duration of ventricular tachycardia. Circulation 1997; 96(8):1–581.

36. Graboys TB, Lown B, Podrid PJ, DeSilva R. Long-term survival of patients with malignant ventricular arrhythmia treated with antiarrhythmic drugs. Am J Cardiol 1982;50:437–443.

37. Swerdlow CD, Winkle RA, Mason JW. Determinants of survival in patients with ventricular tachyarrhythmias. N Engl J Med 1983; 308:1436–1442.

38. Mitchell LB, Duff HJ, Manyari DE, Wyse DG. A randomized clinical trial of the noninvasive and invasive aporaches to drug therapy of ventricular tachycardia. N Engl J Med 1987; 317:1681–1687.

39. Lampert S, Lown B, Graboys TB, Podrid PJ, Blatt CM. Determinants of survival in patients with malignant ventricular arrhythmia associated with coronary artery disease. Am J Cardiol 1988; 61:791–797.

40. Maloney J. CPI AICD Advances. Fourth Quarter 1992; 8–10.

41. Ward DE, Camm AJ. Dangerous ventricular arrhythmias—can we predict drug efficacy? N Engl J Med 1993; 329:498–499.

42. Damle RS, Ehlert FA. The treatment of ventricular tachyarrhythmias. N Engl J Med 1994; 330:286–287.

42a. Winters SL, Rubinstein D, Gomes JA. The treatment of ventricular arrhythmias. N Engl J Med 1994; 330:287 (Letters to the Editor).

43. Biblo LA, Carlson MD, Waldo AL. Insights into the electrophysiology study versus electrocardiographic monitoring trial: Its programmed stimulation protocol may introduce bias when assessing long-term antiarrhythmic drug therapy. J Am Coll Cardiol 1995; 25:1601–1604.

44. Gettes LS. ESVEM and the hazards of clinical trials. Circulation 1995; 91:1908–1909.

45. Mitchell LB, Wyse DG. Interpretation of the results of the electrophysiologic study versus electrocardiographic monitoring (ESVEM) study: programmed ventricular stimulation advacates' view. Coronary Artery Dis 1994; 5:671–676.

46. Winters SL, Curwin JH. Sotalol and the management of ventricular arrhythmias: implications of ESVEM (editorial). Pacing Clin Electrophysiol 1995; 18:377–378.

47. Mason JW for the ESVEM Investigators. (Response to Letters) N Engl J Med 1994; 330:287–288.

48. Lazzara R. Results of Holter ECG guided therapy for ventricular arrhythmias: the ESVEM trial. PACE 1994; 17:473–477.

49. d'Avila A, Fenelon G, Nellens P, Brugada P. Interpretation of the results of the electrophysiologic study versus electrocardiographic monitoring (ESVEM) study: electrocardiographic monitoring advocates' view. Coronary Artery Disease 1994; 5:677–681.

50. Reiffel JA, Reiter MJ, Freedman RA, Mann D, Huang SKS, Hahn E, Hartz V, Mason J and the ESVEM Investigators. Influence of Holter monitor and electrophysiologic study methods and efficacy criteria on the outcome of ventricular tachycardia and ventricular fibrillation patients in the ESVEM trial. Prog Cardiovasc Dis 1996; 38(5): 359–370.

51. Anderson KP, Hartz VL, Hahn EA, Moon TE. Design and analysis of the ESVEM trial. Prog Cardiovasc Dis 1996; 38(6): 489–502.

52. Larsen GC, McAnulty JH, Hallstrom A, Marchant C, Shein M, Akiyama T, Brodsky M, Baessler C, Pinsky SL, Jennings CA, Morris M. Hospitalization charges in the Antiarrhythmics Versus Implantable Defibrillators (AVID) Trial: the AVID economic analysis study. Circulation 1997; 96:1–77 (abstract).

MASOOD AKHTAR

University of Wisconsin Medical School—Milwaukee Clinical Campus, Milwaukee Heart Institute, Sinai Samaritan Medical Center, and St. Luke's Medical Center, Milwaukee, Wisconsin

INTRODUCTION

ESVEM represents a large randomized trial comparing the invasive electrophysiological studies to Holter monitoring for prediction of antiarrhythmic drug efficacy (1–5). Patient Enrollment began on October 1, 1985, and results were published on August 12, 1993, with a total follow-up time of 6.2 years. A maximum of six antiarrhythmic drugs were used in each randomized patient before efficacy or lack thereof was concluded. It was reported that there was no statistically significant difference between the two methods for prediction of drug efficacy in this population with ventricular tachycardia (VT)–ventricular fibrillation (VF) (3).

CRITIQUE

ESVEM's strengths include a relatively large size, randomization of patients, random order of drug utilization, completion of a rigorous protocol with serial drug testing, and long duration of follow-up. However, there are several deficiencies and limitations of both generic and specific nature that need examination to draw meaningful conclusions (6–12). These will be addressed individually.

PATIENT SCREENING

The reason for initiating the screening process is not specified. It is clear that these were not consecutive patients with VT/VF or syncope presenting to the participating centers. Since electrophysiological studies (EPS) were carried out after screening, an ECG-documented arrhythmia probably was the most likely trigger to look for possible eligibility. Potentially this could bias the trial in favor of ambulatory monitoring identifying a higher proportion of patients meeting the eligibility criteria. Infrequent or absent ventricular ectopy at the time of initial encounter may have eliminated many patients who could have benefited from the EPS-guided approach. Comparison of the two methods seems less important than learning which one is clinically more useful in consecutive patients with VT–VF.

Significant center (and investigator) bias can be recognized in this trial. All except one center (Utah) recruited less than 45 patients (3). Over a 6-year period, many of these centers with substantially higher patient volumes were able to enroll only a relatively small proportion of cases. Assuming at least 50 such patients were seen at these sites annually, less than 10% of potential candidates were eventually randomized. While one may consider these numbers adequate as the randomized trials go, it leaves one wondering about the possibility of systematic exclusion by a referring physician or investigator. Possible reasons for exclusion could include:

1. Investigator or referring physician perceptions that the nonpharmacological therapy is more suitable for a given patient.
2. Clinical state of the patient may not permit rigorous testing with one or both methods.
3. The requirement of both 48-h Holter monitoring and serial EPS perceived as time-consuming and costly.
4. Abandonment of practice utilizing multiple drug studies with EPS in the later years of recruitment due to changing trends in arrhythmia management.

The above considerations lead to a highly selected population ultimately recruited into ESVEM trial. Since no systematic information was either gathered or reported to explain nonscreened patients, it is conceivable that the enrolled patients are not representative of VT/VF at large. This makes it difficult to apply ESVEM results to clinical practice of consecutive patients.

ENROLLED POPULATION

ESVEM is predominantly a study of VT population since only 22% had cardiac arrest. The natural history of VT versus VF population is different (3). This issue is further complicated by the fact that out-of-hospital cardiac arrest due to VF has different outcomes in various communities. VF survivorship, for example, in Seattle is >25%, which is vastly different than New York (<5%). Conceivably cardiac arrest survivors from communities with low successful resuscitation rates may contain a higher percentage of natural survivors. This creates the distinct dilemma of how to compare cardiac arrest populations from different communities, let alone lumping VF with VT survivors, as was done in ESVEM. Even among VT patients, hemodynamic stability or lack thereof was not highlighted. If a different proportion of these two categories existed in the two limbs, it could have potentially affected the results. It certainly seems too risky to apply ESVEM results to the VF population.

Patients with coronary artery disease had a significantly greater representation in the Holter versus the EPs limb ($p = 0.036$), among those where drug efficacy was predicted (3). Even though the authors implied this difference did not correlate with recurrence of VT–VF, it is a problem, since EP studies are traditionally less reliable in noncoronary artery substrates for drug efficacy predictions.

Almost two-thirds of the randomized patients had failed at least one antiarrhythmic drug previously and in most cases it was a class I agent (3,4). If the failure was predominantly due to arrhythmia recurrence, a poor outcome with class I drug efficacy prediction was therefore built into the design. This may also have been a factor showing greater drug efficacy with class III agents in comparison (4).

SELECTION OF DRUGS

Seven antiarrhythmic drugs were available in the ESVEM trial and up to six were used in the randomized patients (1–5). All except one (sotalol) had class I properties. There are several problems with this aspect of the design and the antiarrhythmic agents selected.

The practice of serial drug testing using six antiarrhythmic agents was literally abandoned long before the end of recruitment in this trial. This could be ascribed to two main factors:

1. It had become apparent that the highest likelihood of finding an effective agent is at the first trial. With failure of the initial agent, subsequent drug testing yielded poor response rates. At fifth or sixth trial, it will be difficult to distinguish true drug efficacy from noninduction due to variation in the reproducibility of the technique (13–18).
2. Clinical experience had increasingly suggested superiority of implantable defibrillators (ICD) and amiodarone over class I antiarrhythmic drugs for management of high-risk patients with VT–VF (19–24). Consequently, failure of first- or second-drug trial was considered sufficient to resort to ICD therapy.

The main impact of the above was that serial drug testing with multiple agents was being phased out and the drug efficacy prediction using multiple drug trials (as conducted in ESVEM) became obsolete.

Selection of certain antiarrhythmic agents seldom used alone in patients with sustained VT–VF remains debatable. Notwithstanding, the choice of various class I drugs in mostly class-I-refractory population was destined to fail. Clinical practice would have dictated a switch to class III or a combination of agents. In fact, amiodarone was one of the most commonly prescribed agents at the time ESVEM enrollment was still ongoing. The revelation that a class III agent, sotalol, fared better in this population than other drugs was important, but not contrary to clinical expectations. Nonetheless, due to caution regarding the use of sotalol in patients with poor LV function and its proarrhythmic potential, amiodarone continued to remain a commonly prescribed drug for sustained VT–VF, despite the fact it was not used in the ESVEM trial. The evolution of this practice behavior appears justified and independent of ESVEM results.

METHODOLOGY (TESTING PROTOCOLS)

It is well known that many patients with VT/VF do not have sufficient spontaneous ectopy to enable Holter monitoring to be used as a reliable guide. Furthermore, to subject patients to a 48-h Holter monitor and EPS before ESVEM results can be applied severely hampers practical utility of the trial (6). Since neither of the methods used predicted the outcome reliably (i.e., unexpected high VT/VF recurrence rate), one can argue whether either of the tests was applied appropriately.

Less controversy surrounds the Holter protocol, which suggests that under acceptable Holter methodology, the technique is unreliable for drug efficacy prediction. The EPS stimulation protocol, on the other hand, was arguably less aggressive in some cases (only up to two extrastimuli) resulting in overestimation of drug efficacy (8). Class I and class III antiarrhythmic drugs prolong local myocardial refractory periods and, therefore, shorter coupling intervals (S_1S_2, S_1S_3, or S_1S_4) that induced VT/VF in the baseline would be required postdrug before one can declare true noninducibility (25). Intuitively this would have necessitated a more aggressive pacing protocol after the drug compared to the baseline. If this was followed, it is likely that very few drug responders would have been identified using the EPS technique, a more realistic outcome in this drug-refractory group and ultimately evidenced by the high drug failure rate.

FOLLOW-UP AND RESULTS

Perhaps the most disturbing aspects of ESVEM are the disappointing outcomes.

1. High VT/VF recurrence rate ($\geq 38\%$ at 1 year) in patients with drug

efficacy prediction suggests flawed methodology. With these high recurrence rates it appears that neither one of the techniques was predictive of drug efficacy. The authors, in fact, pointed out that the recurrence rates among the 190 patients with no drug efficacy prediction were similar to the 296 with prediction of drug efficacy (3). A more intriguing thought is that the class I drugs were ineffective and the methodology employed was inadequate to differentiate the true responders from nonresponders. The ESVEM trial, therefore, is not a meaningful comparison of Holter versus EPS-guided therapy, but a verdict on the failure of class I drug therapy in this population.

2. When one combines 190 patients for whom no drug efficacy was predicted with those who discontinued the drugs predicted to be effective, a significant number of cases were outside the protocol. By intention-to-treat analysis of arrhythmia recurrence and mortality, 47% and 64% of patient–years, respectively, were outside the protocol. With these figures, it is difficult to apply clinical or statistical relevance of ESVEM to current practice (6).

3. Overall arrhythmia-related mortality in off-protocol patients is expected to be higher (i.e., nondrug responder) than those with predicted drug efficacy. Since the mortality in nonresponders was indeed higher than drug responders, it may be indicative of a lower risk population recruited into the ESVEM trial. A 10% 4-year nonarrhythmic cardiovascular mortality supports this view point (6,26). One can argue that if all ESVEM enrollees were treated with amiodarone and/or ICD, survival in patients with efficacy prediction could have been improved.

4. It has been suggested that the 10% first-year sudden cardiac death (SCD) mortality in the ESVEM population is low. SCD mortality was actually too high for a VT population who did not have significant nonarrhythmic cardiovascular risk. Since SCD mortality could be reduced to <2% a year with ICD, results of ESVEM trial highlight the futility of antiarrhythmic drugs in comparison. It is difficult to visualize the return of antiarrhythmic agents as the primary therapeutic choice for prevention of arrhythmic SCD in VT/VF population.

SUMMARY AND CONCLUSION

The ESVEM trial highlights the pitfalls of a large randomized trial. The key points are as follows:

1. While the population randomized is highly selected, the practicing physician is asked to apply the outcome to consecutive patients—an unjustifiable recommendation.
2. Individual investigator and institution bias should be minimal for a true multicenter representation, which was not the case in the ESVEM trial.
3. It is primarily a VT trial in patients with prior failure to class I antiar-

rhythmic agents. In the same population, a class III agent (sotalol) shows lower long-term VT recurrence rates.

4. Holter and EPS are complimentary and neither is currently utilized according to the protocols used in the ESVEM trial (i.e., 48-h Holter and up to six drug studies).
5. Since ICD therapy is superior to any antiarrhythmic drug, the practice of serial drug testing is irrelevant to today's practice (27,28).
6. Since clinical environments are constantly changing due to rapid innovation, a trial spanning over several years is likely to have limited application as acknowledged by the authors.
7. The suggestion that the academic community might require prior counseling before the perceived unpopular results of trials are revealed seems an overcautious posture and somewhat humorous (29). Results of randomized trials are not sacred and are open to scrutiny from the academic community. Unfortunately, the weaknesses of ESVEM at multiple levels have left a lot of unanswered questions for which the designers and investigators of ESVEM must accept responsibility.

REFERENCES

1. The ESVEM Investigators. The ESVEM trial. Electrophysiologic study versus electrocardiographic monitoring for selection of antiarrhythmic therapy of ventricular therapy of ventricular tachyarrhythmias. Circulation 1989; 79:1354–1360.
2. The ESVEM Investigators. Determinants of predicted efficacy of antiarrhythmic drugs in the electrophysiologic study versus electrocardiographic monitoring trial. Circulation 1993; 87:323–329.
3. Mason JW for the Electrophysiologic Study Versus Electrocardiographic Monitoring (ESVEM) Investigators. A Comparison of Electrophysiologic Testing with Holter Monitoring to Predict Antiarrhythmic-Drug Efficacy for Ventricular Tachyarrhythmias. N Engl J Med 1993; 329:445–451.
4. Mason JW for the Electrophysiologic Study Versus Electrocardiographic Monitoring (ESVEM) Investigators. A Comparison of Seven Antiarrhythmic Drugs in Patients with Ventricular Tachyarrhythmias. N Engl J Med 1993; 329:452–458.
5. Mason JW, Marcus FI, Bigger JT, et al. A summary and assessment of the findings and conclusions of the ESVEM trial. Prog Cardiovasc Dis 1996; 38:347–358.
6. Ward DE, Camm AJ. Dangerous ventricular arrhythmias—can we predict drug efficacy? N Engl J Med 1993; 329:498–499.
7. Damle RS, Ehlert FA. The treatment of ventricular tachyarrhythmias. N Engl J Med 1994; 330:286–287.
7a. Winters SL, Rubinstein D, Gomes JA. The treatment of ventricular arrhythmias. N Engl J Med 1994; 330:287 (letters to the editor).
8. Biblo LA, Carolson MD, Waldo AL. Isights into the electrophysiology study versus elelctrocardiographic monitoring trial: Its programmed stimulation protocol may in-

troduce bias when assessing long-term antiarrhytmic durg therapy. J Am Coll Cardiol 1995; 25:1601–1604.

9. Gettes LS. ESVEM and the hazards of clinical trials. Circulation 1995; 91:1908–1909.

10. Mitchell LB, Wyse DG. Interpretation of the results of the electrophysiologic study versus electrocardiographic monitoring (ESVEM) study: programmed ventricular stimulation advocates' view. Coronary Artery Dis 1994; 5:671–676.

11. Winters SL, Curwin JH. Sotalol and the management of vetnricular arrhythmias: implications of ESVEM (editorial). Pacing Clin Electrophysiol 1995; 18:2377–378.

12. Mason JS for the ESVEM Investigators. N Engl J Med 1994; 330:287–288. (Response to letters.)

13. Kavangh K, Wyse DG, Duff H, Gillis A, Sheldon R, Mitchell LB. Drug therapy for ventricular tachyarrhythmias: How many electropharmacologic trials are appropriate? J Am Coll Cardiol 1991; 17:391–6.

14. Estes M, Garan H, McGovern B, Ruskin J. Influence of drive cycle length during programmed stimulation on induction of ventricular arrhythmias: Analysis of 403 patients. Am J Cardiol 1986; 57:108–112.

15. Rosenbaum M, Wilber D, Finkelstein D, Ruskin J, Garan H. Immediate reproducibility of electrically induced sustained monomorphic ventricular tachycardia before and during antiarrhythmic therapy. J Am Coll Cardiol 1991; 17:133–138.

16. Beckman K, Velasco C, Krafchek J, Lin H, Magro S, Wyndham C. Significant variability in the mode of ventricular tachycardia induction and its implications for interpretation of acute drug testing. Am Heart J 1988; 116:718–726.

17. McPherson C, Rosenfeld L, Batsford W. Day-to-day reproducibility responses to right ventricular programmed electrical stimulation: implantations for serial drug testing. Am J Cardiol 1985; 55:689–695.

18. Kudenchuk P, Kron J, Walance C, Cutler J, Griffith K, McAnulty. Day-to-day reproducibility of antiarrhythmic drug trials using programmed extrastimulus techniques for ventricular tachyarrhythmias associated with coronary artery disease. Am J Cardiol 1990; 66:725–30.

19. The CASCADE Investigators. Randomized antiarrhythmic drug therapy in survivors of cardiac arrest (the CASCADE study). Am J Cardiol 1993; 72:280–287.

20. Rae AP, Greenspan AM, Spielman SR, et al. Antiarrhythmic drug efficacy for ventricular tachyarrhythmias associated with coronary artery disease as assessed by electrophysiologic studies. Am J Cardiol 1985; 55:1494–99.

21. Winkle RA, et al: Long-term outcome with the automatic implantable cardioverter-defibrillator. J Am Coll Cardiol 1989; 13:1353.

22. Saksena S, Camm AJ. Implantable defibrillators for prevention of sudden death: Technology at a medical and economic crossroad. Circulation 1992; 83(6):2316–2321.

23. Tchou PJ, et al. Automatic implantable cardioverter defibrillators and survival of patients with left ventricular dysfunction and malignant ventricular arrhythmias. Ann Intern Med 1988; 109:529.

24. Kelly PA, et al. The automatic implantable cardioverter defibrillator: Efficacy, complications and survival in patients with malignant ventricular arrhythmias. J Am Coll Cardiol 1988; 11:1278.

25. Shenasa M, Gilbert CJ, Krebs A, Akhtar M, Denker S. Increased ventricular refracto-

riness as the predictor of ventricular tachycardia control following Class I antiarrhythmic therapy. Clin Res 1981; 29(4):753A.

26. Akhtar M, Jazayeri M, Sra J, Dhala A, Deshpande S, Blanck Z, Axtell K. Role of implantable cardioverter-defibrillators in the management of patients with ventricular tachycarida and ventricular fibrillation. In: Akhtar M, Myerburg R, Ruskin J, eds. Sudden Cardiac Death: Prevalence Mechanisms, and Approaches to Diagnosis and Management. Philadelphia: Williams & Wilkins, 1994.

27. Moss A, Hall WJ., Cannom D, Daubert J, Higgins J, Higgins S, Klein H, Levine J, Saksena S, Waldo A, Wilber D, Brown Mary and Moonseong, H for the Multicenter Automatic Defibrillator Implantation Trial Investigators. Improved survival with an implanted defibrillator in patients with coronary disease at high risk for ventricular arrhythmia. N Engl J Med 1996; 335:1933–1940.

28. The Antiarrhythmics Versus Implantable Defibrillators (AVID) Investigators. A comparison of antiarrhythmic-drug therapy with implantable defibrillators in patients resuscitated from near-fatal ventricular arrhythmias. N Engl J Med 1997; 337;22: 1576–1583.

5

The Grupo de Estudio de la Sobrevida en la Insuficiencia Cardiaca en Argentina (GESICA) Trial

HERNÁN C. DOVAL

Heart Institute, Italian Hospital, Buenos Aires, Argentina

INTRODUCTION

Despite the major advances in the knowledge of the pathophysiology of congestive heart failure (CHF) and the new therapeutic modalities for this disease, its prevalence and the associated mortality continue to be a significant medical problem.

Patients with severe heart failure have a high frequency of ventricular ectopic activity [multiform ventricular premature beats, couplets, and nonsustained ventricular tachycardia (NSVT)]. Sudden death, presumably due to cardiac arrhythmias, accounts for more than 40% of the total deaths in these patients. However, a more optimistic view arises from a recent report showing that overall mortality—including sudden death—is decreasing in patients waiting for heart transplantation. The use of angiotensin converting enzyme (ACE) inhibitors, warfarin, and digitalis for the treatment of CHF has substantially increased over the last 10 years.

While the prescription of class I antiarrhythmic agents has dramatically decreased, we find of utmost interest that low-dose amiodarone utilization has experienced a fivefold rise over the same period of time. One possible explanation for amiodarone replacing class I antiarrhythmic drugs in subjects with CHF might be better suppression of serious arrhythmias leading to sudden death. However, there was no evidence that prophylactic antiarrhythmic treatment might improve survival.

Amiodarone is most useful in symptomatic complex arrhythmias when other antiarrhythmic treatments fail. In low doses, amiodarone is well tolerated and maintains long-term suppression of arrhythmias.

Until the publication of GESICA, the few amiodarone studies carried out in patients with chronic heart failure had insufficient statistical power, some reports were retrospective, nonrandomized, and did not stratify patients by severity of disease. The primary hypothesis of GESICA might have been that low-dose amiodarone could reduce overall mortality, through a reduction of sudden death. However, amiodarone's multiple pharmacological actions make it more than a simple antiarrhythmic drug.

METHODS AND PATIENTS

Study Design

GESICA was a prospective, parallel, randomized, controlled study, carried out in 26 hospitals in Argentina. Patients were randomized in a stratified manner according to the presence of NSVT in the 24-h admission Holter recording, with the intention of having balanced populations with complex ventricular arrhythmias.

An independent scientific and ethics committee monitored the progress of the study, which was approved by the institutional review board of each hospital. Informed consent was obtained for every patient. The trial hypothesis was that, in patients with severe heart failure, low-dose amiodarone would reduce by 33% the total mortality risk. We estimated a 1-year mortality rate of 30% and 20% for control and treated subjects, respectively [risk reduction (RR) 33%]. A sample size of 710 patients was required to obtain an α significance of 0.05 for two-sided test, and a power of 0.85 (for one tail). Losses or crossover cases would increase the necessary sample size by 10% to 780 patients.

In order to increase the statistical power of our sample, we decided upon a 2-year follow-up period. Analysis was carried out by intention to treat. The primary endpoint was total mortality. Secondary endpoints were subgroup mortality, sudden death, or death due to progressive heart failure (with and without the presence of NSVT in the admission Holter), and decrease in hospital admissions due to heart failure. The scientific and ethics committee reviewed the data at the inclusion of one-third and two-thirds of the planned number of patients. An $\alpha = 0.022$ at the moment of the revision or at the end of the trial was to be considered significant with a Cox regression proportional hazards model.

Inclusion Criteria

1. Severe and stable chronic heart failure (class II advanced, III, and IV of the NYHA scale), despite full treatment, including a low-sodium diet, diuretics, digitalis, and angiotensin converting enzyme inhibitors, but without any antiarrhythmic treatment.
2. At least two of the following indexes of marked systolic myocardial dysfunction: (a) ejection fraction measured by radioisotopes equal to or lower than 35%; (b) end-diastolic echocardiographic diameter equal to or greater than 3.2 cm/m^2 of body surface; and (c) chest x-ray cardiothoracic ratio of more than 0.55.

Exclusion Criteria

1. Amiodarone treatment during the last 3 months.
2. Clinical thyroid dysfunction.
3. Severe respiratory failure.
4. Aortic or mitral stenosis and/or hypertrophic or restrictive cardiomyopathy.
5. Recent angina, myocardial infarction, heart failure onset, or syncope (within the last 3 months).
6. Atrioventricular conduction disorders.
7. History of sustained ventricular tachycardia or ventricular fibrillation, and asymptomatic ventricular tachycardia greater than 10 beats with an R-R shorter than 600 ms.
8. Patients with any concomitant serious disease.

Randomization, Treatment, and Follow-Up

The clinical history on admission and Holter monitoring tapes of eligible patients were submitted to and analyzed by the coordinating center. Randomization was stratified according to hospital and NSVT in the 24-h admission Holter. Patients assigned to amiodarone received 600 mg daily for 14 days, and then 300 mg daily for 2 years. Amiodarone withdrawal during the trial was left to the discretion of the patient's physician.

When a patient required cardiac surgery or transplantation, the follow-up was discontinued at the day of the surgical procedure. The endpoints of our trial were total mortality, cardiopulmonary resuscitation, and symptomatic sustained ventricular tachycardia. Double-blinding was not deemed necessary for these patients, and this facilitated recruitment. Death was classified as due to progressive heart failure; sudden (death occurring within 1 h of presentation of new symptoms); unknown (no means of establishing with certainty the cause of death); and noncardiac death. The report and information given by the principal investigator were approved or reclassified in the coordinating center, blind to the assigned group.

The Kaplan-Meier method was used to delineate life-table curves and log-rank test for statistical analysis. The percentage reduction in mortality was reported as: (1-RR) $\times$ 100, where RR is the estimated relative risk of an event in the amiodarone group as compared with the control group, as estimated from the life-table. A correction adjustment was done for the other variables considered by the likelihood-ratio test on the basis of the proportional hazards model (Cox regression model).

RESULTS

GESICA trial included 516 patients, 256 in the control group and 260 in the amiodarone branch. The study was ended by the Steering Committee on the advice of the Scientific and Ethics Committee after the second prespecified analysis. Baseline clinical features were similar in both groups (Table 1); and the follow-up ranged from 2 to 24 months.

Mortality

There were 106 deaths in the control group and 87 in the amiodarone group [risk reduction (RR) of 28% (95% CI: 4%–45%; $p = 0.024$)]. Adjustment by the proportional hazards Cox model gave an RR of 31% (95% CI: 9%–48%; $p <$ 0.01) (Table 2).

The survival curve shows a lower overall mortality for the amiodarone group. The difference in mortality rate appeared after 3 months, increased at 6 months, and was maintained at the end of the follow-up period, as shown in Figure 1.

These results could be presented in an analogous way to that employed by oncologists in discussing trial outcomes. A hypothetical patient with history of severe CHF could have a 35% chance of death by the first year without amiodarone. Conversely, if he were on amiodarone (300 mg daily), this patient would have a 6 months "death-free interval." In our study, the "number of patients needed to treat" (NNT) to prevent one death per year was only 13.

Amiodarone use reduced both sudden death and death related to progressive heart failure (RR = 27% and 23%, respectively). Given the small number of deaths in each group, these differences failed to reach statistical significance ($p = 0.16$) (Table 2). Deaths of unknown causes and the noncardiac deaths were equally distributed.

Table 1 Clinical Characteristics at Entry

Characteristics	Control (n = 266)	Amiodarone (n = 260)
Age (years)	60.1	58.5
Sex (male)	82.4	79.3
Class II (%)	20.4	21.5
Class III (%)	48	48.5
Class IV (%)	31.6	30
Ejection fraction (%)	20	19
Diastolic diameter (cm/m^2)	3.8	3.8
Cardiothoracic ratio	0.61	0.61
Heart rate (beats/min)	90.6	88.7
Blood pressure (mmHg)	116/73	117/74
Serum sodium (mmol/L)	137.5	137.5
Serum potassium (mmol/L)	4.2	4.2
Serum creatinine (mg/dL)	1.31	1.24
Myocardial infarction (%)	38.3	39.6
Hypertension (%)	39.8	40.4
Idiopathic cardiomyopathy (%)	19.5	23.1
Chagas disease (%)	10.5	8.1
Drink alcohol(%)	34.8	31.2
Atrial fibrillation (%)	30	27.7
VPB more than 10/h (%)	71.2	71.5
Couplets (%)	56.1	57.6
NSVT (%)	33.2	33.8
Digitalis (%)	75.8	76.9
Diuretics (%)	92.2	90.8
Enalapril (%)	89.1	91.5
Anticoagulants (%)	31.6	30

Hospital Admission for Heart Failure

Of 256 patients in the control group, 149 died (58.9%) or were admitted to hospital due to worsening heart failure, significantly more than 119/260 (45.8%) of those allocated to amiodarone. Hospital admissions were reduced by 31% (13%–46%; p = 0.0024) (Table 2).

Subgroups Analysis

The effect of amiodarone was analyzed in different subgroups according to the presence or absence of NSVT, functional capacity, and sex.

Table 2 Deaths and Hospitals Admissions for Congestive Heart Failure

Variable	Control n (%)	Amiodarone n (%)	Risk reduction (95% CI)	Two-sided (p)
Patients	256 (100)	260 (100)		
Deaths	106 (41.4)	87 (33.5)	28 (4 to 45)	0.024
Deaths and hospital admission for CHF	149 (58.2)	119 (45.8)	31 (13 to 46)	0.0024
Cardiovasc. deaths				
Sudden death	39 (15.2)	32 (12.3)	27 (−17 to 54)	0.16
Progressive H.F.	52 (20.3)	44 (16.9)	23 (−15 to 48)	0.16
Unknown or other	15 (5.9)	11 (4.3)		

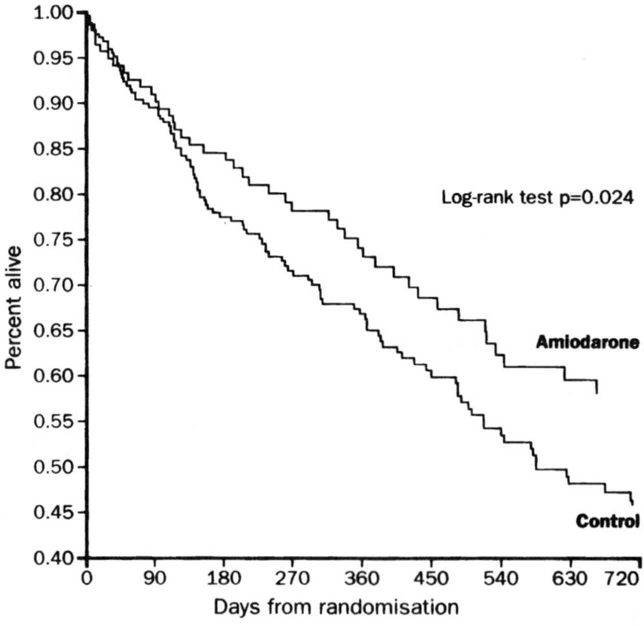

Figure 1 Total mortality.

Table 3 Number of Deaths and Number of Patients with Death or Hospital Admission in Subgroups

Variable	Total mortality		Death and/or hospital admission	
	R.R. (95% CI)	*p* [two-sided]	R.R. (95% CI)	*p* [two-sided]
Sex				
Male	26 (−2 to 46)	0.10	31 (10 to 47)	0.006
Female	48 (0 to 75)	0.076	30 (−25 to 62)	0.262
Heart Failure				
Class II	41 (−39 to 75)	0.224	48 (−1 to 74)	0.078
Class III	24 (−14 to 50)	0.178	21 (−11 to 44)	0.168
Class IV	26 (−14 to 52)	0.178	37 (5 to 27)	0.018
NSVT (Holter 24 h)				
Absent	24 (−12 to 48)	0.16	32 (7 to 51)	0.016
Present	34 (0 to 57)	0.056	30 (0 to 52)	0.056

Table 3 shows that the effect of amiodarone was consistent in the various subgroups considered.

Functional Capacity

The effect of amiodarone in reducing deaths or deaths and/or hospital admissions was similar for the different functional classes. There was a higher proportion of patients in a better functional class (FC I-II 47% vs. 35%) in the amiodarone group at final follow-up assessments (Table 4). In addition, more patients in the amiodarone branch improved by at least one functional class ($p < 0.03$).

Table 4 Functional Capacity at Final Follow-Up

Functional capacity[a]	Amiodarone	Control
Class I–II	124 (47%)	90 (35%)
Class III–IV	136 (53%)	166 (65%)
Total	260 (100%)	256 (100%)

χ^2 $p < 0.03$
[a] Patients who died before the first follow-up were assessed by admission functional class.

Nonsustained Ventricular Tachycardia

In this subgroup, amiodarone use was associated with a RR of 34% (95% CI 0% – 57%; $p = 0.056$), and a similar RR of 30% was observed for the secondary endpoint of death/hospital admission (0%–52%; $p = 0.056$) (Table 3). A similar trend was observed in patients without NSVT, although this failed to reach statistical significance (Table 3).

Heart Rate Changes

Baseline heart rate was of 88.7 (SD 14.6) beats/min in the amiodarone group. Heart rate was significantly reduced at 3 months [83.3 bpm (SD 12.0)] and at 6 months [82.7 bpm (SD 13.5); $p < 0.001$ for both cases]. Baseline and follow-up heart rate in the control group were similar.

Amiodarone and Desethyl-Amiodarone Serum Concentrations

We analyzed the serum concentrations in 20 randomly selected patients, amiodarone concentrations were 0.40 µg/mL to 2.65 µg/mL (1.43 SD 0.65), and desethyl-amiodarone concentrations were 0.30 to 2.05 µg/mL (1.1 SD 0.49). Desethyl-amiodarone concentration was <1.0 µg/mL in nine patients. Five of them had amiodarone concentration <1.0 µg/mL, which suggests that these patients might have been in a subtherapeutic range. Three-quarters (15 patients) were within what is considered the therapeutic range.

Side Effects

Amiodarone-related side effects were reported in 17 patients (6.1%). It led to interruption of treatment in only 12 (4.6%), the majority due to slow heart rate.

RETROSPECTIVE ANALYSIS OF HEART RATE (BASELINE AND AT 6 MONTHS) AND DECREASE IN MORTALITY WITH AMIODARONE IN GESICA

GESICA reported a 28% mortality reduction that was due not only to a decrease in sudden death, but also to a reduction in death from progressive heart failure. The reduction in mortality was independent of the presence of ventricular arrhythmias, and was associated with a decrease in hospital admissions and an improvement of functional class. These results suggest a benefit beyond that expected solely from an antiarrhythmic effect. Amiodarone slows the sinus rate. The precise cause, albeit unclear, may be due to a depression of both sinus node automaticity and atrioventricular node conduction (in atrial fibrillation). Amiodarone exerts these actions, at least in part, by a noncompetitive beta-blockade effect.

Because an inappropriate rapid heart rate in CHF may reflect abnormal activation of the sympathetic system, the clinical benefit of amiodarone may also be mediated by a reduction in heart rate. With this in mind, we sought to analyze the mortality reduction produced by amiodarone relative to the "baseline heart rate" (BHR) and its reduction during treatment.

Methods

Heart rate was determined from a physical examination and, in the presence of atrial fibrillation, the average heart rate for 1 min was assessed. The effect of BHR was evaluated by stratifying each group—amiodarone and control—according to a mean BHR ≥ 90 and <90 beats/min, respectively. In addition, 367 patients completed 6 months of follow-up, when heart rate at rest was reassessed. We considered that a reduction of heart rate could have occurred at follow-up, when it was lower than at baseline.

Results

Clinical Characteristics and Baseline Heart Rate

Of the total group of 516 patients, 254 had a BHR ≥ 90 beats/min and 262 patients had a BHR <90 beats/min. Baseline characteristics differed among the groups (Table 5).

It is clear that patients with a BHR ≥ 90 had worse heart failure, as indicated by a lower systolic blood pressure, serum sodium concentration, and left ventricular ejection fraction. Conversely, these subjects had a worse functional class, right heart failure, and diuretic requirement. All this is summarized in the 2-year mortality rate, which was higher in patients with a BHR ≥ 90 beats/min (50.8%) compared with patients with a BHR <90 beats/min (44.8%) ($p < 0.01$). However, there were no differences between control and amiodarone-treated patients, either in the group with BHR ≥ 90 beats/min or in the group with a BHR <90 beats/min.

Baseline Heart Rate, Mortality, and Amiodarone Treatment

In patients with a BHR <90 beats/min, patients allocated to amiodarone had a mortality rate similar to that of the control patients (RR 1.0, 95% CI 0.74 to 1.45; $p = 0.97$). For patients with a BHR ≥ 90 beats/min, amiodarone strikingly decreased the mortality rate compared with controls (38.4% vs. 62.4% RR 0.55, 95% CI 0.35%–0.95%; $p < 0.002$) (Table 6) (Fig. 2).

In order to analyze this relationship in greater detail, we divided the whole

Table 5 Baseline Heart Rate and Clinical Characteristics

	HR ≥90 beats/min (n = 254)	HR <90 beats/min (n = 262)	p Value
Age (yr)	57.8	60.5	0.01
Male (%)	83	73.3	0.02
HR (beats/min)	102	77.6	0.0001
SBP (mmHg)	113.9	119.2	0.005
Serum Na (mmol/L)	136.9	138.1	0.007
Serum K (mmol/L)	4.2	4.2	0.96
Serum urea (mg/dL)	46.9	47	0.95
LVEF (%)	17.5	20.3	0.003
Diastolic diam (cm/m^2)	3.8	3.83	0.53
NYHA class (%)			0.0001
II	15.4	26.3	
III	46	50.4	
IV	38.6	23.3	
Previous MI (%)	39.4	41.6	0.6
Right HF (%)	57.5	31.3	0.0001
AF (%)	27.1	22.5	0.24
NSVT (%)	36.2	30.9	0.23
Drug therapy			
Digitalis (%)	77.6	75.2	0.52
Furosemide (mg/day)	42.2	36.4	0.003
Enalapril (mg/day)	10.2	9.3	0.01
Nitrites (%)	39.4	30.2	0.03
Anticoagulants (%)	33.1	28.5	0.27

AF = atrial fibrillation; diam = diameter; HF = heart failure; HR = heart rate; LVEF = left ventricular ejection fraction; MI = myocardial infarction; NSVT = nonsustained ventricular tachycardia; NYHA = New York Heart Association; SBP = systolic blood pressure.

Table 6 Initial Baseline Heart Rate ≥90 Beats/Min, Mortality, and Cause of Death

	Control n (%)	Amiodarone n (%)	R.R. (95% C.I.)	p Value
Randomized	132 (100)	122 (100)		
Mortality	65 (49.2)	39 (32.0)	0.55 (0.35–0.95)	0.002
Sudden death	26 (19.7)	13 (10.7)	0.46 (0.24–0.90)	0.02
Progressive HF	34 (25.8)	22 (18.0)	0.60 (0.30–1.03)	0.06

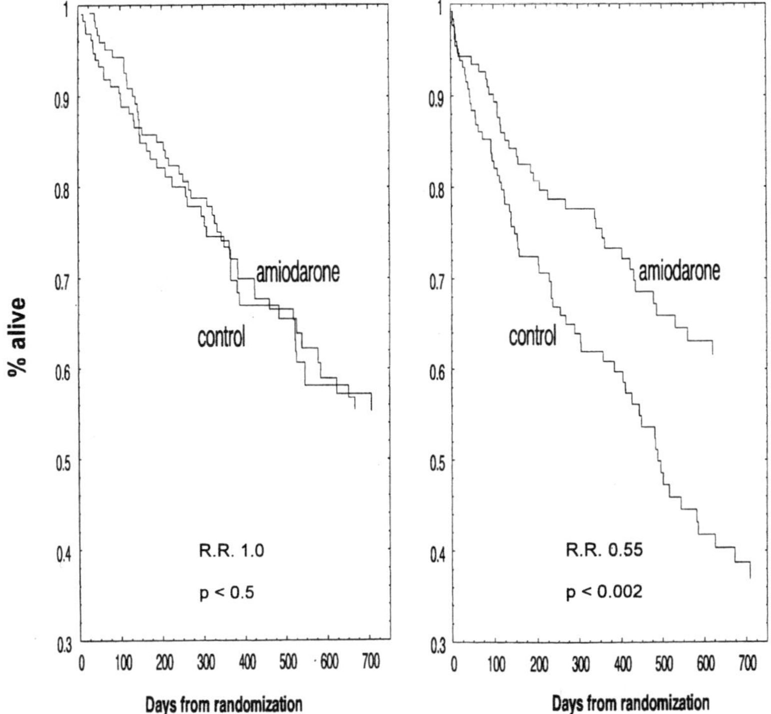

Figure 2 Kaplan–Meier curves showing differences between amiodarone-treated and control patients according to (left) BHR <90 beats/min and (right) BHR ≥90 beats/min.

population into quintiles according to the heart rate on admission. In the first quintile, which considered the patients with the lowest BHR (<76 beats/min), there was a trend against the use of amiodarone (RR 1.34, 95% CI 0.68% to 2.67%; $p < 0.35$). At the opposite end, in the higher quintile (BHR >99 beats/ min), the mortality reduction with amiodarone was highly significant (RR 0.35, 95% CI 0.19% to 0.67%; $p < 0.001$). The higher the heart rate at admission, the greater the benefit from amiodarone observed (Fig. 3). Of interest is the fact that a certain adrenergic stimulation as expressed by an increased heart rate might be necessary for amiodarone to improve survival.

Baseline Heart Rate, Amiodarone Treatment, and Mode of Death

A dual reduction of both sudden and progressive heart failure deaths was seen in patients with BHR ≥90 beats/min treated with amiodarone. These findings

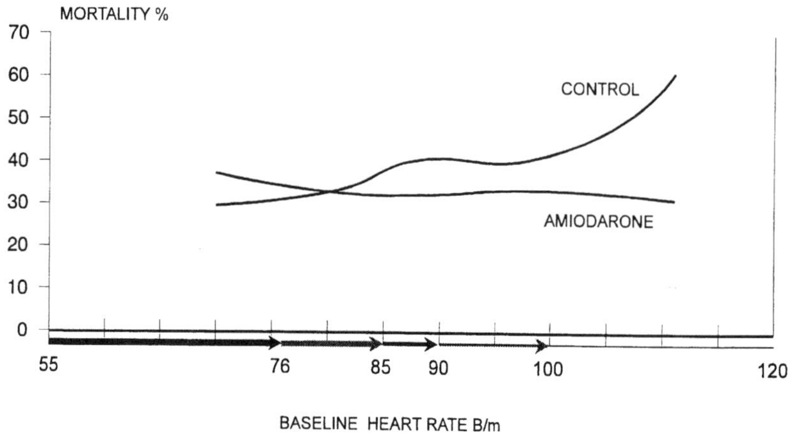

Figure 3 Patient division in quintiles according to BHR and 2-year actuarial mortality in amiodarone-treated and control patients. The arrows on the abcissa indicate the BHR range in each quintile. This graph shows that the higher the BHR, the greater the mortality reduction in the amiodarone group. B/m = beats/min.

showed a definite statistical significance for sudden death (RR 0.46, 95% CI 0.24% to 0.90%; $p < 0.02$), and a clear trend for death due to progressive heart failure (RR 0.60, 95% CI 0.30% to 1.03%; $p < 0.06$) (Table 6).

This dual reduction in the main GESICA study was reported as a trend without statistical significance. However, even when fewer patients were included in this substudy, a highly significant result was observed. These results highlighted the group of patients who obtained the greatest benefit from treatment. In patients with a BHR <90 beats/min, no significant differences in sudden or death from progressive heart failure were observed.

Heart Rate Reduction and Mortality

A total of 367 patients had rest heart rate determined at 6 months of follow-up. Of 188 patients with a BHR ≥90 beats/min, 137 decreased the heart rate at 6 months. In this cohort, the mortality rate was significantly lower with amiodarone (21.7%) compared with controls (53.8%) ($p < 0.002$). In patients whose heart rate was not decreased at 6 months, the mortality rate was similarly high for both amiodarone and control groups (55.2% vs. 55.9%, respectively). Among patients with a BHR <90 beats/min, there were no differences in mortality, regardless of changes in heart rate at 6 months of follow-up.

Baseline Heart Rate and Functional Capacity Modifications

In patients with a BHR $\geq$90 beats/min, the proportion of patients in functional class I or II was greater in the amiodarone group (51.3% vs. 31.5%). Conversely, the proportion of patients with functional class IV was greater in the control group (17.8% vs. 33.7%) ($p < 0.02$). In patients with a BHR $<$90 beats/min, no differences were observed in functional capacity at 6 months between the amiodarone and control patients.

CONCLUSIONS

We found that low-dose amiodarone added to the ''best'' treatment for heart failure at that stage—diuretics, digitalis, and angiotensin converting enzyme inhibitors—reduced 150 deaths and nearly 230 deaths or hospital admissions for congestive heart failure per 1000 patients treated in 2 years. We also observed that only seven patients required treatment in order to prevent one death.

A previous study by Kerin et al. that analyzed patients with NSVT and impaired left ventricular function reported that the suppression of ventricular complex arrhythmias with low-dose amiodarone was not a predictor of survival, results later confirmed by the CHF–STAT study. For this reason, in the GESICA trial we decided that frequent and complex ventricular arrhythmias were not an inclusion criteria. Even more, we did not assess arrhythmias during follow-up.

The decrease of mortality rate with amiodarone was similar for both sudden death and death related to progressive CHF. However, the results failed to reach statistical significance, because the design of the trial did not have enough power for this subgroup analysis. When survival curves were analyzed, it was clear that amiodarone use was associated with a late decrease in mortality due to progressive heart failure, and an early fall in sudden death.

The decrease in mortality and hospital admissions followed the same trend, regardless of the presence or absence of NSVT. This finding validates our decision to include patients without complex ventricular arrhythmias on the Holter recording, and this criterion was the opposite to that used in the CHF–STAT trial. Although patients without NSVT experienced lower mortality compared with those with NSVT, it represented almost two-thirds of all patients included in our study and contributed in over 50% to the reduction of total deaths.

From 1989 to 1995, five randomized clinical trials assessed amiodarone in patients with congestive heart failure, but only two of them, GESICA and CHF–STAT, included more than 200 patients. At first sight, the outcomes of these two studies reported results that seem different. Whilst GESICA yielded a significant decrease of 28% in mortality, CHF–STAT found neutral results. Several editorials ried to explain the differences between the two studies. In this report, we would like to express our point of view regarding this matter, and to show the main clinical differences for both inclusion criteria and follow-up of patients, that may, at least in part, account for the discordant results.

While in the CHF–STAT trial virtually all patients were male, we had a 19% female population. On average, patients were 6 years older in the CHF–STAT study than in GESICA (Table 7). Thus, other diseases might have affected the clinical outcome, as actually occurred. Noncardiac or unknown deaths were only 4% in the GESICA trial versus 22% in the Veterans Affairs trial (Table 7).

In the matter of heart failure severity, 80% of patients were in functional class III–IV in GESICA, which is in disparity with only 43% in CHF–STAT trial. Furthermore, the patients included in GESICA had a lower ejection fraction than those in the CHF–STAT (20% and 26%, respectively) (Table 7). We would also like to comment on the baseline heart rate differences between the two trials (90 beats per minute for GESICA versus 80 beats per minute in the Veterans Affairs trial) (Table 7).

The different patient selection described above may account for the unequal mortality rate at 2 years in the branch without amiodarone. It was higher in GESICA than in CHF–STAT (55% vs. 29%, respectively).

Table 7 Differences Between GESICA and CHF–STAT

Variable	GESICA	CHF–STAT
Inclusion criterion: complex ventricular arrhythmias	NO	YES
Inclusion criterion: active ischemia	NO	YES
Sex (male %)	81	99
Age (years)	59.3	65.5
Functional capacity		
Class I (%)	0	1
Class II (%)	20	65
Class III–IV (%)	80	43
Ejection fraction (%)	20	26
Heart rate (beats/min)	90	80
Overall mortality (%)[a]	55	29
Cardiac death	96	78
Noncardiac death or unknown	4	22
Cause of heart failure (%)		
Ischemic	40	71
Nonischemic	30	29
Unknown	30	0
Withdrawal of the treatment	4.6	41

[a] Mortality at 2 years in the group without amiodarone.

Comparisons between CHF–STAT and GESICA trials had focused on the different proportions of ischemic patients included. This is based on the favorable survival trend observed in the nonischemic patients from CHF–STAT trial. The striking difference in the ischemic cause of heart failure, 71% in the Veterans Affairs trial and only 40% in GESICA trial needs more careful analysis. We did not attempt to classify the cause of heart failure; we just registered the clinical background related to heart failure. Therefore, the patient's history could have involved more than one disease, as was observed in the GESICA report.

In this sense, the GESICA trial had 30% of nonischemic cardiomyopathy, which is comparable to the 29% of CHF–STAT. Nonetheless, the definitions of ischemia were not similar for both studies. While GESICA considered ischemic only those patients with previous myocardial infarction, CHF–STAT established that: ''Ischemic heart disease was documented on the basis of coronary angiographic studies, electrocardiographic changes indicative of myocardial infarction, and chest-pain typical of angina with concomitant electrocardiographic changes or reversible defects on radioisotope perfusion scans.'' It must be remarked that not only was the classification of ischemic heart failure different, but also the CHF–STAT trial included patients with active ischemia, while in the GESICA trial one of the specific exclusion criteria was angina during the last 3 months.

For these reasons, 30% of patients in the GESICA trial remained with unknown cause of heart failure. If we allocated these patients to those already assigned to ischemic or nonischemic cause in the same proportion, the ischemic cause of heart failure in the GESICA trial could have been near that reported in the CHF–STAT trial. Nevertheless, in our trial we did not find etiology differences.

At this point, we would like to consider the most striking difference between the two trials: patient drop out. In the GESICA trial only 4.6% interrupted treatment with amiodarone, while in the Veterans Affairs trial this figure came up to 41% (Table 7). Bias toward the null hypothesis will occur if the contrast between treatment and nontreatment is blurred by nontrial therapy in the placebo or interruption of the drug in the active branch.

Now we can hypothesize that CHF–STAT patients in the amiodarone branch experienced a risk reduction equal to that shown in our trial (28% at 2 years), even when CHF–STAT authors pointed out that 42% mortality in the placebo branch at the end of the study gave enough power to their study. If we take into account the 40% withdrawal, the power decreases to near 45%.

One of the most outstanding effects of amiodarone is heart rate reduction. In patients with baseline heart rate of less than 90 beats per minute, the overall mortality is the same with a R.R. of 1.0; this appears similar to the CHF–STAT results. Nevertheless, when baseline heart rate is equal to or greater than 90 beats per minute, amiodarone strikingly decreased total mortality with a RR of 0.55.

We must remember that the mean BHR in CHF–STAT trial was 80 beats/

min, and eventually, most of the patients had less than 90 beats/min. Moreover, the average heart rate decreased to 70 beats/min during the follow-up. We believe in the importance of this analysis, even more when we consider the CHF–STAT neutral results.

Heart rate appears to be the link between the severity of patients included in both studies, and could explain what, at first sight, looks like dissimilar results. We want to conclude this report with the last phrase of the GESICA report: ''We agree with the SOLVD investigators that there is a need for further treatments to reduce mortality in patients with heart failure, by actions on more that one mechanism of death.

This study shows that the decrease in mortality we obtained is greater than would be expected from a drug which only reduces death through an antiarrhythmic effect. Low-dose amiodarone proved to reduce mortality and hospital admission in patients with severe heart failure, independently of the presence of complex ventricular arrhythmias. These results should not be generalized to patients showing less severe manifestations of heart failure or less impairment of left ventricular systolic function; further investigations are needed in these groups of patients.''

LYNNE WARNER STEVENSON and WILLIAM G. STEVENSON

*Brigham and Women's Hospital, Harvard Medical School,
Boston, Massachusetts*

The GESICA trial described the largest benefit shown in any multicenter trial of amiodarone (1). To put the GESICA trial in perspective both among amiodarone trials and among heart failure trials, it is necessary to consider the patient population and the trial design. Furthermore, this trial exemplifies the challenge of extending trial results to clinical practice, which involves patients who differ from the trial population and who receive therapies that can be individually adjusted before clinical endpoints are reached.

SEVERITY OF HEART FAILURE

The characteristics of the GESICA trial population describe patients with more severe heart failure than studied in any other antiarrhythmic trial to date and, in fact, more severe than in most heart failure trials, with mean left ventricular ejection fraction less than 20% and over 75% of patients classified as class III or class IV. Even the CONSENSUS trial, described as all New York Heart Association class IV patients, studied patients with a serum sodium and systolic blood pressure that indicated less compromise than the GESICA patients (2). The control group mortality of 41% with a mean follow-up of 13 months in GESICA is comparable to that observed in the enalapril-treated arm of CONSENSUS. In fact, the baseline medical therapy of the GESICA group was according to current standards, with over 90% of patients receiving ACE inhibitors, over 90% receiving diuretics, and over 75% receiving digitalis.

This difference in disease severity may explain some of the difference between the GESICA results and the results of CHF–STAT, which was conducted in patients with mild to moderate heart failure (3). Patients with the most severe heart failure may be more likely to derive benefit from amiodarone, or perhaps less likely to experience detectable adverse events. This distinction is supported by the uncontrolled UCLA experience in 307 patients referred for transplantation, approximately half of whom received amiodarone for symptomatic atrial or ventricular arrhythmias or for high-grade ventricular ectopy (4). Among the patients who were class IV at the time of referral, those who subsequently received amiodarone had significantly lower mortality, even though the greater baseline ectopy in the amiodarone-treated patients would have been expected to predict a higher mortality. In this particular population, the major benefit of amiodarone was attributable to a decrease in heart failure endpoints of death and urgent transplantation. In contrast, there was no benefit in the class III patients. The impact of amiodarone specifically on heart failure endpoints was seen in GESICA, with a 31% decrease in the rate of death or hospitalization for heart failure.

SIGNIFICANCE OF HEART RATE REDUCTION

That benefit is more likely in severe heart failure may relate in part to the role of elevated heart rate in heart failure decompensation. The altered force–frequency relationship in failing myocardial segments has been well described in vitro, with rates above 70 associated with less efficient contraction in contrast to normal myocardium. Even a modestly elevated heart rate may contribute to further depression of contractility in chronic heart failure. Amiodarone therapy slows heart rate by an average of 6 to 10 beats, with greater changes sometimes seen from higher baseline rates (1,5,6). The importance of heart rate effects is supported by the post hoc analysis of heart rate in GESICA, in which the benefit from amiodarone appeared to be confined to patients with a resting heart rate above 90 beats per min after stabilization of heart failure therapy (6). In contrast, the mean heart rate in CHF–STAT was only 80 beats per min. It is intriguing that the benefit of amiodarone in CHF–STAT to improve left ventricular ejection appeared to relate to heart rate reduction (5).

Another potential mechanism of benefit may relate to atrial fibrillation, present in 20 to 30% of patients with heart failure. In some patients, amiodarone allows successful cardioversion and maintenance of sinus rhythm. Improvement in left ventricular ejection fraction and exercise performance has anecdotally been described in such patients (7). Even in patients remaining in atrial fibrillation, amiodarone often provides effective rate control without the potential deleterious effects of high-dose digoxin or calcium channel blockers. Furthermore, amiodarone may prevent the first development of atrial fibrillation. The impact of amiodarone on atrial fibrillation was not assessed in the GESICA trial.

ETIOLOGY OF HEART FAILURE

Etiology of heart failure may influence the risks and benefits of certain therapies. Coronary artery disease was less common in the GESICA population than in most U.S. trials, with only 40% of patients having a history of prior myocardial infarction. Alcohol intake was implicated in approximately 33% of patients and Chagas' disease in approximately 10%, known to be particularly associated with ventricular tachycardia. In the CHF–STAT trial there was a trend toward benefit in the nonischemic population. Such differences in etiology and benefit have also been suggested from trials of beta-blockers and in one trial of amlodipine (8,9).

WITHDRAWAL AND BLINDED DESIGN

The GESICA trial, although randomized, was not blinded. Patients and investigators knew who was receiving active therapy. This could have influenced the outcome importantly. The control group was deprived of an antiarrhythmic placebo. The importance of a placebo effect is well known. Although it seems unlikely to be able to improve survival in the control group, it cannot be completely dismissed. The GESICA trial had an extremely low rate of withdrawal from active therapy. Only 12 (4.6%) patients discontinued therapy during the trial. This number is in marked contrast to the withdrawal rate of 41% in placebo-controlled, randomized trials of amiodarone (10). Knowing that the patient was receiving active therapy may have allowed physicians to assess risks and side effects more confidently. In addition, the maintenance dose of amiodarone was 300 mg/day for the 2-year follow-up period, in contrast to 400 mg/day during the first year in CHF–STAT (3). The lower maintenance dose may have contributed to fewer side effects and the relatively low rate of withdrawal. It is also possible that patients who were known to be receiving amiodarone were followed by their physician more carefully in subtle ways, as compared to patients who were not receiving amiodarone.

In summary, several factors may have come together in the GESICA trial to contribute to the benefit observed: the severity of heart failure, predominance of nonischemic causes of heart failure, lack of a placebo group, and low withdrawal rate from therapy. Some of these are limitations of the trial, but identification of features associated with benefit will help to target therapy to those patients most likely to benefit and to aid in the design of future trials.

ROLE OF AMIODARONE IN THERAPY FOR HEART FAILURE

Previous experience has demonstrated amiodarone to be a safe and effective therapy for symptomatic ventricular and atrial arrhythmias in heart failure. It remains unclear whether there is an additional specific effect of amiodarone to decrease the sudden deaths related to tachyarrhythmias in this population. There also remains a concern that amiodarone might increase risk of the largely unexplained bradycardias that can cause sudden death in heart failure. Expanding indications for implantable defibrillators have not eliminated the need for amiodarone for ventricular arrhythmias; it is often required to prevent frequent, disabling defibrillator shocks.

In heart failure without specific arrhythmias that require antiarrhythmic drug therapy, what is the role of amiodarone? There are striking similarities between the effects of amiodarone and beta-blockers in heart failure. Both decrease heart rate and improve left ventricular ejection fraction to similar degrees. Both have been associated with a decrease in heart failure endpoints that is more apparent than any specific decrease in sudden death. There is a suggestion from some, but not all, beta-blocker trials that patients with a nonischemic etiology of heart failure may derive greatest benefit, a surprising finding in view of the positive experience in postinfarction patients. Trials with the beta-blocking agents bisoprolol and carvedilol have both shown greater benefits in patients with more elevated resting heart rates (8,11). Unlike beta-blockers, however, the initiation of amiodarone at a moderate loading dose and low maintenance dose has not been associated with an increased need for diuretics or other evidence of heart failure exacerbation seen with beta-blocking agents, and which is of particular concern in patients with advanced heart failure. One strategy suggested by GESICA, other amiodarone trials, and the beta-blocker experiences is that patients with heart rates above 90 beats per min be considered for adjunctive therapy with either amiodarone or beta-blocking agents. Those patients with relatively compensated heart failure may receive cautious initiation of therapy with beta-blocking agents, while those at high risk for exacerbation of heart failure should be considered for amiodarone therapy.

REFERENCES

1. Doval HC, Nul DR, Grancelli HO, Perrone SV, Bortman GR, Curiel R, for Grupo de Estudio de la Sobrevida en la Insuficiencia Cardiaca en Argentina (GESICA). Randomized trial for low-dose amiodarone in severe congestive heart failure. Lancet 1994; 344:493–498.
2. The CONSENSUS Trial Study Group. Effects of enalapril on survival in patients with reduced left ventricular ejection fraction and congestive heart failure. N Engl J Med 1987; 316:1429–1435.
3. Singh SN, Fletcher RD, Fisher SG, Singh BN, Lewis HD, Deepwania PC, Massie BM, Colling C, Lazzeri D, for the Survival Trial of Antiarrhythmic Therapy in Congestive Heart Failure. Amiodarone in patients with congestive heart failure and asymptomatic ventricular arrhythmias. N Engl J Med 1995; 333:77–82.

4. Stevenson LW, Stevenson WG, Fonarow GC, Middlekauff H, Saxon LA, Hamilton MA, Walden J, Woo M. Survival after hospitalization for Class IV heart failure: Evidence that amiodarone improves outcome. Circulation 1996; 94:1–21.

5. Massie BM, Fisher SG, Deedwania PC, Singh BN, Fletcher RD, Singh SN, for the CHF-STAT Investigators. Effect of amiodarone on clinical status and left ventricular function in patients with congestive heart failure. Circulation 1996; 93:2128–2134.

6. NUL DR, Doval HC, Grancelli HO, Varini SD, Soifer S, Perrone SV, Prieto N, Scapin O. Heart rate is a marker of amiodarone mortality reduction in severe heart failure. J Am Coll Cardiol 1997; 29:1199–1205.

7. Middlekauff HR, Wiener I, Stevenson WG. Low-dose amiodarone for atrial fibrillation. Am J Cardiol 1993; 72:75F–81F.

8. Packer M, Bristow MR, Cohn JN, Colucci WS, Fowler MB, Gilbert EM, Shusterman NH for the U.S. Carvedilol Heart Failure Study Group. The effect of carvedilol on morbidity and mortality in patients with chronic heart failure. N Engl J Med 1996; 334:1349–1355.

9. Packer M, O'Connor CM, Ghali JK, Pressler ML, Carson PE, Belkin RN, Miller AB, Neurberg GW, Frid D, Wertheimer JH, Cropp AB, DeMets DL for the Prospective Randomized Amlodipine Survival Evaluation Study Group. Effect of amlodipine on morbidity and mortality in severe chronic heart failure. Prospective randomized Amlodipine Survival Evaluation Study Group. N Engl J Med 1996; 335:1107–1114.

10. Amiodarone Trials Meta-Analysis Investigators. Effect of prophylactic amiodarone on mortality after acute myocardial infarction and in congestive heart failure: meta-analysis of individual data from 6500 patients in randomized trials. Lancet 1997; 350:1417–1424.

11. CIBIS Investigators and Committees. A randomized trial of beta-blockade in heart failure: The Cardiac Insufficiency Bisoprolol Study (CIBIS). Circulation 1994; 90: 1765–1773.

The Congestive Heart Failure–Survival Trial of Antiarrhythmic Therapy (CHF–STAT)

STEVEN N. SINGH and ROSS D. FLETCHER
Georgetown University and Veterans Affairs Medical Centers,
Washington, D.C.

SUSAN G. FISHER
Veterans Affairs Cooperative Studies Program, Hines, Illinois.

Patients with congestive heart failure (CHF) have an excessive mortality that ranges from 15 to 20%, depending on functional class (1–4). It is estimated that almost 50% of such deaths will be classified as sudden arrhythmic deaths (1). Ventricular arrhythmias such as premature ventricular contractions (PVCs) and nonsustained ventricular tachycardia (NSVT) are frequently found on ambulatory electrocardiogram (ECG) in patients with CHF (5). Therefore, assuming that these arrhythmias are harbingers of sudden cardiac death (SCD), it seems very logical that suppression of such arrhythmias might lead to an improvement in survival. It should be kept in mind, however, that such an improvement in survival will only be seen if the risk of an antiarrhythmic agent is much less than the risk of the warning arrhythmias. As shown in the CAST (Cardiac Arrhythmia Suppression Trial) trials, flecainide and encainide were associated with the unexpected finding of harmful effects (6). Nevertheless, this did not prevent the enthusiasm of testing other antiarrhythmic compounds. Based on several small studies, amiodarone was shown to have powerful antiarrhythmic effects. It was found to be safe with little or no proarrhythmia and positive hemodynamic effects (7–10). We therefore tested the hypothesis that amiodarone can improve survival in patients with heart failure and complex ventricular arrhythmias.

METHODS

The design of the trial has been described elsewhere (11). Patients were screened at 24 centers (listed in the Appendix). The protocol was approved by an Institutional Review Board at each center, and all patients gave informed consent. The conduct of the study was monitored by an external Data and Safety Monitoring Board and by the Human Rights Committee of the Hines Veterans Affairs Cooperative Studies Program Coordinating Center.

Patients with a documented history of congestive heart failure, whether ischemic or nonischemic in origin, and at least 10 ventricular premature beats per hour, unaccompanied by symptoms, were eligible for the study. All patients had shortness of breath on exertion or paroxysmal nocturnal dyspnea, an echocardiogram showing a left ventricular internal diameter of at least 55 mm or a cardiothoracic ratio higher than 0.50, and a left ventricular ejection fraction of 40% or less. All patients received vasodilator therapy. Digoxin and diuretics were administered as deemed appropriate by the treating physicians.

Women of childbearing age were excluded from the study. Other criteria for exclusion were myocardial infarction within the 3 months prior to enrollment, symptomatic ventricular arrhythmia, a history of aborted sudden cardiac arrest or sustained ventricular tachycardia, uncontrolled thyroid disease, the need for antiarrhythmic therapy, electrocardiographic changes in QRS interval ($\geq$180 ms) or QTc interval ($\geq$500 ms), a serious disease other than heart disease that was likely to be fatal within 3 years, and symptomatic hypotension or systolic blood pressure under 90 mmHg.

Before randomization, the patients were stratified according to the cause of their heart disease (ischemic or nonischemic), the ejection fraction ($<$30% or 30–40%), and the participating hospital at which the patient was receiving care. Ischemic heart disease was documented on the basis of coronary angiographic studies, electrocardiographic changes indicative of myocardial infarction, and chest pain typical of angina with concomitant electrocardiographic changes or reversible defects on radioisotope perfusion scans. Each patient was randomized to receive amiodarone (800 mg once a day for 14 days, then 400 mg once a day for 50 weeks, and then 300 mg once a day until the end of the study) or placebo throughout the trial. Clinic visits were made after 2 weeks and then monthly until the end of the study (maximal follow-up, 4.5 years). At each visit, a complete history was taken and a physical examination performed, with documentation of side effects and use of concomitant drugs.

A 24-h continuous electrocardiogram was obtained at baseline; at 2 weeks; at months 1, 3, 6, 9, and 12; and then every 6 months. Chest films (with the cardiothoracic ratio calculated), blood gas values, and pulmonary function values were determined annually. The left ventricular ejection fraction was determined by radionuclide ventriculography at baseline and at months 6, 12, and 24. Echocardiograms were obtained at baseline and at months 12 and 24. Deaths and aborted cardiac arrests were reviewed in a blinded manner by a committee and classified as sudden or nonsudden deaths from cardiac causes or deaths from other causes. In patients with sustained ventricular tachycardia (≥ 30 s), symptomatic unsustained ventricular tachycardia, or intolerable side effects, the study drug was withdrawn, but the patients were followed and included in the statistical analyses.

Patients were recruited for the study over a period of 3.5 years, and all patients were followed for 1 additional year after the enrollment period. Compliance was ensured by means of frequent clinic visits, telephone calls, and pill counts.

The study endpoints were overall mortality and sudden death from cardiac causes. Other factors examined included the effects of amiodarone on the left ventricular ejection fraction and on the suppression of ventricular arrhythmias.

STATISTICAL ANALYSIS

All patients were followed until the completion of the study and were included in the statistical analysis according to the intention-to-treat principle. Continuous and categorical patient characteristics were compared between treatment groups at baseline by the t-test and chi-square test, respectively. Differences in survival were analyzed with the Kaplan–Meier method. Data on surviving patients were censored at the date of the last follow-up visit. For the analysis of sudden deaths, data on deaths from other causes were censored on the date of the death. A two-sided alpha level less than or equal to 0.05 was considered to indicate statistical significance.

RESULTS

Patient Characteristics

During a 3.5-year period, a total of 1303 patients were screened and 674 (52%) were randomized to either placebo (338) or amiodarone (336). The baseline characteristics are shown in Table 1. The mean age of the entire group was 66 years. The median period of follow-up was 45 months (range 0 to 54).

Overall Mortality and Sudden Death

There was no significant beneficial effect on survival in patients assigned to amiodarone over those assigned to placebo. There were 274 deaths throughout the study: 131 (39%) on amiodarone and 143 (42%) in the placebo group. The actuar-

Table 1 Baseline Characteristics of Randomized Patients

Characteristic	Placebo group (*n* = 338)	Amiodarone group (*n* = 336)
Age–year	66.1 ± 8.1	65.0 ± 8.5
Sex–No. (%)		
Men	334 (98.8%)	333 (99.1%)
Women	4 (1.2%)	3 (0.9%)
Cause of heart failure–No. (%)		
Ischemic	239 (70.7)	242 (72.0)
Nonischemic	99 (29.3)	94 (28.0)
Left ventricular ejection fraction–No. (%)		
<30%	222 (65.7)	226 (67.3)
30–40%	116 (34.3)	110 (32.7)
New York Heart Association class–No. (%)		
I	4 (1.2)	4 (1.3)
II	179 (54.7)	179 (56.3)
III or IV	144 (44.0)	135 (42.4)
Premature ventricular contractions/h	279 ± 387	254 ± 370
Episodes of ventricular tachycardia/24 h	85 ± 281	77 ± 352
Atrial fibrillation–No.(%)	52 (15.4)	51 (15.2)
Medication use		
Beta-blocker–No.(%)	16 (4.7)	13 (3.9)
Digitalis–No.(%)	240 (71.0)	230 (68.5)
Vasodilator–No.(%)	320 (95.7)	306 (91.1)
Dose–mg. (No. of patients)		
Enalapril	22.6 ± 8.4 (37)	14.5 ± 9.9 (41)
Captopril	79.8 ± 79.7 (233)	75.7 ± 49.1 (217)
Hydralazine	139.0 ± 54.0 (13)	133.0 ± 67.0 (14)
Furosemide	80.5 ± 64.5 (279)	75.6 ± 61.2 (282)
Systolic blood pressure (mmHg)	127 ± 20	127 ± 18
Heart rate (beats/min)	80 ± 12	80 ± 14
Cardiothoracic ratio >0.50–No.(%)	279 (82.5)	289 (86.0)
Left ventricular internal diameter ≥ 55 mm by echo–No. (%)	305 (90.2)	306 (91.1)

ial survival at 2 years was 69.4% in the amiodarone group and 70.8% in the placebo group (p = 0.6) (Fig. 1).

With respect to sudden cardiac death, 64 and 75 occurred in the amiodarone and placebo groups, respectively (p = 0.43) (Fig. 1). Deaths classified as pump failure were seen in 34 patients on amiodarone and 40 in the placebo group. Twenty-two patients in the amiodarone group and 23 in the placebo group died

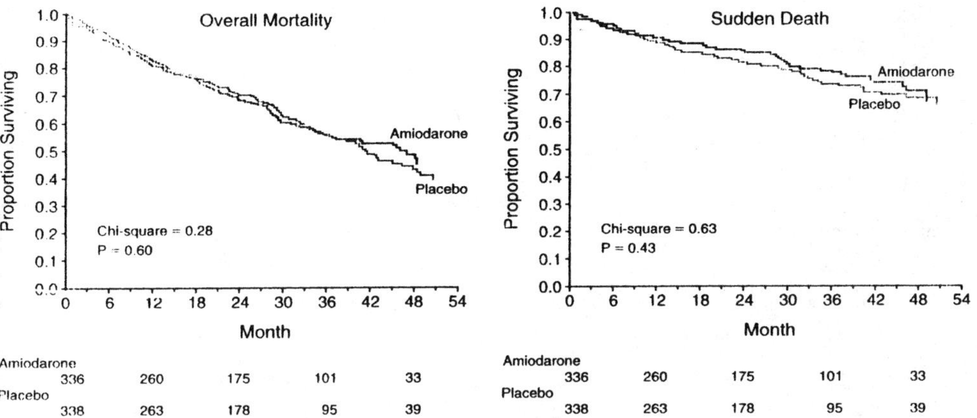

Figure 1 Amiodarone had no significant effect, as compared with placebo, on either overall mortality or time to sudden death. The numbers below the figures are the numbers of patients at risk.

from noncardiac causes. Deaths could not be classified in 11 patients on amiodarone and 5 on placebo.

Outcome According to Etiology of Heart Failure

Survival curves according to ischemic versus nonischemic etiology of heart disease are shown in Figure 2. Compared with placebo, amiodarone had no significant effect ($p = 0.61$) on overall mortality among patients with ischemic cardiomyopathy. However, in patients with nonischemic cardiomyopathy, there was a beneficial trend in favor of amiodarone over placebo ($p = 0.07$).

Suppression of Arrhythmias

At baseline prior to randomization, the mean frequency of PVCs in the amiodarone group was 254 ± 370/h and 279 ± 387/h in the placebo group. At 2 weeks, the average PVC/h was 266 ± 412 in the placebo group and 66 ± 156 in the amiodarone group ($p < 0.001$). Whereas 76% of the patients continued to have episodes of NSVT at 2 weeks on placebo (no different from baseline), only 33% had NSVT episodes on amiodarone (77% at baseline) ($p < 0.001$). Throughout the study NSVT events were significantly lower in patients on amiodarone as compared to those on placebo. There was no difference in overall survival in patients with suppression defined as 80% reduction in the frequency of PVCs compared to those in whom there was no suppression ($p = 0.93$). Figure 3 shows

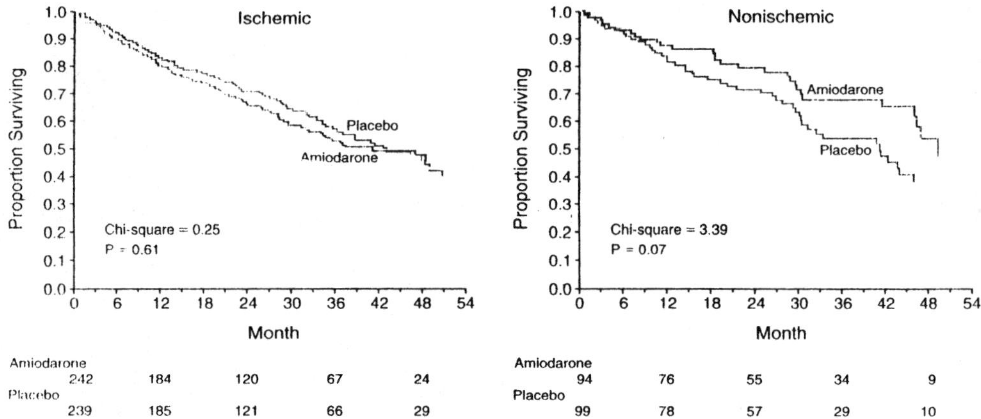

Figure 2   Among the patients with ischemic cardiomyopathy, amiodarone had no significant effect on mortality, as compared with placebo; among those with heart failure of nonischemic origin, there was a trend toward a reduction in overall mortality induced by amiodarone. The numbers below the figures are the numbers of patients at risk.

the survival effects of amiodarone with respect to suppression of PVCs. Similarly, there was no survival benefit in the group of patients whose NSVT episodes were suppressed at 2 weeks by amiodarone ($p = 0.36$).

Effect on Left Ventricular Fraction

At randomization, the mean ejection fraction (EF) in the amiodarone group was 24.9% ± 8.3 compared to 25.7% ± 8.2 in the placebo group. At 6 months, there was a significant increase in EF in those on amiodarone versus those on placebo (33.7% ± 11.0 vs. 29.2% ± 10.7; $p < 0.001$). At 1 and 2 years, the mean EFs were 33.4% ± 11.9 and 35.4% ± 11.5 in the amiodarone group and 29.7% ± 11.0 and 29.8% ± 12.2 on placebo ($p < 0.001$). Amiodarone had no survival benefit in the patients with EF greater or less than 30%. However, the overall survival rate was lower in patients with EF <30% compared to those with EF >30%.

Side Effects

Thyroid abnormalities were observed in four patients on amiodarone (1.2%) and in two on placebo (0.6%). Hepatic enzyme elevation (2 × normal) was seen in four patients on amiodarone (1.2%) and in two patients on placebo (0.6%). Diag-

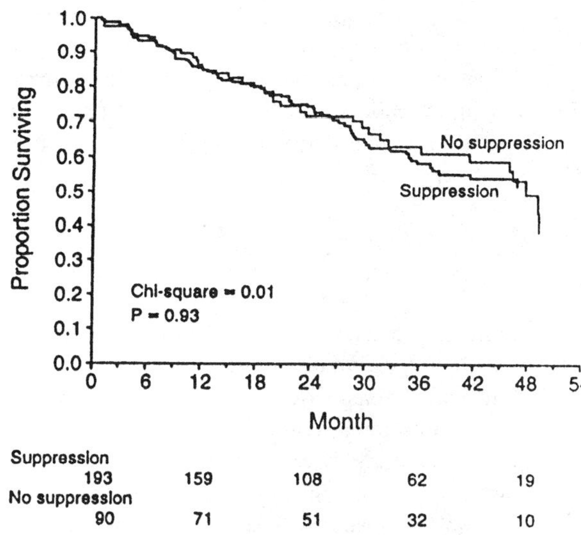

Figure 3   The comparison is between the patients in whom premature ventricular contractions were suppressed by 80% or more and the patients in whom this level of suppression was not achieved. For the purpose of the analysis, runs of ventricular tachycardia are included. There was no significant difference between the group with suppressed contractions and the group with unsuppressed contractions. A similar analysis revealed no significant difference in overall mortality between the group in which runs of ventricular tachycardia were present after 2 weeks of therapy and the group in which such runs were absent. The numbers below the figure are the numbers of patients at risk.

Table 2   Differences Between GESICA and CHF–STAT Trials

	GESICA ($n = 516$) Open-label	CHF–STAT ($n = 674$) Double-blind
Ischemic heart disease (%)	40	72
NYHA class III-IV (%)	80	43
LVEF (%)	20	25
PVC ($>$10/h)%	71	100
NSVT	34	80
2-year mortality control group (%)	44	29
2-year mortality amiodarone group	35	31
Maintenance dose (mg) of amiodarone during the first year	300	400
(%) of patients on amiodarone at the end of study	95	60

nosis of pulmonary fibrosis was made on four patients (1.2%) on amiodarone and three patients (0.9%) on placebo. No case of torsades de pointes was seen in either group. Study medication was discontinued because of intolerance in 90 patients on amiodarone (27%) and in 78 patients on placebo (23%) ($p = 0.1$ between groups). In addition, 46 patients on amiodarone and 32 patients on placebo withdrew or were lost to follow-up.

DISCUSSION

The results of this trial show that amiodarone had no beneficial effect on total and sudden death mortality in patients with congestive heart failure, reduced ejection fraction, and frequent premature ventricular beats. However, in patients with non-ischemic cardiomyopathy, there was a trend toward an improvement in survival.

Amiodarone has been shown to have significant antiarrhythmic activity. However, the survival rates for patients whose arrhythmias were suppressed ($\geq$80% reduction of PVCs) were similar to those in whose arrhythmias were not adequately suppressed. This finding, in light of the results of CAST, questions the importance of using PVC suppression in an attempt to improve survival. Certainly, unlike CAST, where the active drugs possess harmful effects, amiodarone has little or no potential for proarrhythmia and yet failed to improve survival.

Even though amiodarone improved ejection fraction in our study, this effect was not translated into an overall beneficial effect. Indeed, it is well known that certain inotropic agents (phosphodiesterase inhibitors, beta agonists) may increase mortality in patients with heart failure (13,14). There seems to be no relationship between changes in left ventricular ejection fraction and survival with amiodarone or other cardiotonic agents.

Unlike other antiarrhythmic agents, amiodarone was shown to be safe with little or no potential for arrhythmia aggravation. The incidence of noncardiac severe side effects that required drug discontinuation was acceptable and low.

In summary, amiodarone failed to improve survival in patients with congestive heart failure and asymptomatic PVCs despite the suppression of these arrhythmias. Amiodarone is associated with an improvement in left ventricular function and minimal side-effect profile. The trend toward a beneficial effect in nonischemic cardiomyopathy needs to be explored prospectively.

Doval et al. reported the findings of the GESICA (Grupo de Estudio de la Sobrevida la Insufficencia Cardiaca en Argentina) trial in which 516 patients with class III and IV heart failure were prospectively randomized in an open-label design to amiodarone or a control group (600 mg $\times$ 14 days, 300 mg daily thereafter) (15). They found a significant reduction in all-cause mortality (risk reduction 25%, 95% Cl 4% to 45%, log rank test $p = 0.024$). Sudden and progressive heart failure deaths were reduced (27% and 23%, respectively; $p = 0.16$). In the group with nonsustained ventricular tachycardia, amiodarone significantly improved survival ($p = 0.05$). There was a trend toward improvement in survival in the group without this arrhythmia ($p = 0.16$). In a subsequent analysis, patients whose heart rate exceeded 90 beats per minute had a worsened survival than those with heart rate <90 beats per minute (16). A reduction in heart rate by amiodarone correlated with an improvement in survival at 6 months.

Two other large trials involving the use of amiodarone after myocardial infarction are worth mentioning. The first is CAMIAT (Canadian Amiodarone Myocardial Infarction Arrhythmia Trial). This trial included 1202 patients with prior myocardial infarction and PVCs (17). The primary endpoint of resuscitated ventricular fibrillation or arrhythmic death using the intent-to-treat analysis was significantly reduced ($p = 0.029$). There was a trend in the reduction of all-cause mortality, but this was not significant ($p = 0.13$). It should be kept in mind that the study was not powered to detect a difference in all-cause mortality. The second study is EMIAT (European Myocardial Infarct Amiodarone Trial). This study included 1486 patients with prior myocardial infarction and reduced left ventricular function (18). Ventricular arrhythmia was not a prerequisite in order to enter the trial. As with CAMIAT, there was a significant reduction in sudden arrhythmic death ($p = 0.05$) but not in all-cause mortality ($p = 0.96$).

What have we learned from these trials? Undoubtedly, amiodarone appears to be safe and proarrhythmia is uncommon in both heart failure and myocardial infarction. Since GESICA included patients mostly with nonischemic cardiomyopathy and showed a benefit in overall survival, and with a trend of such an effect in CHF–STAT, perhaps there is a potential role for this antiarrhythmic agent. However, such an effect needs to be tested prospectively. It is very intriguing to think that such benefit may be related to the beta-blocking property of amiodarone, especially since in this subset of patients (i.e., without ischemia) the beta-blockers have shown beneficial effects. After all, the GESICA investigators have shown amiodarone benefited those especially with higher heart rates reflecting enhanced sympathetic tone. Table 2 summarizes the differences between the GESICA and CHF–STAT trials. Of interest, in both EMIAT and CAMIAT, patients receiving beta-blockers and amiodarone fared better than those on beta-blockers alone, suggesting the need for more sympathetic blockade. Clearly, amiodarone also improves left ventricular performance. This effect may be due to the beta-blocking property and perhaps to the prolongation of the action potential duration. Was the improvement in survival seen in GESICA and a trend in CHF–STAT related to an improvement in ejection fraction in patients with nonischemic heart disease? If this is the case, then one needs to question the ''protective'' antiarrhythmic property of the drug, since in both GESICA and CHF–STAT, sudden death rates were not significantly reduced. Will an improvement in ventricular performance in itself lead to freedom from arrhythmia over time as is the case with the angiotensin converting enzyme inhibitors? If the two major mechanisms of death in heart failure patients relate to arrhythmia and pump failure, then why aren't the positive effects of amiodarone, a drug that can markedly suppress arrhythmia (and without proarrhythmic effects) and improve ventricular function, not clearly seen. The blame cannot be placed on noncardiac deaths, since this is not the case. Moreover, how can two large trials (EMIAT and CAMIAT) show a reduction in sudden death rates and no impact on overall mortality? Is it a definition problem? Obviously, we can no longer rely on sudden death as an endpoint. Is it possible that the arrhythmias are merely markers of a dying ventricle and any attempt to suppress them might be an exercise in futility.

Finally, is there compliance with the drug? In GESICA, almost 95% of the patients took their medications until the end of the study. Amazingly, in all 3 of these studies—CHF–STAT, EMIAT, and CAMIAT—over 40% of the patients were not receiving amiodarone by the time the trials had ended. Since the results are analyzed by the intent-to-treat principle rather than the efficacy analysis, there might be some potential and (we repeat potential) bias against the drug.

Is there any way to resolve these results? The Sudden Cardiac Death Heart Failure Trial (SCD HeFT) will provide some answers. The intent of this trial is to randomize heart failure patients to either placebo, amiodarone, or implantable defibrillators. This study may provide the final answer as to the role of amiodarone in heart failure patients.

APPENDIX: CHF–STAT INVESTIGATORS

Clinical Centers	Personnel
Bronx, NY	Paul Scweitzer, M.D.
	Pross Patascil, R.N.
Chicago–West Side	James Cumming, M.D.
	Towanda Redmond, R.N.
Dallas, TX	Paul Grayburn, M.D.
	Susan Dougherty, R.N.
Fresno, CA	Prakash C. Deedwania, M.D.
	Rebecca Kanefield, R.N.
Jackson, MS	T.N. Srivastava, M.D.
	Tom King, R.N.
Kansas City, KS	Daniel Lewis, M.D.
	Ruth Corbett, R.N.
Loma Linda, CA	David R. Ferry, M.D.
	Karen Okubo, R.N.
Long Beach, CA	Robert Wesley, M.D.
	Sandra Saniga

APPENDIX: Continued

Clinical Centers	Personnel
Louisville, KY	Abraham Joseph, M.D.
	Nancy Zettwoch, R.N.
Madison, WI	Peter Kosolcharoen, M.D.
	Kathy Cox, M.S.
Miami, FL	C. Simon Chakko, M.D.
	Juanita Johnson
Newington, CT	Martha J. Radford, M.D.
	Debbie Roth, R.N.
North Chicago, IL	Rajindar Singh, M.D.
	Andrea Skillman, R.N.
Oklahoma City, OK	Ralph Lazzara, M.D.
	Tammy Deaton, R.N.
Pittsburgh, PA	Morteza Amidi, M.D.
	Julie Pulman, R.N.
Providence, RI	Satish Sharma, M.D.
	Elizabeth Coccio, R.N.
Richmond, VA	Kenneth A. Ellenbogen, M.D.
	Edith Early, R.N.
Salem, VA	Douglas Russell, M.D.
	Michael Judd, R.N.
Salt Lake City, UT	Richard Klein, M.D.
	Lynn Morrison, R.N.
San Francisco, CA	Barry Massie, M.D.
	Elaine Derr, R.N.
Sepulveda, CA	Vasant N. Udhoji, M.D.
	Patrick Pekale
Syracuse, NY	Robert Warner, M.D.
	Paul Lilja, R.N.
Washington, D.C.	Robert Hall, M.D.
	Diane Lazzeri, M.H.A.
West Haven, CT	Ira Cohen, M.D.
	Louisa Canestri, R.N.

Co-Chairmen:	
Washington, D.C.	Steven N. Singh, M.D.
Washington, D.C.	Ross D. Fletcher, M.D.
Study Pharmacist:	
Albuquerque, N.M.	Cindy L. Colling, R.Ph.,M.S.
Central Holter Monitor Laboratory:	
Washington, D.C.	Ross D. Fletcher, M.D.
Nurse Coordinator:	
Washington, D.C.	Diane Lazzeri, R.N., M.H.A.

APPENDIX: Continued

Hines Cooperative Studies Program Coordinating Center:
Director	William G. Henderson, Ph.D.
Biostatistician	Susan Gross Fisher, Ph.D.
Study Programmer	Laura Weber, M.S.
Study Coordinators	Deanna Cavello
	Mary Biondic

Data Monitoring Board:
  J. Thomas Bigger, M.D.
  Jeffery Anderson, M.D.
  Debra Echt, M.D.
  Milton Packer, M.D.
  Joel Morganroth, M.D.
  George Williams, Ph.D.

Department of Veterans Affairs Headquarters:
Chief Research and Development Officer	John Feussner
Program Assistant	Joe Gough
Staff Assistant	Ping Huang, Ph.D.

REFERENCES

1. Cohn JN. Current therapy of the failing heart. Circulation 1988; 78:1099–1107.
2. Meinertz TE, Hofman T, Kasper W, et al. Significance of ventricular arrhythmias in idiopathic dilated cardiomyopathy. Am J Cardiol 1984; 53:902–907.
3. von Olshausen K, Schafer A, Mehmel HC, Schwarz F, Senges J, Kubler W. Ventricular arrhythmia in idiopathic dilated cardiomyopathy. Br Heart J 1984; 51:195–201.
4. Unverferth DV, Magorien RD, Moeschberger ML, Baker PB, Fetters JK, Leier CV. Factors influencing one-year mortality of dilated cardiomyopathy. Am J Cardiol 1984; 54:147–152.
5. Massie B, Francis G, Tandon P, et al. Asymptomatic ventricular arrhythmias do not identify patients with severe heart failure at risk for sudden death. J Am Coll Cardiol 1993; 21(suppl A):6A–13A.
6. The Cardiac Arrhythmia Suppression Trial II Investigators. Effect of antiarrhythmic agent moricizine on survival after myocardial infarction. N Engl J Med 1992; 327: 227–233.
7. Cleland JGF, Dargie HJ, Findlay IN, et al. Clinical, hemodynamic and antiarrhythmic effects of long term treatment with amiodarone of patients in heart failure. Br Heart J 1987; 57:436–445.
8. Ceremuzynski L, Kleczar E, Krzeminska-Pakula M, et al. Effect of amiodarone on mortality after myocardial infarction: a double-blind, placebo-controlled pilot study. J Am Coll Cardiol 1992; 20:1056–1062.

9. Pfisterer M, Kiowski W. Burckhardt D, Follath F, Burkart F. Beneficial effect of amiodarone on cardiac mortality in patients with asymptomatic complex ventricular arrhythmias after acute myocardial infarction and preserved but not impaired left ventricular function. Am J Cardiol 1992; 69:1399–1402.

10. Singh BN. Amiodarone: historical development and pharmacologic profile. Am Heart J 1983; 106:788–797.

11. Singh SN, Fletcher R, Fisher S, Deedwania P, Lewis D, Massie B, Singh B, Colling C, and the CHF-STAT Investigators. Congestive Heart Failure: Survival Trial of Antiarrhythmic Therapy (CHF-STAT). Controlled Clin Trials 1992; 13(5):339–350.

12. Doval HC, Nul DR, Vancelli HO, et al. Randomized trial of low-dose amiodarone mortality reduction in severe heart failure. Lancet 1994; 344:493–498.

13. Packer M, Carver SR, Rodenheffer RJ, et al. Effect of oral milrinone on mortality in severe chronic heart failure. N Engl J Med 1991; 325:1468–1475.

14. Yusuf S, Teo K. Inotropic agent increase mortality in patients with congestive heart failure. Circulation 1990; (suppl III):III-673 (abstr).

15. Doval HC, Nul DR, Vancelli HO, et al. Randomised trial of low-dose amiodarone in severe congestive heart failure. Lancet 1994; 344:493–498.

16. Cairns J, Connolly S, Roberts R, Gent M for the Canadian Amiodarone Myocardial Infarction Arrhythmia Trial Investigators. Randomised trial of outcome after myocardial infarction in patients with frequent or repetitive ventricular premature depolarizations: CAMIAT. Lancet 1997; 349:675–682.

17. Julian DG, Camm AJ, Frangin G, Janse MJ, Munoz A, Schwartz PJ, Simon P for the European Myocardial Infarction Amiodarone Trial Investigators. Randomised trial of effect of amiodarone on mortality in patients with left ventricular dysfunction after recent myocardial infarction: EMIAT. Lancet 1997; 349:667–674.

MICHAEL J. DOMANSKI and DEREK V. EXNER

National Heart, Lung and Blood Institute,
National Institutes of Health, Bethesda, Maryland

CHF–STAT: A PERSPECTIVE

This discussion presents a perspective on the contribution of CHF–STAT to the field of sudden cardiac death (SCD) prevention in patients with left ventricular dysfunction and symptomatic heart failure.

Tools for SCD Prevention

A substantial research effort has been directed to the prevention of SCD in patients with and without symptomatic heart failure. Many of these studies have been restricted to populations with a history of prior myocardial infarction (MI). A number of conceptions about what is and what is not effective in SCD prevention have been derived from this research including:

1. None of the nonamiodarone antiarrhythmics studied to date have been effective in preventing SCD and, in fact, most have increased the risk of fatal ventricular arrhythmias in patients post-MI or with significant left ventricular dysfunction (1–4). One agent that has not increased mortality is dofetilide (5,6). This agent appears to be an alternative to amiodarone for treating patients with significant left ventricular dysfunction and supraventricular arrhythmias.
2. In post-MI patients, beta-blockers reduce both mortality and SCD (7,8). The efficacy of beta-blockers in heart failure appears similar (9,10).

119

3. The implantable cardioverter defibrillator (ICD) is highly effective in reverting ventricular tachyarrhythmias to sinus rhythm (11).
4. Amiodarone appears to exert a small protective effect in the prevention of malignant ventricular arrhythmias (12–15).
5. The ICD is more effective than amiodarone in preventing mortality in patients with resuscitated life-threatening ventricular arrhythmias and in post-MI patients with depressed left ventricular systolic function and inducible, but nonsuppressible, ventricular tachycardia (16,17).

The Population with Left Ventricular Dysfunction

A population gains importance as a target for SCD prevention based upon the degree to which SCD contributes to total mortality and the size of the population. Heart failure is the most frequent discharge diagnosis in older Americans (18) and its incidence and prevalence are increasing (19). In North America, a majority of these patients (~70%) have ischemic heart disease with or without a prior MI (20). Approximately half of these patients will die suddenly (21); therefore, the prevention of SCD would be expected to reduce overall mortality.

Arrhythmia Qualifiers (Risk Stratification)

In considering CHF–STAT and discussing ongoing trials, it is useful to first define the concept of an *arrhythmia qualifier*. An arrhythmia qualifier is a characteristic that allows the selection of members of a population at higher risk for SCD than the population as a whole.

Apart from a reduced left ventricular ejection fraction and symptomatic heart failure, both of which increase the risk of SCD (22), a variety of arrhythmia qualifiers have been advocated to further identify which patients are at highest risk. These have included the presence of frequent premature ventricular contractions (PVCs), altered heart rate variability, late potentials on signal-average electrocardiography, altered QT dispersion, and others (23–26). The *strength* of an arrhythmia qualifier is the degree to which possessing it increases a patient's risk of SCD. The importance of an arrhythmia qualifier is related not only to its ability to select members of a population likely to die suddenly, but also to the size of the resultant population subset that it identifies (Fig. 1). A strong arrhythmia qualifier loses importance if it identifies only a few patients. A potent arrhythmia qualifier that selects a very small, though extremely high-risk, population may be less desirable than another that identifies a larger population that is at a moderately increased risk of SCD. As studies are discussed, it is useful to consider how the investigators have tried to *enrich* their left ventricular dysfunction populations to select those individuals at higher risk for SCD.

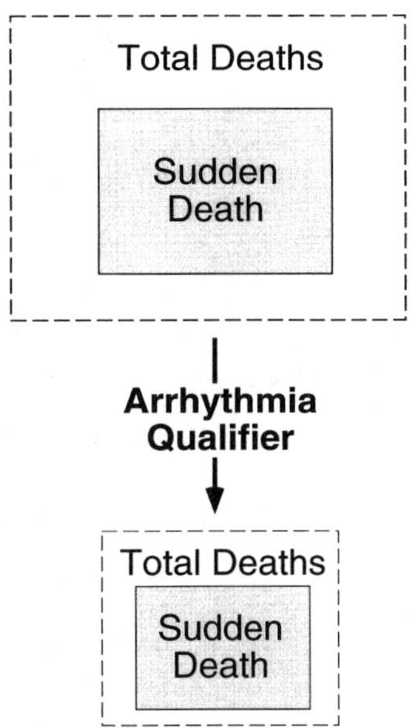

Figure 1 Schematic representation of the total number of deaths, and those attributable to a sudden cardiac demise. Patients with symptomatic heart failure and reduced left ventricular ejection fraction values are presented on the upper portion, while a selected subset of these patients who additionally possess the arrhythmia qualifier (see text) are presented in the lower portion. Using the arrhythmia qualifier results in an increase in the proportion of sudden deaths in the study population, but the absolute number of sudden deaths is reduced.

CHF–STAT

The Congestive Heart Failure-Survival Trial of Antiarrhythmic Therapy (CHF–STAT) was a multicenter, randomized, double-blind, placebo-controlled study that evaluated the effectiveness of amiodarone in reducing total mortality (27). A total of 674 patients with moderate-to-severe symptoms of heart failure, a left ventricular ejection fraction (LVEF) of ≤ 0.40 and ≥ 10 PVCs per hour were randomized to amiodarone ($n = 336$) or matching placebo ($n = 338$). The requirement of frequent ventricular ectopy on Holter was the arrhythmia qualifier in CHF–STAT. Patients with low (LVEF 0.30–0.40) and very low (LVEF $<$ 0.30) ejection fractions were evaluated separately, as were those with ischemic and nonischemic causes of their heart failure.

No statistically significant difference in survival was found between the amiodarone and placebo groups during 45 months of average follow-up ($p =$

Table 1 Comparison of the CHF–STAT and GESICA Trials

Characteristic	CHF–STAT	GESICA
Design	Blinded	Unblinded
Number	674	516
Mean age (years)	65.6	59.3
Female	1%	19%
Mean heart rate (per min)	80.0	89.6
Presumed ischemic etiology	71%	39%
Arrhythmia qualifier	> 10 PVCs per hour	None
Functional class > II	43%	79%
Mean ejection fraction	0.25	0.20
Frequent PVCs (>10 per hour)	100%	71%
Amiodarone discontinuation	40.5%	5.8%
Placebo annual mortality rate	9.4%	21.0%
Mortality reduction (absolute)	0.7%	7.9%
Mortality reduction (relative)	7%	38%

PVC = premature ventricular contractions.

0.6) (Table 1). However, a trend toward reduced mortality in patients with non-ischemic cardiomyopathy ($p = 0.07$), but not in patients with ischemic cardiomyopathy ($p = 0.6$) was observed. No difference in the effect of amiodarone on mortality in patients with low versus very low ejection fractions was found. Furthermore, there was no significant difference in the frequency of SCD in the amiodarone versus placebo groups ($p = 0.4$).

Why Did Amiodarone Fail to Show an Overall Therapeutic Benefit in CHF–STAT?

There are a number of possible explanations but no definite answer to this question. One possibility is that amiodarone is simply not effective in preventing death or SCD in this patient population. However, we know that amiodarone has a significant, though small, protective effect against fatal arrhythmias in post-MI patients with frequent PVCs or LVEF values ≤ 0.40 (13,14). It is possible that the weakly protective effect of amiodarone may not exist in populations like CHF–STAT, or that the number of patients in CHF–STAT was insufficient to detect such a small difference. It is also possible that the presence of frequent PVCs was an insufficient arrhythmia qualifier (i.e., it did not identify patients at higher risk for SCD). Due to the inclusion of severely symptomatic patients (NYHA class IV) in CHF–STAT, competing risks of death, particularly from progressive pump failure, may have decreased amiodarone's potential impact on reducing SCD. Previous studies have shown that patients with the most advanced symptoms of heart failure tend to die from progressive pump failure, rather than SCD (10,28).

The strong trend towards a mortality reduction with amiodarone in the non-ischemic, but not in the ischemic, cardiomyopathy patients, suggests that the etiology of the left ventricular dysfunction may be important. However, it is often difficult to accurately identify a single cause of heart failure in many patients. For example, it would not be reasonable to attribute an ischemic etiology of heart failure to a patient with single-vessel coronary artery disease and global ventricular dysfunction, but the coronary artery disease may have contributed to the left ventricular dysfunction. A recent study suggests that the severity of coronary artery disease, rather than its presence or absence, has greater prognostic importance (29).

A significant problem in CHF–STAT is that 41% of patients on amiodarone were withdrawn from the drug. The combination of amiodarone's relatively weak protection from ventricular tachyarrhythmias, its potential toxicity, and its high rate of discontinuation may have resulted in an insufficient number of patients taking amiodarone to definitively know if it was effective or not.

CHF–STAT VERSUS GESICA

Superficially, the results of CHF–STAT are at variance with the Grupo de Estudio de la Sobrevida en la Insuficiencia Cardiaca en Argentina (GESICA), another large trial of amiodarone in heart failure patients (30). The GESICA trial was an unblinded study performed in South America. They randomized 516 patients with moderate-to-severe symptoms of heart failure (CCS class II–IV) and left ventricular dysfunction to standard medical therapy with or without the addition of open-label amiodarone. A significant reduction in morality was observed over 24 months of follow-up ($p = 0.02$) (Table 1).

Why was there a difference in the results of CHF–STAT and GESICA? A clear answer is unavailable, but some important differences exist between these studies (Table 1). The unblinded nature of GESICA cannot exclude the possibility of unrecognized bias in the assessment or follow-up of these patients. As well, the CHF–STAT population was essentially all men; therefore, a difference in the results on the basis of gender cannot be excluded. Similarly, differences in baseline heart rate, the frequency of PVCs, the severity of symptoms, or LVEF values may, in part, explain the discrepant results. An important distinction between the CHF–STAT and GESICA populations is the greater frequency of no prior MI history in GESICA. Given the strong trend toward a reduction in mortality in the nonischemic group in CHF–STAT ($\sim$20% relative risk reduction; $p = 0.07$), it is possible that the etiology of left ventricular dysfunction may have been important. Another possible reason for CHF–STAT failing to show the same benefit as GESICA is the different withdrawal rate from amiodarone in these two studies. In CHF–STAT almost half (41%) of the patients assigned to amiodarone were withdrawn from the drug, while only 6% were withdrawn in GESICA. This suggests that the borderline significant result in the nonischemic CHF–STAT subgroup may have been due to an insufficient number of patients on amiodarone to truly know whether amiodarone was, or was not, beneficial.

FUTURE DIRECTIONS

So where do these results leave us? The negative result of CHF–STAT suggests that amiodarone is unlikely to have a substantially favorable effect in the North American heart failure population, but the results of GESICA prevent our drawing this conclusion with certainty. Also, the role of the implantable cardioverter defibrillator and the relative role of amiodarone versus ICD therapy have not been adequately addressed in these patients. In addition, the identification of suitable arrhythmia qualifiers in this population remains an important endeavor.

Several ongoing studies will help to address these issues (Table 2). These trials are evaluating the effect of the ICD (all) and amiodarone (SCD-HeFT) therapy on total mortality in symptomatic heart failure patients with reduced LVEF values.

The Sudden Cardiac Death in Heart Failure Trial (SCD-HeFT) will randomize 2500 patients with moderate heart failure symptoms (class II–III) and LVEF values $\leq$0.35 to ICD, amiodarone, or placebo. This study has no additional arrhythmia qualifier. Consequently, its results will apply to the majority of heart failure patients (Fig. 1). However, the absence of an arrhythmia qualifier will

Table 2 Ongoing Sudden Death Prevention Trials in Heart Failure

Trial	Number	LVEF	NYHA class	Arrhythmia qualifier(s)
SCD-HeFT	2500	$\leq$0.35	II-III	None
MADIT 2	1200	$\leq$0.30	I-III	Previous MI
DINAMIT	525	$\leq$0.35	I-III	Recent MI/depressed HRV
DEFINITE	440	$\leq$0.35	I-III	Nonischemic/frequent PVCs or NSVT

HRV = heart rate variability; LVEF = left ventricular ejection fraction; MI = myocardial infarction; NYHA = New York Heart Association functional class; NSVT = nonsustained ventricular tachycardia; PVCs = premature ventricular contractions.

lead to a greater proportion of deaths due to competing risks, mostly progressive heart failure. To address this potential problem, a large number of patients are being randomized so that a small, but significant, reduction in mortality with either amiodarone or the ICD is not overlooked.

The Second Multicenter Automatic Implantable Defibrillator Trial (MADIT II) will randomize 1200 post-MI patients with mild-to-moderate heart failure symptoms and LVEF values ≤ 0.30 to ICD or standard care. The arrhythmia qualifier used in this study is the presence of a prior MI. This qualifier, along with a lower ejection fraction requirement, should identify a somewhat higher risk subgroup of patients.

The Defibrillators in Non-Ischemic Cardiomyopathy Treatment Evaluation (DEFINITE) will randomize 400 nonischemic cardiomyopathy patients with mild-to-moderate heart failure symptoms and LVEF values ≤ 0.35 to ICD or standard therapy. The arrhythmia qualifier used in this trial is presence of nonsustained ventricular tachycardia or ≤ 10 PVCs per hour within the previous 6 months.

The Defibrillators in Acute Myocardial Infarction Trial (DINAMIT) will randomize 525 patients with mild-to-moderate heart failure symptoms and LVEF values ≤ 0.35 to ICD or usual care. Two arrhythmia qualifiers are being used: (1) recent MI (within 6 to 31 days) and (2) depressed heart rate variability (SDNN <70 ms) or elevated resting heart rate (mean RR interval ≤ 750 ms) on Holter monitoring. These criteria should identify a subgroup of heart failure patients at very high risk for SCD.

The completion of MADIT II, DEFINITE, and DINAMIT will help to clarify the effect of ICD therapy on total mortality in these select heart failure populations. Additionally, SCD-HeFT will assess amiodarone and ICD therapy in a less selected, but more symptomatic, heart failure population.

REFERENCES

1. Echt DS, Liebson PR, Mitchell LB, Peters RW, Obias-Manno D, Barker AH, Arensberg D, Baker A, Friedman L, Greene HL. Mortality and morbidity in patients receiving encainide, flecainide, or placebo. The Cardiac Arrhythmia Suppression Trial. N Engl J Med 1993; 324:781–788.
2. Waldo AL, Camm AJ, deRuyter H, Friedman PL, MacNeil DJ, Pauls JF, Pitt B, Pratt CM, Schwartz PJ, Veltri EP. Effect of d-sotalol on mortality in patients with left ventricular dysfunction after recent and remote myocardial infarction. The SWORD Investigators. Survival With ORal d-Sotalol. Lancet 1996; 348:7–12.
3. Siebels J, Cappato R, Ruppel R, Schneider MA, Kuck KH. Preliminary results of the Cardiac Arrest Study Hamburg (CASH). CASH Investigators. Am J Cardiol 1993; 72:109F–113F.

4. Teo KK, Yusuf S, Furberg CD. Effects of prophylactic antiarrhythmic drug therapy in acute myocardial infarction. An overview of results from randomized controlled trials. JAMA 1993; 270:1589–1595.

5. Moller M. DIAMOND antiarrhythmic trials. Danish Investigations of Arrhythmia and Mortality on Dofetilide. Lancet 1996; 348:1597–1598.

6. Moller M. Danish Investigations of Arrhythmia and Mortality on Dofetilide (DIAMOND). Circulation 1997; 96:3820.

7. Norwegian Timolol Multicenter Study Investigators. Timolol-induced reduction in mortality and reinfarction in patients surviving acute myocardial infarction. N Engl J Med 1981; 304:801–807.

8. Beta-Blocker Heart Attack Trial Investigators. A randomized trial of propranolol in patients with acute myocardial infarction. I. Mortality results. JAMA 1982; 247:1707–14.

9. CIBIS-II Investigators. The Cardiac Insufficiency Bisoprolol Study II (CIBIS-II): a randomised trial. Lancet 1999;353:9–13.

10. MERIT-HF Investigators. Effect of metoprolol CR/XL in chronic heart failure: Metoprolol CR/XL Randomised Intervention Trial in Congestive Heart Failure (MERIT-HF). Lancet 1999;353:2001–2007.

11. Saksena S, Madan N, Lewis C. Implanted cardioverter-defibrillators are preferable to drugs as primary therapy insustained ventricular tachyarrhythmias. Prog Cardiovasc Dis 1996; 38:445–454.

12. Ceremuzynski L, Kleczar E, Krzeminska-Pakula M, Kuch J, Nartowicz E, Smielak-Korombel J, Dyduszynski A, Maciejewicz J, Zaleska T, Lazarczyk-Kedzia E. Effect of amiodarone on mortality after myocardial infarction: a double-blind, placebo-controlled, pilot study. J Am Coll Cardiol 1992; 20:1056–1062.

13. Julian DG, Camm AJ, Frangin G, Janse MJ, Munoz A, Schwartz PJ, Simon P. Randomised trial of effect of amiodarone on mortality in patients with left-ventricular dysfunction after recent myocardial infarction: EMIAT. European Myocardial Infarct Amiodarone Trial Investigators. Lancet 1997; 349:667–674.

14. Cairns JA, Connolly SJ, Roberts R, Gent M. Randomised trial of outcome after myocardial infarction in patients with frequent or repetitive ventricular premature depolarisation: CAMIAT. Canadian Amiodarone Myocardial Infarction Arrhythmia Trial Investigators. Lancet 1997; 349:675–682.

15. Amiodarone Trials Meta-Analysis Investigators. Effect of prophylactic amiodarone on mortality after acute myocardial infarction and in congestive heart failure: meta-analysis of individual data from 6500 patients in randomised trials. Lancet 1997; 350:417–1424.

16. The Antiarrhythmics Versus Implantable Defibrillators (AVID) Investigators. A comparison of antiarrhythmic-drug therapy with implantable defibrillators in patients resuscitated from near-fatal ventricular arrhythmias. N Engl J Med 1997; 337:1576–1583.

17. Moss AJ, Hall WJ, Cannom DS, Daubert JP, Higgins SL, Klein H, Levine JH, Saksena S, Waldo AL, Wilber D, Brown MW, Heo M. Improved survival with an implanted defibrillator in patients with coronary disease at high risk for ventricular arrhythmia. Multicenter Automatic Defibrillator Implantation Trial Investigators. N Engl J Med 1996; 335:1933–1940.

18. Graves EJ, Gillum BS. Detailed diagnoses and procedures, National Hospital Discharge Survey, 1995. Vital Health Stat 13 1997; 130:1–146.

19. Schocken DD, Arrieta MI, Leaverton PE, Ross EA. Prevalence and mortality rate of congestive heart failure in the United States. J Am Coll Cardiol 1992; 20:301–306.

20. SOLVD Investigators. Effect of enalapril on survival in patients with reduced left ventricular ejection fractions and congestive heart failure. N Engl J Med 1991; 325:293–302.

21. Kannel WB, Sorlie P, McNamara PM. Prognosis after initial myocardial infarction: the Framingham study. Am J Cardiol 1979; 44:53–59.

22. Gradman A, Deedwania P, Cody R, Massie B, Packer M, Pitt B, Goldstein S. Predictors of total mortality and sudden death in mild to moderate heart failure. Captopril-Digoxin Study Group. J Am Coll Cardiol 1989; 14:564–570.

23. Bigger JT Jr, Fleiss JL, Kleiger R, Miller JP, Rolnitzky LM. The relationships among ventricular arrhythmias, left ventricular dysfunction, and mortality in the 2 years after myocardial infarction. Circulation 1984; 69:250–258.

24. Hartikainen JE, Malik M, Staunton A, Poloniecki J, Camm AJ. Distinction between arrhythmic and nonarrhythmic death after acute myocardial infarction based on heart rate variability, signal-averaged electrocardiogram, ventricular arrhythmias and left ventricular ejection fraction. J Am Coll Cardiol 1996; 28:296–304.

25. Bigger JT Jr, Fleiss JL, Steinman RC, Rolnitzky LM, Kleiger RE, Rottman JN. Frequency domain measures of heart period variability and mortality after myocardial infarction. Circulation 1992; 85:164–171.

26. Waspe LE, Seinfeld D, Ferrick A, Kim SG, Matos JA, Fisher JD. Prediction of sudden death and spontaneous ventricular tachycardia in survivors of complicated myocardial infarction: value of the response to programmed stimulation using a maximum of three ventricular extrastimuli. J Am Coll Cardiol 1985; 5:1292–1301.

27. Singh SN, Fletcher RD, Fisher SG, Singh BN, Lewis HD, Deedwania PC, Massie BM, Colling C, Lazzeri D. Amiodarone in patients with congestive heart failure and asymptomatic ventricular arrhythmia. Survival Trial of Antiarrhythmic Therapy in Congestive Heart Failure. N Engl J Med 1995; 333:77–82.

28. Luu M, Stevenson WG, Stevenson LW, Baron K, Walden J. Diverse mechanisms of unexpected cardiac arrest in advanced heart failure. Circulation 1989; 80:1675–1680.

29. Bart BA, Shaw LK, McCants CB Jr, Fortin DF, Lee KL, Califf RM, O'Connor CM. Clinical determinants of mortality in patients with angiographically diagnosed ischemic or nonischemic cardiomyopathy. J Am Coll Cardiol 1997; 30:1002–1008.

30. Doval HC, Nul DR, Grancelli HO, Perrone SV, Bortman GR, Curiel R. Randomised trial of low-dose amiodarone in severe congestive heart failure. Grupo de Estudio de la Sobrevida en la Insuficiencia Cardiaca en Argentina. Lancet 1994; 344:493–498.

7

The Survival With ORal D-Sotalol (SWORD) Trial

ALBERT L. WALDO
Case Western Reserve University, Cleveland, Ohio

CRAIG M. PRATT
Baylor College of Medicine, Houston, Texas

THE DESIGN AND RESULTS OF SWORD

Introduction

It is well recognized that survivors of myocardial infarction (MI) face an increased risk of sudden cardiac death. Identification of those patients most at risk is still evolving, and therapies that could favorably impact the incidence of sudden cardiac death clearly are most welcome. At the time of the initiation of the Survival With ORal D-sotalol (SWORD) trial in August 1992, it was recognized that depressed left ventricular function (1), ventricular ectopic activity (2), signal-averaged late potentials (3), low heart rate variability (4), and low baroreflex sensitivity (5) identified patients at highest risk when an MI was recent. When an MI was remote, the risk of sudden cardiac death remained substantial (6), but identification of high-risk patients was still not well characterized. For these "remote" MI patients, left ventricular dysfunction was regarded as the best predictor of total mortality. However, with the increased use of improved treatment strategies for these patients (e.g., coronary artery bypass graft surgery, afterload reduction, etc.), the actual incidence of sudden arrhythmic death in patients with depressed left ventricular dysfunction was uncertain and a moving target. Furthermore, the true incidence of sudden cardiac death due to ventricular tachyarrhythmia in "remote" MI patients had not been well characterized.

In addition, very little was known at this time about the efficacy of pure class III antiarrhythmics in the primary prevention of sudden cardiac death in this patient population. Beta-adrenergic blockers had been shown to provide some protection from all-cause mortality and sudden cardiac death after MI (7). However, data from numerous clinical trials showed and still show that these drugs are used rather infrequently in patients with impaired ventricular function (8,9). Results with class IC agents in the Cardiac Arrhythmia Suppression Trials (CAST I and II) (8,10,11), together with meta-analysis of data from the use of class I antiarrhythmic drugs in this patient population (12), had shown that sodium channel-blocking agents were associated with increased rather than decreased all-cause mortality and sudden cardiac death, despite suppression of frequent and complex ventricular ectopy. Results with class III antiarrhythmic drugs were expected to be different, although the potential for proarrhythmia in the form of torsades de pointes was appreciated (13–15). However, in 1992, the post-MI experience with class III agents only included several small trials with amiodarone, which had provided encouraging results (13,14,16). However, amiodarone had important limitations related to its multiple (class I, II, and IV as well as class III) antiarrhythmic effects, complicated kinetics, and potentially very serious adverse effects (17). Because of the high worldwide incidence of coronary artery disease, the continued desire to reduce mortality in high-risk patients, the promise of class III antiarrhythmic agents, and the limitations of available drugs, investigation of new class III antiarrhythmic agents seemed warranted.

d-Sotalol was among the new class III agents available in 1992. It had been the most widely used and was expected to be well tolerated by patients with severe left ventricular dysfunction. d-Sotalol, the dextrorotatory isomer of the racemate d,l-sotalol, is a class III antiarrhythmic drug that prolongs the action potential duration and refractoriness of cardiac tissue by blocking the Ik_r (delayed rectifier) channel (18). It was shown to be antifibrillatory in an ischemic model (19), but not in models that are associated with sympathetic hyperactivity (20). Unlike d,l-sotalol, d-sotalol has no clinically significant β-blocking activity in humans (21). In clinical trials prior to SWORD, d-sotalol had been well tolerated, with a low incidence of reported adverse events. Torsade de pointes had occurred in approximately 1.2% of those exposed to the drug (data on file, Bristol-Myers Squibb, Princeton, NJ), with a still lower incidence on ≤200 mg bid. It is in the above context that the SWORD trial was initiated. It was a multinational, multicenter, randomized, double-blind, placebo-controlled trial to test the hypothesis that d-sotalol, a drug with pure potassium channel blocking action, reduced all-cause mortality in patients with previous MI and left ventricular dysfunction.

Methods

The SWORD trial (22) was performed at 546 centers, although only 406 centers actually enrolled patients. Eligible patients were men and women ≥18 years of age who had a left ventricular ejection fraction of ≤40% determined within 6 months of randomization. In addition, to be eligible, patients must have had evidence of a prior MI. Eligible patients were divided into two groups. Group 1 (recent group) consisted of patients with an MI 6 to 42 days before randomization with or without overt heart failure. Group 2 (remote group) consisted of patients with an MI occurring > 42 days before randomization and a history of overt heart failure (New York Heart Association functional class II or III). Eligible women had to be either surgically sterile, postmenopausal, or using an acceptable method of contraception. Women of childbearing potential must have had a negative pregnancy test before randomization.

Major exclusion criteria included: corrected QT (QT_c) interval > 460 ms; recent (within 14 days) coronary angioplasty or coronary artery bypass graft surgery; unstable angina; history of life-threatening arrhythmia unrelated to an MI; nonischemic or severe (class IV) heart failure; sick sinus syndrome or high-grade heart block without a pacemaker; concomitant antiarrhythmic agents or drugs that prolong the QT interval; and specific electrolyte (serum potassium < 4.0 mEq/L or serum magnesium < 1.5 mEq/L), renal, or liver abnormalities.

The study consisted of a screening and a double-blind phase (Fig. 1). During screening, a three-channel 24-h ambulatory ECG recording identified baseline characteristics, including supraventricular and ventricular rhythm disturbances, heart rate variability, and the presence or absence of signal-averaged electrocardiographic abnormalities. Randomization was not contingent upon the results of the ambulatory ECG.

Eligible patients who consented to participate were enrolled in the study. They were randomly assigned to receive a titrated dose of either d-sotalol or placebo. Doses could not exceed 200 mg twice daily for the duration of the study. Patients were initially assigned oral d-sotalol 100 mg twice daily or matching placebo for 1 week. If this dose was tolerated with a QT_c < 520 ms, the dose was increased to 200 mg twice daily or matching placebo for a further week. If tolerated with a QT_c of < 560 ms, this dose was given for the duration of the study. If the QT_c exceeded 560 ms at any time during the follow-up, the dose was reduced. If the QTc was still above this value at the 100-mg twice-daily dose, the study drug was discontinued. During follow-up, concomitant treatment with beta-blockers (except d,l-sotalol), digoxin, angiotensin-converting enzyme inhibitors, and calcium antagonists was allowed.

Follow-Up

Except for weekly visits for the first 2 weeks, patients were followed every 3 months for the first year and every 4 months thereafter. Periodic clinical evaluations and laboratory studies were obtained during the follow-up clinic visits. At month 3, a three-channel, ambulatory ECG recording was repeated. Patients who discontinued the study medication were followed for the duration of the study. The minimal follow-up period was set at 18 months.

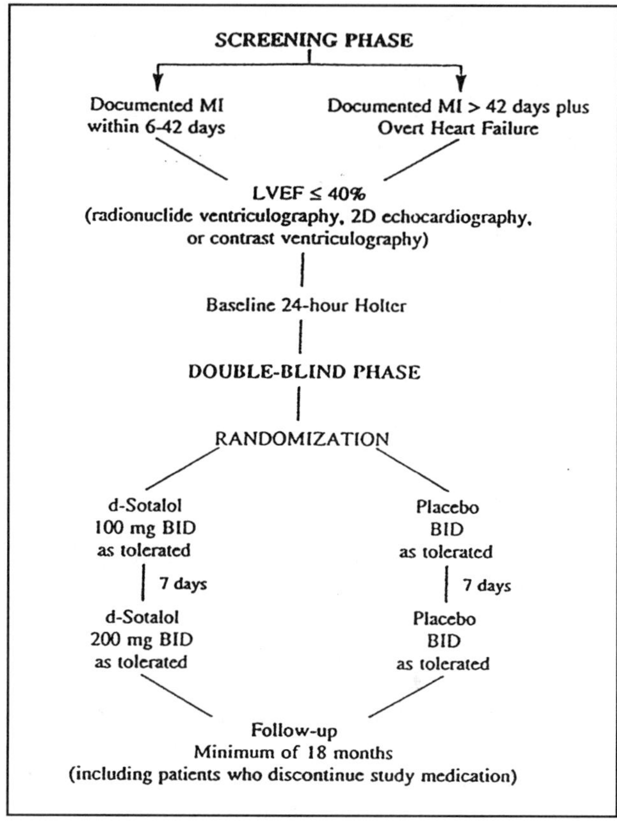

Figure 1 Protocol for the Survival With ORal D-sotalol trial. High-risk survivors of a myocardial infarction are randomized to receive either d-sotalol or placebo and followed for 18 months. BID = twice daily; 2D = two-dimensional; LVEF = left ventricular ejection fraction; MI = myocardial infarction. From Ref. 22, with permission.

Endpoints

The primary efficacy endpoint was all-cause mortality. Cardiac mortality was a secondary endpoint. tertiary endpoints were cardiovascular mortality, presumed arrhythmic death, nonfatal severe arrhythmic events, hospitalizations for cardiovascular causes and composites of these endpoints. An events committee blinded to treatment assignment reviewed all deaths, and nonfatal severe arrhythmic events to verify the investigators' interpretation. The final classification of an event was the responsibility of the events committee.

Statistical Considerations

The goal of the study was to enroll 6400 patients, all of whom would be in the final analysis. In estimating sample size, the following assumptions were made: (1) the trial duration would be 3 years, with a minimal patient follow-up of 18 months and an average follow-up of 2.25 years; (2) group 1 (recent group) and group 2 (remote group) patients would be entered in a ratio of 2:1; (3) the cumulative average mortality would be 17.7% in the placebo-treated patients; (4) a 20% reduction in all-cause mortality would be associated with d-sotalol therapy; (5) a two-sided significance level of 0.05 would be present; (6) a power of 90% would be present; and (7) 10% dropouts in the d-sotalol group (patients who stopped taking study medication) and 5% drop-ins in the placebo group (patients who start taking another antiarrhythmic agent) would occur. A calculated sample size of 6374 patients provided power for the log-rank test of at least 0.90 under the hypothesis that d-sotalol would lower mortality by 20%. The sample size estimate was based on the assumption that there would be one intention-to-treat analysis at the conclusion of the trial. However, during the study, the Data and Safety Monitoring Committee would make periodic assessments with defined stopping rules that permitted termination of the trial before its completion, if appropriate (23).

For each interim analysis, the assessment of efficacy was based on a critical boundary value determined by the procedure of Lan and DeMets (24). Interim assesssments of safety used an advisory statistical boundary as described by DeMets (25). In addition, the committee used the stochastic curtailment procedure described by Pawitan and Hallstrom (26) to assess the likelihood that the study would find a favorable result if carried to completion.

SWORD used a group sequential design so that early termination of the study was possible for either efficacy or safety concerns (23). The data for interim analyses were unblinded by an independent third party, who carried out the analyses and presented the results to the Data and Safety Monitoring Committee. For efficacy, a monitoring protocol used one-sided boundary values determined from an α-spending function (24) approximating those of O'Brien-Fleming (27), with overall $\alpha = 0.025$. This approach gave boundary values that were extremely conservative early in the study, and it did not require either the number or the timing of the interim analyses to be specified in advance. For safety, the trial applied an advisory, rather than a formal statistical boundary using a Z value -2.25 or less from the log-rank test comparing survival curves (25,28).

For the results presented here, baseline values were analyzed by t test or χ^2 with a p of 0.05 or less for significance. For mortality or other endpoints, Kaplan–Meier survival curves (29) were compared by log-rank tests with nominal two-tailed p values. The relative risks associated with d-sotalol treatment were estimated within various clinically defined subgroups by proportional haz-

Table 1 Prerandomization Characteristics of Treatment Groups

	d-Sotalol ($n = 1549$)	Placebo ($n = 1572$)
Demography		
Male	86%	86%
White	93%	93%
Age (years)*	60.4 (10.1)	59.9 (9.8)
Medical history (%)		
MI before index MI	34%	32%
Hypertension	37%	35%
CABG	23%	22%
PTCA	14%	16%
Chronic atrial fibrillation	4%	3%
Recent MI (6–42 days)	29%	29%
Weeks from index MI		
Recent MI stratum	3.2 (1.6)	3.2 (1.6)
Remote MI stratum	213 (247)	225 (263)
LVEF		
<30%	43	44
31–40%	57	56
Mean LVEF*	31.0 (6-8)	30.8 (7-0)
NYHA class		
I	7%	8%
II	72%	72%
III	22%	21%
12-lead ECG		
Heart rate*	73.0 (13-6)	73.2 (13-5)
QT (ms)*	386 (40)	385 (41)
QT_c (ms)*	417 (31)	416 (32)
Abnormal Q waves	78%	78%
LVH	14%	12%
Pacemaker	2%	1%
24 h ECG	($n = 1452$)	($n = 1480$)
No VPD	2%	3%
<6 VPD per h	42%	43%
>6 VPD per h	56%	54%
Mean VPD per h	54 (130)	59 (148)
VT runs	36%	36%
Concomitant medications at randomization		
Diuretics	48%	50%
Digoxin	27%	26%

Table 1 Continued

	d-Sotalol ($n = 1549$)	Placebo ($n = 1572$)
ACE inhibitors	71%	72%
Nitrates	54%	53%
Beta-blockers	33%	32%
Calcium blockers	19%	19%
Aspirin	64%	66%

CABG = coronary artery bypass graft; PTCA = percutaneous transluminal coronary angioplasty; LVEF = left ventricular ejection fraction; NYHA = New York Heart Association; LVH = left ventricular hypertrophy; VPD = ventricular premature depolarizations; VT = ventricular tachycardia; ACE = angiotensin converting enzyme. Data are % of group or *mean (SD).
Source: Ref. 31.

ard regression (30). The same method was used to explore the consistency of the drug's subgroup effects with its overall trial effect by testing treatment-by-subgroup interactions.

Results

By Nov 1, 1994, after 2.3 years of recruitment, the SWORD trial had enrolled 3121 patients with a mean follow-up of 148 days. At that time, the Data and Safety Monitoring Committee recommended termination of the trial because an interim analysis showed an increased mortality in patients assigned d-sotalol that crossed the prespecified advisory statistical boundary (observed $Z = -2.75$) (31).

The trial originally intended to recruit two patients with a recent MI (recent group) for each one with a remote MI (remote group). This was because of concerns for potential differences in cause-specific mortality between patients in each group. However, and importantly, at the time of termination of the study, the ratio was reversed (31). There were 915 patients with a recent MI and 2206 with a remote MI (ratio 1:2.04); 1549 patients had been assigned d-sotalol and 1572 placebo. The baseline characteristics of the two treatment groups were similar (Table 1). There was little difference in the important prognostic variables of left ventricular ejection fraction, New York Heart Association heart failure class, and use of concomitant medications. The time from the index MI and proportion of patients with ventricular arrhythmias were similar in the two groups (31).

When the study was terminated, there had been 30 excess deaths in d-sotalol-assigned compared with placebo-assigned patients (78/1549 [5.0%] versus 48/1572 [3.1%]; relative risk 1.65 [95% CI 1.15–2.36]; $p = 0.006$) (31).

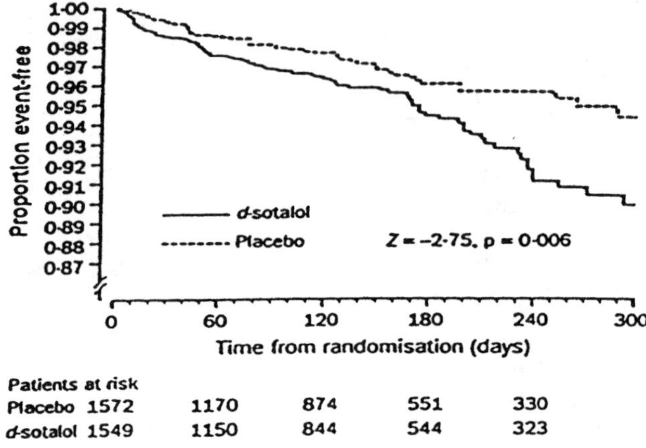

Figure 2 Survival among 3121 patients randomly assigned d-sotalol or placebo. From Ref. 31, with permission.

Table 2 Cause-Specific Mortality

	Number of deaths			
	d-Sotalol ($n = 1549$)	Placebo ($n = 1572$)	Log-rank p^*	Relative risk (95% Cl)
All causes	78	48	0.006	1.65 (1.15-2.36)
Cardiac deaths				
All cardiac	73	45	0.008	1.65 (1.14-2.39)
Arrhythmic (presumed)	56	32	0.008	1.77 (1-15-2-74)
Nonarrhythmic	17	13	—	—
Progressive CHF	10	8	—	—
Acute MI	6	5	—	—
Other	1	0	—	—
Other				
Cerebrovascular	2	2	—	—
Noncardiovascular	3	1	—	—

CHF = congestive heart failure.
*Nominal two-sided significance level of log-rank test.
Source: From Ref. 31.

Survival curves are shown in Figure 2. Significantly greater numbers of cardiac and arrhythmic deaths accounted for this increased mortality (Table 2). Rates of nonfatal cardiac events were similar in the d-sotalol-treated and placebo-treated groups (31). In particular, there were no excess serious arrhythmic events in the d-sotalol group. The reported incidence of torsades de pointes in these patients was low (3/1549 [0.2%]). One of these events was fatal. During the trial, 100 patients assigned to d-sotalol and 82 assigned to placebo discontinued study medication because of adverse events (31). Discontinuations for worsening heart failure and serious arrhythmic events were infrequent, and there were similar numbers in the two groups.

Exploratory subgroup analyses generally showed a consistency of drug effect on mortality (Fig. 3) (31). In all subgroups of interest, patients assigned to d-sotalol had a higher death rate than patients assigned to placebo. The observed increased risk with d-sotalol was present regardless of age, sex, time from index

Prerandomisation characteristic		n	Number of deaths		Relative risk (95% CI)
			d-sotalol	Placebo	
All patients		3121	78	48	
Sex	Male	2684	64	45	
	Female	437	14	3	
Age (years)	<60	1368	23	17	
	>60	1753	55	31	
Days from MI	6–42	915	23	13	
	>42	2206	55	35	
LVEF (%)	<30	1361	45	40	
	31–40	1760	33	8	
VPD per h	<6	1325	13	8	
	>6	1598	55	35	
QTc (ms)	<420	1699	38	22	
	420–460	1334	37	20	
Potassium (mmol/L)	<4·5	1767	40	29	
	>4·5	1300	37	17	
Creatinine (µmol/L)	<97·2	1397	31	16	
	>97·2	1670	46	30	
Diuretic use	Yes	1487	55	43	
	No	1560	18	5	
Digoxin use	Yes	817	37	25	
	No	2230	36	23	
Beta-blocker use	Yes	983	16	10	
	No	2064	57	38	
Calcium-blocker use	Yes	575	15	12	
	No	2472	58	36	
ACE inhibitor use	Yes	2171	55	38	
	No	876	18	10	
Aspirin use	Yes	1980	37	26	
	No	1067	36	22	

0·5   1   2   4   8

Figure 3 Effect of d-sotalol on mortality in subgroups: Squares of area proportional to number of deaths in that subgroup indicate relative risk; solid vertical line corresponds to a finding of no effect and dashed vertical line to effect observed in full sample. Deviations of subgroup relative risks from overall relative risk assessed by testing for interaction by proportional hazards regression. $\chi^2 = 7.27$ ($p = 0.007$) for interaction of effect of d-sotalol on mortality over subgroups of ejection fraction. Tests for interaction with other characteristics not significant. From Ref. 32, with permission.

MI, left ventricular ejection fraction, or concomitant therapy. However, the adverse effect associated with d-sotalol was more pronounced in patients with relatively better ventricular function (ejection fraction 31–40%) than in those with lower ejection fractions, and in women rather than in men, although few women were studied. Concomitant therapy with beta-blockers, diuretics, or calcium channel blockers did not alter the adverse effect.

WHY WAS THERE AN EXCESS MORTALITY ASSOCIATED WITH d-SOTALOL?

Introduction

One of the obvious possible explanations of the SWORD trial data was that the excess deaths on d-sotalol were due to ventricular proarrhythmia, particularly torsades de pointes. However, from the initial analysis, this was not at all obvious. There were only three reported cases of torsades de pointes, and, with the exception of the more pronounced risk of death in women on d-sotalol (although few women [14%] participated in the study), other baseline characteristics likely to favor torsades de pointes were not associated with the increased mortality. Therefore, an additional analysis was performed to gain insight into the nature of the d-sotalol-associated mortality risk (32). Despite the above, this analysis examined the hypothesis that because of the known association of drugs (such as d-sotalol) that prolong repolarization time with torsades de pointes, d-sotalol-associated mortality in the SWORD trial was due to this proarrhythmic mechanism (33–38).

Analysis Methods

For the purposes of this additional analysis, the two original SWORD MI groups—recent (6 to 42 days) and remote (> 42 days)—were further stratified into those with poor (LVEF 31% to 40%) and very poor (LVEF ≤30%) ventricular function. The two LVEF groups and the two index MI groups then became the four major subgroups of this additional analysis. Variables of known prognostic importance (age, LVEF, heart failure class) (39–41) as well as variables known to be related to torsades de pointes (gender, temporal relation to initiation of trial medication, QT_c, bradycardia, serum potassium and magnesium, and diuretic use) were assessed (38). Interactions between treatment and baseline arrhythmia were investigated by examining the frequency of premature ventricular complexes and the presence of nonsustained ventricular tachycardia on a baseline ambulatory electrocardiogram. The potential interactions between these four major index MI and LVEF subgroups and medications at baseline (beta-blockers, calcium blockers, angiotensin-converting enzyme inhibitors, digoxin, aspirin, nitrates) were also examined. The contribution of ischemia was indirectly assessed by the patient's history of coronary artery bypass graft surgery or percutaneous transluminal coronary angioplasty, the presence or absence of a Q-wave MI, and baseline nitrate use. In all of the comparisons, separate assessments of total mortality and presumed arrhythmic death mortality were performed. Assessments of heart rate on the 24-h ambulatory ECG (analyzed blinded to treatment assignment by a certified private facility) obtained at baseline were also related to mortality in the index MI groups. The influence of the d-sotalol dose (100 mg twice daily or 200 mg twice daily) on mortality was also examined.

Treatment-specific Kaplan–Meier survival curves were constructed within the four major subgroups defined by MI group (recent or remote) and degree of ventricular dysfunction (LVEF ≤30% or 31% to 40%) (29). A fully hierarchical Cox model containing effects for MI type, LVEF category, treatment assignment, and each two- and three-way interaction was fitted to the data to explore the effect of d-sotalol's influence on survival in the four major subgroups and to explore the uniformity of this effect (30). This was performed both for total mortality and for presumed arrhythmic death mortality, treating the latter case, nonarrhythmic deaths, as censored events.

A final series of exploratory analyses were conducted to evaluate the ability of salient baseline variables that could possibly modify the effect of d-sotalol on mortality among the four major LVEF and index MI subgroups. A pair of Cox models was constructed, initially using the full hierarchical model described above (30). The first examined the ability of the covariant to modify the effect of d-sotalol on survival across the two LVEF and two index MI major subgroups (by adding covariant treatment by index MI and adding covariant by treatment by LVEF terms to the full model with additional terms for covariant main effect and its interaction with treatment). The second examined effect modification due to the covariant across the four major LVEF and index MI subgroups by adding a covariant by treatment, by index MI, and by LVEF term to the first model. A significance level of $p = 0.10$ was used for tests of covariant by treatment interactions, and a p value of 0.05 was used for tests of higher order interactions.

Analysis Results

Baseline Characteristics: Relation to Index Myocardial
Infarction and Ventricular Function

Although there were no significant differences in baseline characteristics known to be of prognostic importance between d-sotalol- and placebo-assigned patients as previously described (31), there were many differences in the baseline characteristics of the two distinct prospectively defined index MI groups, recent and remote (Table 3) (32). The significant differences were consistent with the greater degree of systolic ventricular dysfunction and symptomatic heart failure in the remote MI group. Furthermore, the d-sotalol-associated total mortality risk and presumed arrhythmic death varied widely (1.0–7.9 and 1.2–20.7, respectively) among the groups, and was greatest in the remote MI group with a LVEF of 31% to 40% (Table 4). The effect of d-sotalol was not uniform among the four subgroups.

Treatment-specific survival curves for total mortality in these four subgroups are shown in Figure 4. The remote MI, LVEF 31% to 40% group, had a strikingly low placebo mortality. The curves also indicate that the d-sotalol-associated risk was not confined to the period early after the initiation of treatment. In fact, only six d-sotalol- and two placebo-treated patients died in the first week after receiving therapy.

Relation of Baseline Characteristics to Mortality

Many of the well-characterized risk factors were associated with an increased risk of death. Aspirin and beta-blocker administration were associated with a decreased risk of death. These patterns of association were observed for the entire SWORD population, and were also evident within each treatment group. Patients presenting with frequent ventricular premature complexes ($\geq$ 6/h) or with non-sustained ventricular tachycardia had a significantly higher risk of death than those without (32). For ventricular premature complexes, this risk was evident regardless of treatment assignment. However, the magnitude of the risk associated with nonsustained ventricular tachycardia tended to be greater ($p = 0.09$) among d-sotalol-assigned patients (3.6-fold) than placebo-assigned patients (1.8-fold). The increased risk of baseline nonsustained ventricular tachycardia, either alone or in combination with d-sotalol therapy, was derived chiefly from the remote MI group ($p = 0.02$ for the interaction of ventricular tachycardia by index MI and treatment assignment).

Gender Influence

Although men and women were at a similar risk of death in SWORD, within the d-sotalol group, women tended to be at higher risk than men, whereas in the placebo group, the reverse was true (32). Relative to placebo, d-sotalol was associated with a 4.7-fold increased risk of death in women and 1.4-fold increase in men (32). In women, the total number of d-sotalol-associated deaths was small (14 of 219 [6.4%]), and only 2 of 14 d-sotalol-associated deaths in women occurred in the first 2 weeks. Most (10 of 14 [71%]) occurred in the recent MI group despite the fact that most (133 of 219 [61%]) of the women receiving d-sotalol were in the remote index MI group ($p = 0.005$).

Table 3 Baseline Characteristics by Index Myocardial Infarction

| | Index MI | | |
Characteristic	Recent ($n = 915$)	Remote ($n = 2206$)	p Value
Men (%)	83	87	0.007
Caucasian (%)	91	93	0.01
Age (yrs) (mean, SD)	59.5 (10.6)	60.4 (9.7)	0.01
Medical history (%)			
MI, before index MI	29	35	<0.001
Hypertension	37	36	0.51
CABG	9	28	<0.001
PTCA	15	15	0.97
Chronic AF	2	4	<0.001
Weeks from index MI (mean, SD)	3.2 (1.6)	219 (255)	—
LVEF (%)			
≤30%	37	47	
31%–40%	63	54	
Mean (SD)	31.9 (6.4)	30.5 (7.0)	<0.001
NYHA class (%)			
I	25	0	
II	56	78	<0.001
III	19	22	
12-Lead ECG			
Heart rate (mean, SD)	73.9 (13.7)	72.8 (13.6)	0.03
QT (ms) (mean, SD)	385 (43)	386 (40)	0.42
QTc (ms) (mean, SD)	415 (32)	416 (31)	0.44
Abnormal Q waves (%)	70	81	<0.001
LVH (%)	7	16	<0.001
Pacemaker (%)	1	1	0.34
LBBB (%)	4	7	0.01
RBBB (%)	5	6	0.08
24-h ECG			
Number of patients	875	2057	
PVC/h (%)			
None	4	2	
Present (<6)	58	37	
≥6	39	61	
Mean (SD)	35 (101)	65 (152)	<0.001
Paired PVCs	47	67	<0.001
VT runs (%)	27	40	<0.001

Table 3 Continued

| | Index MI | | |
Characteristic	Recent (n = 915)	Remote (n = 2206)	p Value
Concomitant medications at randomization (%)			
Diuretics	36	54	<0.001
Digoxin	17	31	<0.001
ACE inhibitors	69	72	0.11
Nitrates	52	54	0.43
Beta-blockers	41	29	<0.001
Calcium blockers	12	22	<0.001
Aspirin	71	62	<0.001

AF = atrial fibrillation; CABG = coronary artery bypass graft surgery; LBBB = left bundle branch block; LVH = left ventricular hypertrophy; NYHA = New York Heart Association; PTCA = percutaneous transluminal coronary angioplasty; PVC = premature ventricular complex; RBBB = right bundle branch block; VT = ventricular tachycardia.
Source: Ref. 32.

Analysis of Other Electrocardiographic and Clinical Baseline Variables

Exploratory analyses of other selected baseline variables failed to reveal any additional significant interactions (32). By protocol design, patients with a QT_c > 460 ms at baseline were excluded from the SWORD trial. Overall, patients in the SWORD trial with a baseline QT_c > 420 ms were at similar risk of death with those with a shorter QT_c (RR = 1.2), a pattern that was similar in each treatment group. Among the four major index MI and LVEF groups, the presence of a longer baseline QT_c did not have a significant impact on the mortality effect associated with d-sotalol (p > 0.05 for treatment by QT_c interaction). A similar conclusion was reached when the QT_c interval measured after 2 weeks of treatment was evaluated. The presence of ischemia, ascertained in several ways, including concomitant nitrate use, a history of revascularization, or a non-Q-wave index MI, showed no significant relation to survival in the overall study, or within the individual treatment group. Neither minimum nor average heart rate, as measured on the 24-h baseline ambulatory ECG, were found to alter the risk of death associated with d-sotalol. At the completion of the 2-week drug titration phase, > 88% of d-sotalol-treated patients were receiving the 200-mg twice-daily dose; a limited analysis of the two doses at that time revealed no relation to mortality.

Table 4 Total and Arrhythmic Deaths in Patients Given Placebo Compared with Those Given d-Sotalol: Relation to Ejection Fraction and Index Myocardial Infarction

	d-Sotalol				Placebo				
Index MI	n	Death type	No. of deaths	%	n	Death type	No. of deaths	%	RR ($\pm$95% CI)
LVEF ≤30%	160	Total	14	8.8	175	Total	8	4.6	2.0 [0.84–4.79]
Recent MI		Arrhythmic	8	5.0		Arrhythmic	8	4.6	1.1 [0.43–3.1]
LVEF 31%–40%	296	Total	9	3.0	284	Total	5	1.8	1.7 [0.56–5.0]
Recent MI		Arrhythmic	4	1.4		Arrhythmic	3	1.1	1.3 [0.28–5.6]
LVEF ≤30%	510	Total	31	6.1	516	Total	32	6.2	1.0 [0.6–1.6]
Remote MI		Arrhythmic	23	4.5		Arrhythmic	20	3.9	1.2 [0.65–2.2]
LVEF 31%–40%	583	Total	24	4.1	597	Total	3	0.5	7.9 [2.4–26.2]
Remote MI		Arrhythmic	21	3.6		Arrhythmic	1	1.7	20.7 [2.8–153.7]
Total cohort	1,549	Total	78	5.0	1,572	Total	48	3.1	1.65 [1.15–2.36]
		Arrhythmic	56	3.6		Arrhythmic	32	2.0	1.77 [1.15–2.74]

Source: Ref. 32.

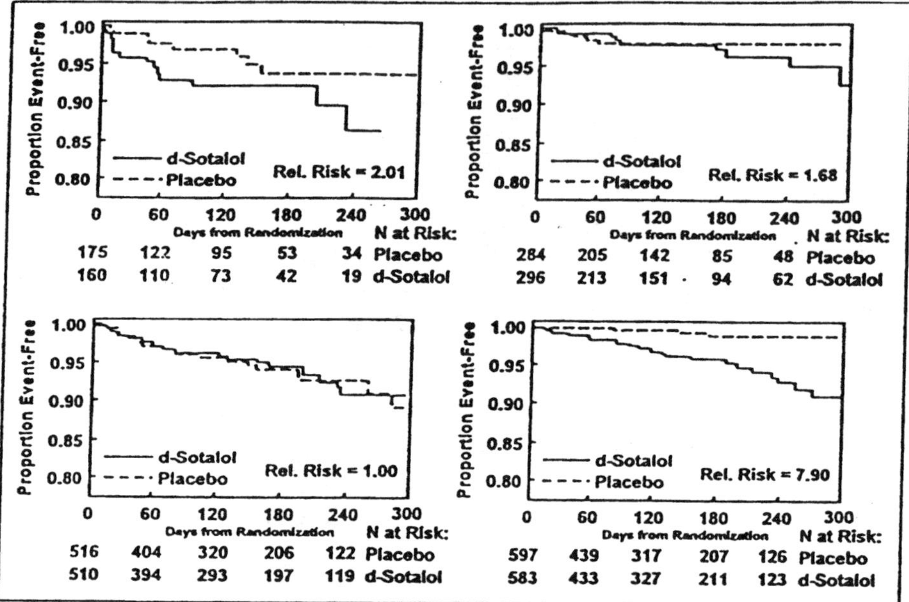

Figure 4 Survival curves by treatment group for *total mortality*. The four major subgroups are represented. Recent MI, LVEF ≤30% (top left); recent MI, LVEF 31% to 40% (top right); remote MI, LVEF ≤30% (bottom left); remote MI, LVEF 31% to 40% (bottom right). The d-sotalol-treated patients in this latter group exhibit a progressive increased mortality risk compared with a nearly event-free, placebo-assigned group (RR = 7.9). From Ref. 32, with permission.

Fatal and Serious Nonfatal Arrhythmic Events with Electrocardiographic Documentation

There was only one d-sotalol-treated patient with arrhythmic death directly attributable to electrocardiograph documented torsades de pointes (31,32). Only 2 of 132 of the nonfatal cardiac events in the 1549 patients receiving d-sotalol (vs. 0 of 118 in the 1572 patients receiving placebo) were documented as torsades de pointes. Nonfatal serious arrhythmic events occurred in < 1% of patients treated with either d-sotalol or placebo. Other serious nonfatal arrhythmias were uncommon, both in patients receiving d-sotalol and placebo: resuscitated cardiac arrest (4 vs. 4), ventricular fibrillation (7 vs. 3), and sustained ventricular tachycardia (3 vs. 4), respectively, for the two treatment groups.

Discussion of Analysis

The primary observations from these analyses included the following.

1. Most of the d-sotalol-associated mortality risk was greatest in patients very remote from their MI (mean = 4.1 years) who had an LVEF of 31% to 40%, whereas comparable placebo-treated patients had an extremely low mortality risk.
2. There was a relation between d-sotalol-associated mortality risk and gender: women with a recent MI tended to have a higher d-sotalol-associated mortality risk than men.
3. The d-sotalol-associated mortality was not related to the severity of heart failure, baseline measures of heart rate, or indirect measures of ischemia.
4. The increased d-sotalol-associated mortality risk was not accentuated in the first weeks of drug administration; rather, it was evenly distributed throughout the entire trial interval for both women and men.

Is Torsades de Pointes the Culprit?

Based on this detailed analysis, data supporting the hypothesis that d-sotalol-associated mortality in the SWORD trial is due to torsades de pointes are limited. In fact, the data provide no support for any proarrhythmic mechanism. Because torsades de pointes is an electrocardiographic entity, it can only be diagnosed by recording an ECG during the event (33–38). It is possible that many cases of d-sotalol-associated torsades de pointes were missed because they were rare, or common but fleeting, or sustained and nearly uniformly fatal. In this study, all of the information available on factors known to be associated with torsades de pointes were assessed (33–38,42,43). The only major factor supporting torsades de pointes as the d-sotalol-associated proarrhythmic mechanism was that women tended to have a greater risk than men (42). There was no relation of d-sotalol-associated mortality to the QT_c at baseline, QT_c after 2 weeks of drug therapy, d-sotalol dose, serum potassium, or serum creatinine (33–37). There was also no support for torsades de pointes based on the analysis of baseline heart rate. If reverse use dependence was a significant contributor to initiating episodes of torsades de pointes, excessive d-sotalol-associated mortality would be expected to be more prevalent in patients with the lowest heart rates (33,38), but this was not found. The temporal pattern of the d-sotalol-associated mortality in the SWORD trial did not resemble the temporal profile of torsades de pointes–associated mortality reported for quinidine or racemic sotalol, both of which occurred early after drug initiation or dose escalation (37,38,43). Torsades de pointes and other proarrhythmias usually occur more frequently with worsening LV function (37,38,43–45). In contrast, in the SWORD trial, an inverse relation was identified between d-sotalol-associated arrhythmic death and the LVEF, isolated primarily to patients with a LVEF of 31% to 40%. The association of baseline nonsustained ventricular tachycardia to subsequent d-sotalol-associated mortality risk is consistent with an unidentified proarrhythmic mechanism.

The excessive d-sotalol-associated mortality risk was predominantly classified as presumed arrhythmic. Thus, if the death classification was accurate, it would be difficult to conceptualize lethal mechanisms other than proarrhythmia to explain d-sotalol-associated mortality. In the SWORD trial, deaths presumed to be arrhythmic accounted for approximately two-thirds of the placebo mortality. This high estimate of the proportion of presumed arrhythmic death may be accurate or could reflect inadequacies in the current approaches available to classify death, because 60% of deaths classified ''arrhythmic'' in the SWORD trial were unwitnessed, increasing the likelihood of misclassification (16,46–48). There are many competing cardiovascular and noncardiac risks emulating ''sudden death'' in patients remote from the MI (46). Thus, the clustering of d-sotalol-associated mortality in heart failure patients remote from MI with LVEFs of 31% to 40% is intriguing and remains unexplained.

Implications of the SWORD Trial

The SWORD trial has once again demonstrated the critical importance of placebo-controlled randomized trials. In the SWORD trial, patients receiving placebo who were remote from their MI and had an LVEF of 31% to 40% had an excellent prognosis despite having clinical heart failure. It was this population of patients who received d-sotalol that had most of the d-sotalol-associated risk seen in the total trial. Clearly, identifying the patient population at risk to be studied must be done carefully. We do not wish to treat patients with little need for the potential benefits of a medication because that simply exposes them needlessly to the potential risks of the medication. And patient populations at risk not uncommonly are a moving target. In the case of the SWORD patient population, various new treatment measures likely improved patient outcome, particularly in the remote MI group. In this light, the results of the SWORD trial suggest that the predictive accuracy of classical risk factors such as poor LV function, derived from retrospective data collected over a decade ago in the prethrombolytic–pre-afterload reduction era, must be reevaluated (39–41,49–51).

REFERENCES

1. Mukharji J, Rude RE, Poole K, Gustafson N, Thomas LJ, Jr., Strauss HW, Jaffe AS, Muller JE, Roberts R, Raabe DS, Jr, Croft, CH, Passamani E, Braunwalk E,

Willerson JT, and the Milis Study Group. Risk factors for sudden death after acute myocardial infarction: Two-year follow-up. Am J Cardiol 1984; 54:31–36.

2. Moss AJ, Davis HT, DeCamilla J, Bayer LW: Ventricular ectopic beats and their relation to sudden and nonsudden cardiac death after myocardial infarction. Circulation 1979; 60:998–1003.

3. Steinberg J, Regan A, Sciacca R, Bigger JT Jr, Fleiss J. Predicting arrhythmic events after acute MI using the signal-averaged electrocardiogram. Am J Cardiol 1992; 69: 13–21.

4. Odemuyiwa O, Malik M, Farrell TG, Bashir Y, Poloniecki J, Camm AJ. Comparison of the predictive characteristics of heart rate variability index and left ventricular ejection fraction for all-cause mortality, arrhythmic events and sudden death after acute myocardial infarction. Am J Cardiol 1991; 68:434–439.

5. Schwartz PJ, LaRovere MT, Vanoli E. Autonomic nervous system and sudden cardiac death. Circulation 1992; 85 (suppl I):78–91.

6. SOLVD Investigators. Effect of enalapril on survival in patients with reduced left ventricular ejection fractions and congestive heart failure. N Engl J Med 1991; 325: 293–302.

7. Yusuf S, Peto R, Lewis J, Collins R, Sleight P. Beta blockade during and after myocardial infarction: An overview of the randomized trials. Prog Cardiovasc Dis 1985; 27:335–371.

8. The Cardiac Arrhythmia Suppression Trial (CAST) Investigators: Preliminary report: Effect of encainide and flecainide on mortality in a randomized trial of arrhythmia suppression after myocardial infarction. N Engl J Med 1989; 321:406–412.

9. Schwartz PJ, Camm AJ, Frangin G, Janse MJ, Julian DG, Simon P, on behalf of the EMIAT Investigators. Does amiodarone reduce sudden death and cardiac mortality after myocardial infarction. Eur Heart J 1994; 15:620–624.

10. The Cardiac Arrhythmia Suppression Trial II Investigators. Effect of antiarrhythmic agent moricizine on survival after myocardial infarction. N Engl J Med 1992; 327: 227–233.

11. Echt DS, Liebson PR, Mitchell LB, Peters RW, Obias-Manno D, Barker AH, Arenberg D, Baker A, Friedman L, Greene HL, Huther ML, Richardson DW and the CAST Investigators. Mortality and morbidity in patients receiving encainide, flecainide, or placebo. N Engl J Med 1991; 324:781–788.

12. Teo KK, Yusuf S, Furberg CD. Effects of prophylactic antiarrhythmic drug therapy in acute myocardial infarction: An overview of results from randomized control trials. JAMA 1993; 270:1589–1595.

13. Burkart F, Pfisterer M, Kiowski W, Follath, F, Burckhardt D. Effect of antiarrhythmic therapy on mortality in survivors of myocardial infarction with asymptomatic complex ventricular arrhythmias: Basel Antiarrhythmic Study of Infarct Survival (BASIS). J Am Coll Cardiol 1990; 16:1711–1718.

14. Ceremuzynski L, Kleczar E, Krzeminski-Pakula M, Kuch J, Nartowica E, Smielak-Korombel J, Dyduszynski A, Maciejewica J, Zaleska T, Luzarczyk-Kedzia E, Motyka J, Paczkowska B, Sczaniecka O, Yusuf S. Effect of amiodarone on mortality after myocardial infarction: A double-blind, placebo-controlled, pilot study. J Am Coll Cardiol 1992; 20:1056–1062.

15. Doval HC,Nul DR, Grancelli HO, Perrone SV, Bortman GR, Curiel R, for Grupo

de Estudio de la Sobrevida en la Insuficiencia Cardiaca en Argentina (GESICA). Randomised trial of low-dose amiodarone in severe congestive heart failure. Lancet 1994; 344:493–498.

16. Cairns JA, Connolly SJ, Cent M, Roberts R. Post-myocardial infarction mortality in patients with ventricular premature depolarizations: Canadian amiodarone myocardial infarction arrhythmia trial pilot study. Circulation 1991; 84:550–556.

17. Mason JW. Drug therapy. Amiodarone. N Engl J Med 1987; 316:455.

18. Kato R, Ikeda N, Yabek S, Ramaswamy K, Singh B. Electrophysiologic effects of the levo- and dextrorotatory isomers of sotalol in isolated cardiac muscle and their in vivo pharmokinetics. J Am Coll Cardiol 1986; 7:116–125.

19. Patterson E, Lucchesi BR. Antifibrillatory properties of the beta-adrenergic receptor antagonists nadolol, sotalol, atenolol, and propranolol in the anesthetized dogs. Pharmacology 1984; 28:121–129.

20. Vanoli E, Priori SC, Nakasawa H, Hirao K, Napolitano C, Diehl L, Lazzara R, Schwartz PJ. Sympathetic activation, ventricular repolarization, and Ik_r blockade: Implications for the antifibrillatory efficacy of k^+ channel blockers. J Am Coll Cardiol 1995; 25:1609–1614.

21. Yasuda SU, Barbey JT, Funck-Brentano C, Wellstein A, Woosley RL. d-Sotalol reduced heart rate in vivo through a β-adrenergic receptor-independent mechanism. Clin Pharmacol Ther 1993; 53:436–442.

22. Waldo AL, Camm AJ, DeRuyter H, Friedman PL, MacNeil DJ, Pitt B, Pratt CM, Rodda BE, Schwartz PJ. The SWORD trial. Survival with oral d-sotalol in patients with left ventricular dysfunction after myocardial infarction: Rationale, design and methods. Am J Cardiol 1995; 75:1023–1027.

23. Task Force of the Working Group on Arrhythmias of the European Society of Cardiology. The early termination of clinical trials: Causes, consequences and control with special reference to trials in the field of arrhythmias and sudden death. Circulation 1994; 89:2892–2907.

24. Lan KKG, DeMets DL. Discrete sequential boundaries for clinical trials. Biometrika 1983; 70:659–663.

25. DeMets DL. Practical aspects in data monitoring: A brief review. Stat Med 1987; 6:753–760.

26. Pawitan Y, Hallstrom A. Statistical interim monitoring of the Cardiac Arrhythmia Trial. Stat Med 1990; 9:1081–1090.

27. O'Brien PC, Fleming TR. A multiple testing procedure for clinical trials. Biometric 1979; 35:549–556.

28. DeMets DL, Ware JH. Group sequential methods for clinical trials with a one-sided hypothesis. Biometrika 1980; 67:651–660.

29. Kaplan E, Meier P. Nonparametric estimation from incomplete observations. J Am Stat Assoc 1958; 53:457–481.

30. Cox DR. Regression models and life-tables. J R Stat Soc Ser B 1972; 34:1187–1202.

31. Waldo AL, Camm AJ, deRuyter H, Friedman PL, MacNeil DJ, Pauls JF, Pitt B, Pratt CM, Schwartz PJ, Veltri EP. Effect of d-sotalol on mortality in patients with left ventricular dysfunction after recent and remote myocardial infarction. Lancet 1996; 348:7–12.

32. Pratt CM, Camm AJ, Cooper W, Friedman PL, MacNeil DJ, Moulton KM, Pitt B, Schwartz PJ, Veltri EP, Waldo, AL. Mortality in the Survival With ORal D-Sotalol (SWORD) trial: Why did patients die? Am J Cardiol 1998; 81:869–876.

33. Kay GN, Plumb VJ, Arciniegas JG, Henthorn RW, Waldo AL. Torsades de pointes: the long-short initiating sequence and other clinical features. Am J Cardiol 1983; 2:806–817.

34. Jackman WM, Friday KJ, Anderson JL, Aliot EM, Clark M, Lazzara R. The long QT syndromes: a critical review, new clinical observations and a unifying hypothesis. Prog Cardiovasc Dis 1988; 31:115–172.

35. Schwartz PJ, Locati E: QT interval lengthening and cardiac arrhythmias. In: Singh BN, ed. Control of Cardiac Arrhythmias by Lengthening Repolarization. Mount Kisco, NY: Futura Publishing Co., 1988:129–152.

36. Investigators Brochure. d-Sotalol. Bristol-Myers Squibb, November 1, 1993.

37. MacNeil DJ, Davies RO, Deitchman D. Clinical safety profile of sotalol in the treatment of arrhythmias. Am J Cardiol 1993; 72:44A–50A.

38. Priori SG, Diehl L, Schwartz PJ. Torsade de pointes. In: Podrid PJ, Kowey PR, eds. Cardiac Arrhythmia, Mechanisms, Diagnosis and Management. Baltimore, MD: Williams & Wilkins, 1995:951–963.

39. Ruberman W, Weinblatt E, Goldberg JD, Frank CS, Chaudhary BS, Shapiro S. Ventricular premature complexes and sudden death after myocardial infarction. Circulation 1981; 64:297–305.

40. Moss AJ, Davis HT, DeCamilla J, Bayer LW. Ventricular ectopic beats and their relation to sudden and nonsudden cardiac death after myocardial infarction. Circulation 1979; 60:998–1003.

41. Bigger JT, Fleiss JL, Kleiger R, Miller JP, Rolnitzky LM, and the Multicenter Post-Infarction Research Group. The relationships among ventricular arrhythmias, left ventricular dysfunction, and mortality in the 2 years after myocardial infarction. Circulation 1984; 69:250–258.

42. Makkar RR, Fromm BS, Steinman RT, Meissner MD, Lehmann MH. Female gender as a risk factor for torsades de pointes associated with cardiovascular drugs. JAMA 1993; 270:2590–2597.

43. Bauman JL, Bauernfeind RA, Hoff JV, Strasberg B, Rosen KM. Torsades de pointes due to quinidine observations in 31 patients. Am Heart J 1984; 107:425–430.

44. Pratt CM, Eaton T, Francis M, Woolbert S, Mahmarian J, Roberts R, Young JB. The inverse relationship between baseline left ventricular ejection fraction and outcome of antiarrhythmic therapy: a dangerous imbalance in the risk-benefit ratio. Am Heart J 1989; 118:433–440.

45. Hallstrom A, Pratt CM, Greene HL, Huther M, Gottlieb S, DeMaria A, Young JB. The interrelationships between heart failure, ejection fraction, arrhythmia suppression and mortality: analysis of the Cardiac Arrhythmia Suppression Trial (The CAST). J Am Coll Cardiol 1995; 25:1250–1257.

46. Pratt CM, Greenway PS, Schoenfeld MH, Hibben ML, Reiffel JA. An exploration of the precision of classifying sudden cardiac death: Implications for the interpretation of clinical trials. Circulation 1996; 93:519–524.

47. Bigger JT. Why patients with congestive heart failure die: Arrhythmias and sudden cardiac death. Circulation 1987; 75:IV28–IV35.

48. Zeische S, Rector TS, Cohn JN. Interobserver discordance in the classification of mechanisms of death in studies of heart failure. J Cardiac Failure 1995; 1:127–132.
49. The Cardiac Arrhythmia Pilot Study (CAPS) Investigators. Effects of encainide, flecainide, imipramine and moricizine on ventricular arrhythmias during the year after myocardial infarction: The CAPS. Am J Cardiol 1988; 61:501–509.
50. Hinkle LE Jr, Thaler HT. Clinical classification of cardiac deaths. Circulation 1982; 65:457–464.
51. Marcus FL, Cobb LA, Edwards JE, Kuller L, Moss AJ, Bigger T, Fleiss JL, Rolnitzky L, Serokman R, and the Multicenter Post Infarction Research Group. Mechanism of death and prevalence of myocardial ischemic symptoms in the terminal event after myocardial infarction. Am J Cardiol 1988;61:8–15.

RAYMOND L. WOOSLEY
Georgetown University Medical Center, Washington, D.C.

STEVEN N. SINGH
Georgetown University and Veterans Affairs Medical Centers,
Washington, D.C.

Patients with ischemic heart disease and/or depressed left ventricular function and documented premature ventricular beats are at increased risk of dying prematurely (1). Empiric attempts have been made to suppress these warning arrhythmias hoping to improve survival. However, the results of the Cardiac Arrhythmia Suppression Trial (CAST I) stunned the world in that an unexpected excessive mortality was noted despite arrhythmia suppression (2). Thus, since CAST, it has been generally accepted that sodium channel blockers such as encainide and flecainide, which slow conduction velocity, may lead to arrhythmia aggravation and death in patients with ischemic heart disease. After CAST, there was a new impetus to seek other ways to suppress ventricular arrhythmia's and potassium channel blockers emerged as new antiarrhythmic candidates.

d-Sotalol is a potent blocker of the rapid component of the delayed rectifier potassium current. It prolongs the action potential duration and proportionally increases the refractory period. Even though there was awareness of a propensity of sotalol to cause torsade de pointes, the SWORD (Survival With ORal d-Sotalol) trial was initiated. Thus, the hypothesis that an antiarrhythmic drug can improve survival in patients with prior myocardial infarction was once more to be tested.

Patients with left ventricular ejection fraction (LVEF) less than 40% with a recent MI (6 to 42 days) or remote (>42 days) MI with congestive heart failure (CHF) (class II or III) were prospectively randomized in a double-blind fashion to receive sotalol or placebo. The primary endpoint was all-cause mortality. After 3121 patients were recruited, the trial was prematurely terminated because of

151

excessive deaths in the group assigned to d-sotalol. There was a highly significant difference in mortality with a p value $= 0.006$ (3). This excessive mortality was due to deaths classified as sudden.

The annualized mortality rate in the placebo arm of SWORD was 7.8%, which was identical to that assumed for calculation of the sample size for the study. Therefore, it is obvious that sotalol was truly harmful, resulting in a death rate far greater than the natural occurrence. Since the excessive mortality was classified as sudden arrhythmic death, the proarrhythmic side effect of sotalol was underestimated. While the relative risk of death from sotalol was eight times greater in the group with LVEF between 31 to 40% and remote MI, it was negligible in the group with depressed LVEF <30% (4). Perhaps these divergent effects could be explained by competing risks. The group with the lower LV was at greater risk of ventricular fibrillation for which the drug may have been protective and countering the harmful effects. On the other hand, in patients with little or no risk of dying, only the harmful effects could be observed. This was also seen in the CAST trial in which the relative risk of sudden cardiac death from encainide and flecainide in the group with LVEF >30% was almost twice that with LVEF <30%. Of interest, dofetilide, an IKr blocker somewhat similar to d-sotalol showed no harmful effects in patients with CHF and with LVEF <30% (5). It seems that these drugs have no net beneficial or harmful effects in the population with lower ventricular function.

Since the excessive deaths in SWORD were classified as sudden, there is an assumption that proarrhythmic events were responsible. By prolonging the action potential duration, d-sotalol can lead to early after-depolarizations (EAD) and eventually torsades de pointes. However, only two such cases were documented in SWORD. Moreover, torsade is a bradycardia-dependent arrhythmia. But this phenomenon may not have contributed since the patients with the lowest heart rates did not have a higher mortality. Patients with nonsustained ventricular tachycardia, however, did seem to have had an excessive d-sotalol-associated mortality. It is of interest that the relative risk of d-sotalol was higher in women. This suggests that torsades de pointes could have been responsible for the excessive sudden death because of the female preponderance to this form of toxicity. It is possible that the toxicity of d-sotalol would have been greater if the entry criteria had not resulted in the screening out of those with a long QT, electrolyte disorders, etc.

In summary, the SWORD trial failed to show an improvement in survival with the use of d-sotalol in patients with previous myocardial infarction and left ventricular dysfunction. It was clearly harmful, especially in those patients with remote MI and LVEF between 31 to 40%. While the excessive mortality was classified as sudden death, documented torsades de pointes was rare. In the wake of the disappointing results of CAST and SWORD, the future role of prescribing antiarrhythmic agents to improve survival is questioned.

REFERENCES

1. Bigger JT, Fleiss JL, Kleiger R, Miller JP, Rolnitzky LM, and the Multicenter Post Infarction Research Group. The relationships among ventricular arrhythmias, left ventricular dysfunction and mortality in the 2 years after myocardial infarction. Circulation 1984; 69:250–258.
2. The Cardiac Arrhythmias Suppression Trial (CAST) Investigators. Preliminary report: effect of encainide and flecainide on mortality in a randomized trial of arrhythmia suppression after myocardial infarction. N Eng J Med 1989; 321:406–412.
3. Waldo AL, Camm JA, de Ruyter H, Friedman PL, MacNeil DJ, Pauls JF, Pott B, Pratt CM, Schwartz PI, Veltri EP for the SWORD Investigators. Effect of d-sotalol on mortality in patients with left ventricular dysfunction after recent and remote myocardial infarction. Lancet 1996; 348:7–12.
4. Pratt CM, Camm JA, Cooper W, Friedman PL, Macneil DJ, Moulton KM, Pott B, Schwartz PJ, Veltri AP, Waldo AL. Mortality in the survival with oral d-Sotalol (SWORD) trial: Why did patients die? Am J Cardiol 1988; 81:869–876.
5. Torp-Pedersen C, and the Danish Investigations of Arrhythmia and Mortality on Dofetelide (DIAMOND) Study Group. Dofetilide: A new class III antiarrhythmic drug which is safe in patients with congestive heart failure. J Am Coll Cardiol 1998; 160 (abstr.).

8

The Multicenter Automatic Defibrillator Implantation Trial (MADIT)

Arthur J. Moss

University of Rochester Medical Center, Rochester, New York

INTRODUCTION AND BACKGROUND

The Multicenter Automatic Defibrillator Implantation Trial (MADIT) (1) had its origin back in the 1980s, with the publications that related to the risks posed by left ventricular dysfunction and ventricular ectopic beats (VEBs) in the setting of subacute coronary heart disease. In 1983, the Multicenter Postinfarction Research Group (MPRG) published their findings on the cardiovascular risk factors associated with long-term mortality in patients who had survived an acute myocardial infarction (2). A striking finding was the exponential increase in 1-year mortality as the ejection fraction declined below 0.35 (Fig. 1). This inverse relationship between ejection fraction and mortality has been substantiated in many subsequent studies by other investigators, before and after the introduction of thrombolytic therapy, revascularization procedures, and pharmacological treatment with beta-adrenergic blocking agents and angiotensin converting enzyme inhibitors. A reduced ejection fraction indicates significant and extensive myocardial disease, with an increased propensity for heart failure and scar-related reentrant ventricular tachyarrhythmias.

The MPRG group also reported on the relationship between ventricular arrhythmias recorded on a 24-h Holter and mortality in the 2 years after myocardial infarction (3). Bigger et al. showed a stepwise increase in mortality as one progressed from single, to paired, to three or more VEBs in a row [nonsustained ventricular tachycardia (NSVT)], with a 2-year mortality of almost 30% in patients with NSVT (3). The risk from NSVT was further accentuated in the presence of left ventricular dysfunction with ejection fraction ≤ 0.35.

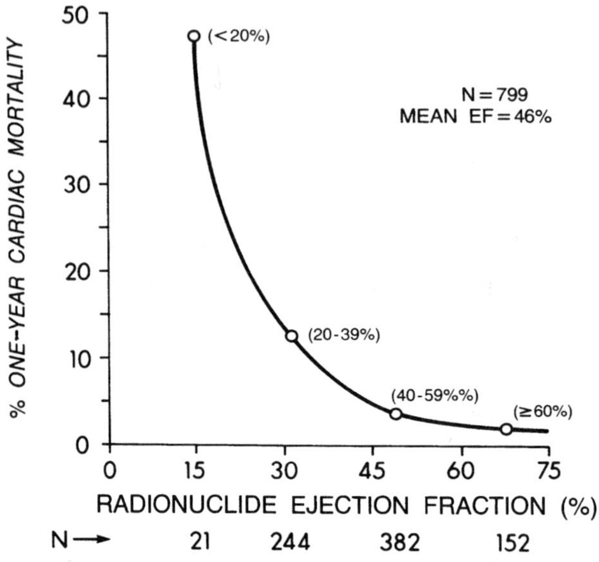

Figure 1   One-year cardiac mortality rate as a function of the radionuclide ejection fraction determined before hospital discharge after an acute myocardial infarction. (Reprinted with permission from Ref. 2.)

Other relevant background for MADIT included the findings from the Cardiac Arrhythmia Suppression Trial (CAST) (4) and the publication by Wilber et al. in 1990 (5). Wilber described the risk implications of induced and nonsuppressed ventricular tachyarrhythmias at electrophysiological testing in patients with NSVT, coronary heart disease, and ejection fraction <0.40. The 1- and 2-year actuarial incidence of aborted cardiac arrest or sudden death was 34% and 50%, respectively, in patients with inducible and sustained (not suppressed by antiarrhythmic challenge) ventricular tachyarrhythmias in this high-risk population.

Antiarrhythmic drug therapy had been widely used in the treatment of frequent and repetitive VEBs, but several trials failed to substantiate improved survival with this treatment (4,6,7). In December 1990, the MADIT investigators initiated a prophylactic trial in which high-risk patients with coronary heart disease and asymptomatic NSVT were randomly assigned to receive an implanted cardioverter-defibrillator (ICD) or conventional medical management. To ensure a population at high risk for malignant ventricular arrhythmias, eligible patients had to have an ejection fraction ≤0.35, NSVT unrelated to an acute coronary event, and an inducible, sustained, nonsuppressible ventricular tachyarrhythmia on electrophysiological testing. The endpoint of the trial was overall mortality during long-term follow-up.

The primary hypothesis of MADIT was that prophylactic ICD therapy in high-risk coronary patients with ejection fraction ≤0.35, NSVT, and inducible, nonsuppressible ventricular tachyarrhythmia would be associated with improved survival when compared to patients managed with conventional treatment not involving ICD therapy.

TARGET PATIENT POPULATION

The eligibility and exclusion criteria for MADIT are presented in Table 1. Eligibility included patients of either sex, aged 25 to 80 years, with a documented Q-wave or enzyme-positive myocardial infarction 3 weeks or more before entry, an episode of asymptomatic NSVT unrelated to an acute myocardial infarction, an ejection fraction ≤0.35, NYHA class I to III, and no indication for coronary revascularization. Patients were excluded from enrollment if they had a previous cardiac arrest, documented sustained ventricular tachycardia, coronary artery by-

Table 1 MADIT Eligibility and Exclusion Criteria

Eligibility Criteria
1. Male or female, aged 25 to 80
2. One or more prior myocardial infarctions
3. Documented episode of nonsustained ventricular tachycardia (run of 3 to 30 VEBs at a rate >120 bpm) within the 3 months prior to enrollment
4. Ejection fraction ≤0.35
5. NYHA Class I to III
6. Inducible, nonsuppressible ventricular tachycardia at electrophysiological study

Exclusion Criteria
1. Aborted cardiac arrest at any time in the past
2. History of sustained ventricular tachycardia unrelated to an acute myocardial infarction
3. Enzyme-positive myocardial infarction in the past 3 weeks
4. Coronary artery bypass graft surgery within the past 8 weeks or coronary angioplasty within the past 12 weeks
5. Indication for coronary revascularization in the foreseeable future
6. Major comorbidity with a reduced likelihood of survival for the duration of the trial
7. Cardiogenic shock, symptomatic hypotension, or NYHA class IV
8. Participation in other clinical trials
9. Patients unwilling to sign a consent form for participation in MADIT

pass graft surgery within the past 2 months, coronary angioplasty within the past 3 months, NYHA class IV, or major noncardiac comorbidity. Patients were referred to MADIT investigators at the discretion of their primary attending physician. Eligible, nonexcluded patients underwent electrophysiological testing according to a prespecified protocol (8) and qualified for enrollment if sustained monomorphic ventricular tachycardia (with two or three extra stimuli) or polymorphic ventricular tachycardia/ventricular fibrillation (with two extra stimuli) were reproducibly induced and not suppressed after intravenous procainamide.

PROTOCOL

Qualifying patients gave informed consent and were randomly assigned to ICD or no ICD therapy. The choice of conventional medical therapy was left to each patient's attending physician. Only medications approved and released by the FDA could be administered to patients in either group. The flow diagram for the protocol is presented in Figure 2.

The trial was designed to have an 85% power to detect a 46% reduction in mortality rate in the ICD patients when compared with a 2-year mortality of 30% among patients randomly assigned not to receive the ICD, with a two-sided significance level of 0.05. A triangular sequential design (9) modified for two-sided alternatives was used with preset boundaries to permit termination of the trial for efficacy, no difference, or inefficacy. The trial was designed to be terminated when the path of the log-rank statistic, measuring imbalance between the survival curves for the two randomized groups, crossed one of the preset termination boundaries of the sequential design. All endpoint analyses were carried out using the intention-to-treat principle. Details of the design and the statistical analyses are presented in the original publication (1).

ENROLLED PATIENT POPULATION

The clinical characteristics of the 196 patients enrolled in MADIT by treatment group are presented in Table 2. The baseline characteristics of the two treatment groups were clinically similar. The MADIT-defined patient was predominantly male, average age 63 years, with an ejection fraction of 0.26. More than half the patients had been treated previously for heart failure and almost half the patients had prior coronary artery bypass graft surgery. Of special note, the average number of repetitive beats in the qualifying run of NSVT was 9 to 10 beats. At electrophysiological study, monomorphic ventricular tachycardia was induced by double or triple extra stimuli in about 90% of the patients, with the remaining 10% induced into either polymorphous ventricular tachycardia or ventricular fi-

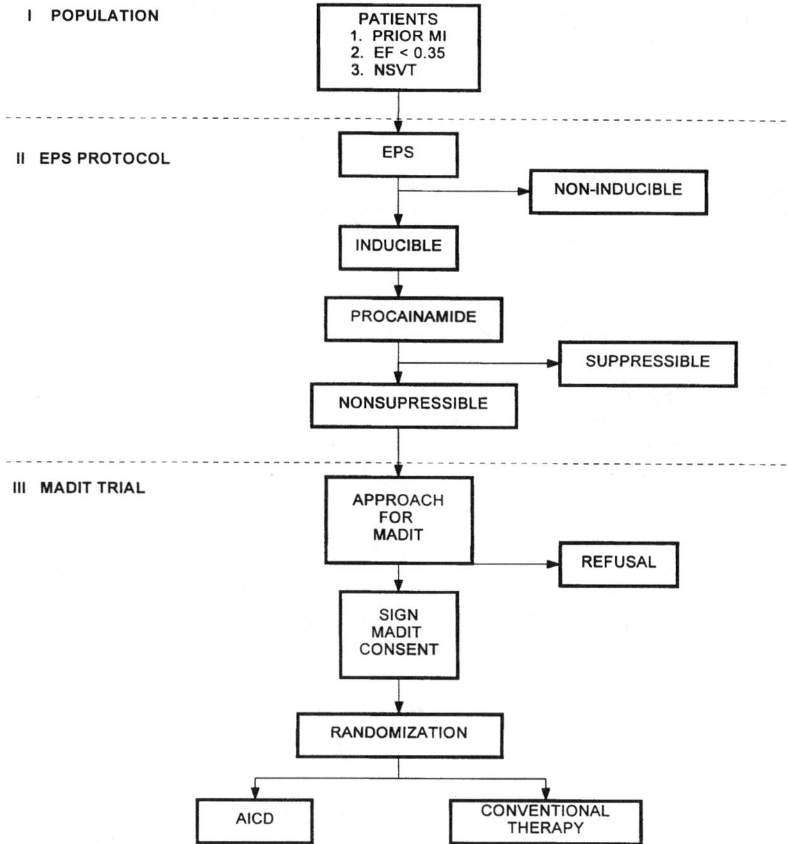

Figure 2   Flow diagram for enrollment of patients into the MADIT protocol.

brillation by double extra stimuli. At the time of enrollment, more than one-half of the patients were receiving angiotensin converting enzyme inhibitors and diuretics, and more than one-third were receiving a digitalis preparation.

RESULTS

During an average follow-up of 27 months per patient, there were 15 deaths in the defibrillator group and 39 deaths in the conventional therapy group. The hazard ratio (ICD:No-ICD) by Cox analyses (10) for overall mortality was 0.46 (95% CI = 0.26–0.82; p = 0.009). The Kaplan–Meier survival analysis by assigned

Table 2 Baseline Characteristics of 196 Patients Randomized to Conventional or Defibrillator Therapy

	Treatment group[a]	
Characteristic	Conventional (*n* = 101)	Defibrillator (*n* = 95)
Mean age (yr)	64 ± 9	62 ± 9
Sex (M/F)	92/8	92/8
Cardiac history		
Two or more prior myocardial infarctions	29	34
Treatment for ventricular arrhythmias	35	42
NYHA class II to III	67	63
Treatment for congestive heart failure	51	52
Treatment for hypertension	35	48
Insulin-dependent diabetes	5	7
Coronary bypass surgery	44	46
Implanted pacemaker	7	2
Cardiac findings at enrollment		
Blood urea nitrogen > 25 mg/dL	21	22
Left bundle branch block	8	7
Mean ejection fraction	0.25 ± 0.07	0.27 ± 0.07
Qualifying nonsustained ventricular tachycardia		
Number of consecutive beats	9 ± 10	10 ± 9

[a] Figures are percentages unless otherwise indicated; plus–minus values are mean ± SD.

treatment is presented in Figure 3. The two mortality curves separate early and remain well separated throughout the 5-year trial, with a significantly lower mortality rate for patients randomized to ICD versus no ICD therapy. Of note, there were no operative deaths due to implantation of the ICD. The cumulative time to the first shock in the ICD group was analyzed, and 40% of the ICD patients had a shock discharge within 1 year after device implantation, 60% within 2 years, and 90% within 5 years.

During clinical follow-up after randomization, the use of prescribed antiarrhythmic medication differed between the two treatment groups (Table 3). At the 1-month postenrollment contact, amiodarone therapy predominated in the nondevice group (74% vs. 2%), and beta-blockers were used more frequently in the ICD group (26% vs. 8%). Class I antiarrhythmic agents were utilized in 11% of the study population, mostly for management of atrial tachyarrhythmias, and the use of these agents was equally divided between the two treatment groups.

Cox regression analyses were used to estimate the hazard ratio after adjustment for relevant covariates and to evaluate interaction effects. The power of

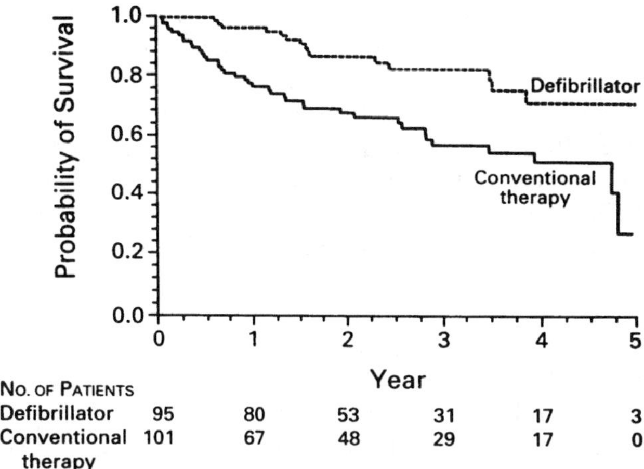

Figure 3 Kaplan–Meier analysis of the probability of survival according to assigned treatment. The difference in the mortality rates between the two treatment groups was significant at $p = 0.009$. (Reprinted with permission from Ref. 1.)

these adjustment and interaction analyses is limited because the sequential design concentrates the power of the study on the primary goal (i.e., the effect of randomized therapy on mortality). There is little that can be derived from the adjustment analyses about the influence of amiodarone on the observed ICD:No-ICD hazard ratio since amiodarone was a surrogate for conventional therapy, with 74% receiving this medication at 1 month in the conventional group and 2% in the ICD

Table 3 Antiarrhythmic Medications at 1 Month After Enrollment According to Treatment Assignment

	Conventional[a] (n = 93)	Defibrillator[a] (n = 93)
	(%)	
Antiarrhythmic medications		
Amiodarone	74	2
Beta-blockers	8	26
Class I antiarrhythmic agents	10	12
Sotalol	7	1

[a] At 1 month after enrollment, eight patients in the conventional therapy group and two patients in the defibrillator group had missing data.

group. However, appropriate adjustment and interaction analyses were performed for beta-blocker use. The beneficial ICD:No-ICD hazard ratio remained significant ($p = 0.02$) after adjustment for beta-blocker use, and there was no significant interaction between beta-blocker use and randomized ICD or no-ICD therapy (11). That is, the beneficial effect of ICD therapy was similar in those receiving and not receiving beta-blocker medication. Additional Cox analyses showed no evidence of differential effects of ICD therapy between patients implanted with transthoracic or transvenous leads, or in any of several relevant subgroups.

CONCLUSIONS

MADIT is the first randomized device trial to evaluate the safety and efficacy of prophylactic ICD therapy in high-risk patients with coronary heart disease. The implanted cardioverter-defibrillator was associated with a 54% reduction in all-cause mortality in this patient population when compared to conventional, non-ICD therapy. We conclude that the ICD saves lives in high-risk coronary patients with left ventricular dysfunction, asymptomatic NSVT, and inducible-sustained ventricular tachycardia at electrophysiological study. The ICD is recommended as prophylactic therapy in MADIT-defined patients. Similar beneficial results with ICD therapy have been reported recently by the investigators from the Antiarrhythmics Versus Implantable Defibrillators (AVID) trial (12). These studies confirm the role of ICDs as the therapy of first choice for specific subsets of patients at high risk for sudden arrhythmic death as identified by criteria utilized in the MADIT and AVID trials.

REFERENCES

1. Moss AJ, Hall WJ, Cannom DS, Daubert JP, Higgins SL, Klein H, Levine JH, Saksena S, Waldo AL, Wilber D, Brown MW, and Heo M for the MADIT Investigators. Improved survival with an implanted defibrillator in patients with coronary disease at high risk for ventricular arrhythmia. N Engl J Med 1996;335:1933–1940.
2. The Multicenter Postinfarction Research Group. Risk stratification and survival after myocardial infarction. N Engl J Med 1983;309:331–336.
3. Bigger JT Jr, Fleiss JL, Kleiger R, Miller JP, Rolnitzky LM, and the Multicenter Post-Infarction Research Group. The relationship among ventricular arrhythmias, left ventricular dysfunction and mortality in the 2 years after myocardial infarction. Circulation 1984;69:250–258.
4. Echt DS, Liebson PR, Mitchell LB, et al., and the CAST Investigators. Mortality and morbidity in patients randomized to receive encainide, flecainide, or placebo in the Cardiac Arrhythmia Suppression Trial. N Engl J Med 1991;324:781–788.
5. Wilber DJ, Olshanksy B, Moran JF, Scanlon PJ. Electrophysiologic testing and non-

sustained ventricular tachycardia: use and limitation in patients with coronary artery disease and impaired ventricular function. Circulation 1990;82:350–358.

6. Singh SN, Fletcher RD, Fisher SG, Singh BN, Lewis HD, Deedwania PC, Massie BM, Colling C, Lazzeri D, for the Survival Trial of Antiarrhythmic Therapy in Congestive Heart Failure. Amiodarone in patients with congestive heart failure and asymptomatic ventricular arrhythmia. N Engl J Med 1995;333:77–82.

7. Julian DG, Camm AJ, Frangin G, et al. Randomized trial of effect of amiodarone on mortality in patients with left-ventricular dysfunction after recent myocardial infarction: EMIAT. Lancet 1997;349:667–674.

8. MADIT Executive Committee. Multicenter automatic defibrillator implantation trial (MADIT): Design and Clinical Protocol. PACE 1991(II):14:920–927.

9. Whitehead J. The Design and Analysis of Sequential Clinical Trials, 2nd ed. Chichester, England: Ellis Horwood Ltd, 1992.

10. Cox DR. Regression models and life-tables. J R Stat Soc B 1972;34:187–220.

11. Moss AJ. Background, outcome, and clinical implications of the multicenter automatic defibrillator implantation trial (MADIT). Am J Cardiol 1997;80(5B):28F–32F.

12. The Antiarrhythmics Versus Implantable Defibrillators (AVID) Investigators. A comparison of antiarrhythmic-drug therapy with implantable defibrillators in patients resuscitated from near-fatal ventricular arrhythmias. N Engl J Med 1997;337:1576–1583.

Eric N. Prystowsky
Northside Cardiology, P.C., and St. Vincent Hospital, Indianapolis, Indiana

RISK STRATIFICATION: WHY BOTHER?

It has been known for decades that the presence of ventricular ectopy after a myocardial infarction (MI), especially in patients with diminished left ventricular function, is associated with increased mortality (1–4). Even in the current era of revascularization during acute MI, whether with drugs or mechanically, the combination of ventricular arrhythmias and left ventricular dysfunction augurs a relatively poor outcome (5). Multiple antiarrhythmic drug trials after MI (reviewed elsewhere in this book) have shown either neutral or detrimental effects on survival, except for beta-blockers. In lieu of any further investigations on methods to diminish sudden death after MI, one could simply take the position that it is reasonable to treat only patients who have an episode of sustained ventricular tachycardia (VT) or survived a cardiac arrest. Unfortunately, there is a great disparity in survival rates for out-of-hospital cardiac arrest in the United States, and some of the largest cities report resuscitation of less than 5% of cardiac arrest victims (6,7). Thus, such an approach would have minimal impact on survival of high-risk patients after MI.

In patients with sustained monomorphic VT and coronary artery disease, electrophysiological testing initiates sustained VT in greater than 90% of patients (8). Because of this high sensitivity, electrophysiological testing has been used for risk-stratification in individuals after MI with nonsustained VT. Two multicenter randomized control trials—the Multicenter Unsustained Tachycardia Trial (MUSTT) and the Multicenter Automatic Defibrillator Implantation Trial (MADIT)—have employed electrophysiological testing for risk stratification

(9,10). The concept is that induction of sustained VT at electrophysiological study can identify a high-risk subgroup of patients for subsequent arrhythmic mortality, and appropriate therapy can improve survival. MADIT results have been published, and a critique of these results follows.

TRIAL DESIGN AND PATIENT SELECTION

MADIT enrolled patients from 32 centers, 30 in the United States and 2 in Europe. Eligible patients were those who had a MI at least 3 weeks before entry; left ventricular ejection fraction 0.35% or less; and nonsustained VT of 3 to 30 beats with a rate >120/min. The target group of patients is well documented to have increased risk of mortality after MI. Major exclusions included coronary artery bypass graft surgery within 2 months, percutaneous transluminal coronary angioplasty within 3 months, and New York Heart Association class IV rank for congestive heart failure. Exclusion of class IV congestive heart failure patients seems appropriate. Unfortunately, restrictions on trial entry of patients after surgery or angioplasty precludes generalization of the results of MADIT to these patient groups who commonly meet entry criteria.

Patients underwent a standard electrophysiological testing protocol for induction of sustained VT or ventricular fibrillation. If either arrhythmia was initiated and not suppressed with intravenous procainamide (or an equivalent drug if procainamide was contraindicated), the patient was eligible for randomization. Patients received either an implantable cardioverter defibrillator (ICD) or ''conventional'' medical therapy, the choice of which was left to the patient's attending physician. No control group was included. There are several potential problems with the electrophysiological study results and subsequent randomization of patients. Failure to suppress inducible sustained VT with antiarrhythmic drugs may preselect patients who are at higher risk for subsequent arrhythmic events. Further, data from earlier investigations of electrophysiological–electropharmacological testing showed that failure to suppress sustained VT with intravenous procainamide predicted subsequent failure to other antiarrhythmic drugs (8). Thus, it is conceivable that the overall randomized patient population was at higher than anticipated risk for subsequent mortality, and that antiarrhythmic drugs would be minimally useful in such patients. The lack of a control group is unfortunate. As one of the designers and active participants in MUSTT, I fully understand the angst of withholding specific antiarrhythmic therapy for patients who have sustained VT induced at electrophysiological study. Many electrophysiologists would consider such patients at high risk for subsequent sudden death. Yet, 50% of such patients enrolled in MUSTT, approximately 350 patients, have been followed long-term without any specific antiarrhythmic treatment. The value of such a control group was evident when the data from MUSTT was recently presented.

MADIT enrolled 196 of 253 (76%) qualified patients. This relatively small number of patients was enrolled over approximately 5 years at 32 institutions, but 2 (6%) of the centers enrolled 63 (32%) patients. The small enrollment from most centers over several years demonstrates the common problems of entry bias including referring physician, investigator, and patient. If participating institutions were selected based on known patient volume and investigator enthusiasm, then one has to assume that either the referring physician or the investigator elected on many occasions not to enroll patients in MADIT. There are no data given regarding the number of patients who met entry criteria but were not enrolled because of either patient refusal, lack of sustained VT initiated at electrophysiological study, or VT that was suppressed with drug therapy. This lack of data precludes any comparison of patients enrolled in MADIT versus those who met criteria but were not included in the study. These deficiencies do not negate the results of MADIT, but make it more difficult for clinicians to generalize the results of this study to their own patient populations.

A flaw in the randomization design of this study was the variable therapy given to patients in the conventional group. The choice of the term "conventional" was unfortunate, since most physicians do not routinely prescribe antiarrhythmic drug therapy for patients with asymptomatic, nonsustained VT after MI. The multiple, nonstandardized therapies chosen in the conventional group make it impossible to analyze the mortality differences for any specific treatment. There is even a minor concern regarding use of class I antiarrhythmic drugs in a small percentage of patients, since these agents may have worsened survival through a proarrhythmic mechanism. I do not think this is a major issue in MADIT.

TRIAL RESULTS

The primary endpoint was overall mortality. MADIT showed a very impressive survival benefit of the ICD versus conventional medical therapy. Analysis of the Kaplan-Meier survival curves reveals an early and substantial separation of the survival curves that remains significant throughout the trial duration. Allowing literary license to use the Latin term *res ipsa loqitur* (the thing speaks for itself) in a much more positive sense, one can simply accept the results of MADIT on face value as a trial that demonstrates superiority of the ICD for survival in high-risk patients. If only life were so simple. Unfortunately, several factors need to be addressed.

The clinical characteristics between patient groups appear balanced. However, there is an apparent significant imbalance in the use of beta-blockers, with

8% use in the conventional medical group compared with 26% in patients receiving an ICD. Sotalol has substantial beta-blocking effects and the use of sotalol or a beta-blocker occurred in 15% of patients in the conventional group, making the disparity less; this also assumes minimal proarrhythmic events due to sotalol, which is reasonable. Amiodarone was prescribed for 74% of patients in the conventional therapy group, but only 45% of patients were receiving such treatment at the last patient contact. In essence, an ICD was superior to a potpourri of therapies. Although 60% of patients with an ICD received a shock within 2 years of enrollment, most devices did not have stored intervals or electrograms. Therefore, it is impossible to know how many patients actually received an appropriate shock for sustained VT. Even assuming that the vast majority did receive an appropriate shock, this is not a surrogate for mortality as an endpoint. It was fortunate that mortality was used as the endpoint, and therefore these data are not necessary regarding the main outcome of the study.

CONCLUSION

MADIT, as is true for all randomized prospective control trials, has blemishes and questions regarding generalization to other patient populations. The patients appear highly selected, a fact supported by the mean of 9 to 10 beats of nonsustained VT in MADIT compared with the typical 4 to 5 beats of nonsustained VT noted in most of post-MI trials. Regardless of all the potential problems of MADIT, the ICD clearly provided a survival benefit for these individuals. The results of MUSTT support the data from MADIT, confirming the demonstrated superiority of ICDs on survival in high-risk patients after MI, a result not witnessed in any of the antiarrhythmic drug trials, including amiodarone. How should the clinician interpret the results of MADIT? When in doubt, I invoke the family-based approach to patient care—I will treat my patients in the same manner I would treat my mother, father, siblings, or myself. I choose an ICD.

REFERENCES

1. Chiang BN, Perlman LV, Ostrander LD, Epstein FH. Relationship of premature systoles to coronary heart disease and sudden death in the Tecumseh epidemiologic study. Ann Intern Med 1969;70:1159.
2. Ruberman W, Weinblatt E, Goldberg JD, Frank CW, Shapiro S. Ventricular premature beats and mortality after myocardial infarction. N Engl J Med 1977;297:750.
3. Moss AJ, David HT, DeCamilla J, Bayer LW. Ventricular ectopic beats and their relation to sudden and nonsudden cardiac death after myocardial infarction. Circulation 1979;60:988.

4. Cannom DS, Prystowsky EN. Modern management of ventricular arrhythmias—detection, drugs and devices. JAMA 1999;281:172–179.

5. Maggioni AP, Zuanetti G, Franzosi MG, Rovelli F, Santoro E, Staszewsky L, Tavazzi L, Tognoni G. Prevalence and prognostic significance of ventricular arrhythmias after acute myocardial infarction in the fibrinolytic era. GISSI-2 results. Circulation 1993;87(2):312–322.

6. Lombardi G, Gallagher J, Gennis P. Outcome of out-of-hospital cardiac arrest in New York City. JAMA 1994;271:678–683.

7. Eisenberg MS, Horwood BT, Cummins RO, Reynolds-Haertle R, Hearne TR. Cardiac arrest and resuscitation: A tale of 29 cities. Ann Emerg Med 1990;19:179–186.

8. Prystowsky EN. Electrophysiologic study versus electrocardiographic monitoring (ESVEM): A critical appraisal. Controlled Clin Trials 1996;17:28S–36S.

9. Buxton AE, Fisher JD, Josephson ME, Lee KL, Pryor DB, Prystowsky EN, Simson MB, DiCarlo L, Echt DS, Packer D, Greer GS, Talajic M and the MUSTT Investigators. Prevention of sudden death in patients with coronary artery disease: The Multicenter Unsustained Tachycardia Trial (MUSTT) Progress in Cardiovascular Diseases 1993;36(3):215–226.

10. Moss AJ, Hall WJ, Cannom DS, Daubert JP, Higgins SL, Klein H, Levine JH, Saksena S, Waldo AL, Wilber D, Brown MW, Heo M, for the Multicenter Automatic Defibrillator Implantation Trial Investigators. Improved survival with an implanted defibrillator in patients with coronary disease at high risk for ventricular arrhythmias. N Engl J Med 1996;335–1933–1940.

9

The Antiarrhythmics Versus Implantable Defibrillator (AVID) Trial

Douglas P. Zipes

*Krannert Institute of Cardiology, Indiana University School of Medicine,
Indianapolis, Indiana*

INTRODUCTION

While numerous studies (1) have shown that the implantable cardioverter defibrillator (ICD) accurately detects and successfully terminates ventricular tachyarrhythmias, and that the ICD therefore "must" save lives, the effect of the ICD on total mortality, particularly when compared against antiarrhythmic agents, was never established in a rigorous fashion by a prospective randomized clinical trial until the Antiarrhythmics Versus Implantable Defibrillator (AVID) study was published (2). Initial studies of the ICD used surrogate endpoints for death such as "appropriate" shocks from a device, or historical or concurrent controls (3). Also, some studies chose arrhythmic mortality as an endpoint rather than total mortality. The latter must be used because accurately determining the cause of death can be very difficult, even with stored electrogram recordings, and therefore total mortality is a more reliable measure of the effectiveness of an intervention such as an ICD (4). Further, to establish the value of the therapy, unless its application so obviously and dramatically alters the natural history of the disease (e.g., penicillin for pneumococcal pneumonia), it must be compared against another therapy in a prospective, randomized fashion. Thus, while ICD efficacy was indisputable (1), it was not known whether the ICD reduced overall or total mortality compared with the best medical therapy until the AVID trial.

Yet, despite this knowledge gap, the ethics of performing a randomized trial of the ICD was challenged, much as the ethics of executing the CAST were

171

questioned (5). The propriety of such a study was a critically important issue and one that the organizers of the National Heart, Lung and Blood Institute (NHLBI) and the participating investigators wrestled with at length during the planning stages of AVID. The general conclusion was that it was unethical not to perform such a study. Until the ICD was randomized against the best medical management, conclusions about which therapy was best in general or for specific patient groups, such as those with preserved left ventricular function versus those without, could not be made. Therefore, randomization was made between two treatments known to be effective in order to find out which one was better, and not to show that treatment was better than no treatment at all.

Contributing to the importance of AVID, and setting it apart from any of the other ICD trials, was the fact that patients who presented with ventricular tachyarrhythmias but were not randomized for a variety of reasons were entered into a registry to judge the adequacy of the population sampling from which the randomized patients were drawn. These patients have been followed up through the National Death Index to allow mortality assessments so that AVID results can be put into proper perspective.

Another important aspect was that, while the choice of ICD was left to the individual investigator, the particular ICD used was always a state-of-the-art device with tiered therapy and bradycardia and antitachycardia pacing options. AVID did not attempt to compare one ICD versus another.

Patients randomized to the drug limb were considered for a subrandomization to receive amiodarone or sotalol, the former empirically and the latter guided by ambulatory recordings or electrophysiological study. Patients who could not receive sotalol because of reduced left ventricular function or because of an adverse response received empiric amiodarone. Only if both drugs were ineffective or not tolerated were class I drugs to be used. While AVID sought to answer the fundamental question of whether drugs were better than devices in high-risk populations, in reality, many patients receive an ICD plus an antiarrhythmic drug. In fact, one could envision AVID II, to test whether an ICD plus an antiarrhythmic drug is better than an ICD alone.

Methods

The objective of the AVID trial was to determine, by a randomized clinical trial, the relative benefit of antiarrhythmic drugs versus ICDs on survival in patients with life-threatening ventricular tachyarrhythmias. The design was based on sequential monitoring at the end of the pilot study and every 6 months thereafter, testing the hypothesis that there was no difference in overall mortality between therapy with an ICD and antiarrhythmic drug therapy. Analysis was performed according to the intention-to-treat principle and significance was based on a two-sided alpha level of 0.05 for comparisons of survival distributions. We estimated a sample size of 1200 patients, assuming an average follow-up of 2.6 years and an event rate of 40% in the antiarrhythmic drug group at 4 years to detect a 30% decrease in mortality. Criteria for termination of the study were based on an O'Brien-Fleming spending function.

Trial Eligibility Criteria

Patients recruited for randomization (Fig. 1) included patients who (1) were resuscitated from ventricular fibrillation; (2) had documented ventricular tachycardia with syncope; (3) had documented sustained ventricular tachycardia with an ejection fracture ≤40% and near syncope, systolic blood pressure less than 80 mmHg, or significant symptoms such as angina or heart failure symptoms.

Principal exclusion criteria were ventricular tachyarrhythmia due to a reversible cause such as acute myocardial infarction, electrolyte imbalance or drug toxicity, contraindication to receiving antiarrhythmic drugs or an ICD, low risk of recurrent arrhythmias, high likelihood of death from comorbidity or obstacles to trial participation. The primary endpoint was total mortality and secondary endpoints included cost and cost-effectiveness and quality of life.

Therapy

Patients could not be considered for placebo treatment and were therefore randomized to the ICD or the best contemporary antiarrhythmic drug therapy, which

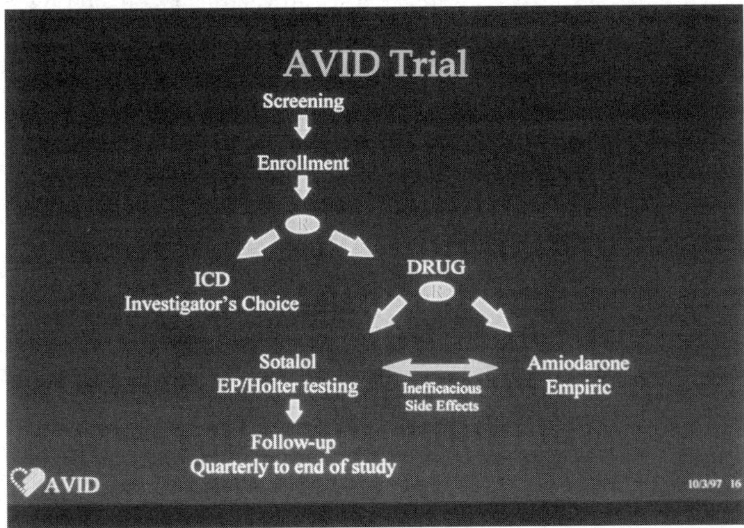

Figure 1   Randomization schema.

was felt to be amiodarone or sotalol. Whether patients assigned to the drug arm were subrandomized to sotalol or amiodarone was left to the judgment of the investigator. Exclusions for not treating with sotalol included a history of asthma, low ejection fraction, history of congestive heart failure or prolonged QT interval. Amiodarone was used empirically while the response to sotalol was guided by electrophysiological testing, Holter recording, or both.

AVID began at the very end of the thoracotomy technique for implantation of ICDs and therefore virtually all patients received a transvenous ICD. Any advanced state-of-the-art ICD that met prespecified criteria could be used if it provided tiered therapy, pacing for tachycardia and bradycardia, memory capabilities, and appropriate outputs of DC shock. The ICDs had received market approval or were implanted under an IDE to permit the use of the newest devices before market approval. ICDs manufactured by Guidant/CPI, Sulzer Intermedics, Medtronic, and Ventritex were the major types used.

The Investigational Review Board of each institution approved the study prior to randomizing patients at that particular institution. All patients gave written, informed consent. AVID began with a pilot study of 200 patients, followed by the main study. Recruitment of patients began on June 1, 1993, and randomization was concluded prematurely at the advice of the Data and Safety Monitoring Board on April 7, 1997. At that time, analysis revealed that the difference in the primary outcome variable between the two groups had crossed the statistical boundary for early termination of the study. By that time, 1016 patients had been randomized.

Prespecified subgroup analyses were for age, left ventricular ejection fraction $\leq 35\%$ versus $>35\%$, etiology of coronary disease versus noncoronary disease, and VF versus VT. There was no intention to evaluate individual ICDs or antiarrhythmic drugs.

RESULTS

Of the 6035 patients who were screened and the 4621 who entered the registry, 1885 were found to be eligible for randomization (Table 1). One thousand sixteen of these patients were randomized to treatment with an ICD (507, 49.9%) or antiarrhythmic drug therapy (509, 50.1%). Except for a history of atrial fibrillation or atrial flutter, which was higher (26%) in the antiarrhythmic drug than in the ICD group (21%) and New York Heart Association class III heart failure, which was higher (12%) in the drug limb than in the ICD limb (7%), baseline characteristics were similar in the two treatment groups. The initial concern that there might be an excessive number of patients with VT rather than VF was not borne out in that 455 patients had VF and 561 had VT. Of these, 216 had syncope and 345 had other symptoms of hemodynamic compromise with a reduced ejection fraction.

Table 1 History and Characteristics of the Patients Assigned to Receive Implantable Cardioverter-Defibrillators or Antiarrhythmic Drugs[a]

Characteristic	Defibrillator group ($n = 507$)	Antiarrhythmic drug group ($n = 509$)
Age (yr)	65 ± 11	65 ± 10
Male sex (%)	78	81
White race (%)	87	86
Index arrhythmia (no.)		
Ventricular fibrillation	226	229
Sustained ventricular tachycardia	281	280
Clinical history before index arrhythmia (%)		
Atrial fibrillation or flutter	21	26
Ventricular fibrillation	5	5
Ventricular tachycardia	14	15
Unexplained syncope	11	15
Coronary artery disease	81	81
Myocardial infarction	67	67
Congestive heart failure	46	47
Hypertension	55	56
Diabetes	25	24
Angina	48	50
Peripheral vascular disease	16	15
Antiarrhythmic drug therapy	16	15
Left ventricular ejection fraction	0.32 ± 0.13	0.31 ± 0.13
Median time from index event to measurement (days)	3	3
Angina at enrollment (%)		
No angina	64	65
CCS class I or II	34	33
CCS class III	2	2
Congestive heart failure or enrollment (%)[b]		
No congestive heart failure	45	40
NYHA class I or II	48	48
NYHA class III	7	12
Findings on baseline electrocardiogram[c]		
Heart rate (beats/min)	77 ± 18	78 ± 17
PR interval (ms)	178 ± 37	183 ± 37
QRS complex (ms)	116 ± 26	117 ± 26
Corrected QT interval (ms)	441 ± 40	445 ± 39
Paced (% of patients)	3	4
Bundle-branch block (% of patients)	23	25

[a] Plus-minus values are means ± SD. CCS, Canadian Cardiovascular Society: NYHA, New York Heart Association.
[b] Patients with class IV congestive heart failure were excluded from the study.
[c] The baseline electrocardiogram was recorded when patients were taking no antiarrhythmic drugs and without cardiac pacing.

There was a minor difference in ejection fraction between the two limbs in that patients with VF who received an ICD had a somewhat higher (36 ± 15%) ejection fraction than those in the drug limb (33 ± 15%). The left ventricular ejection fraction was identical (29%) among the patients with VT in the two treatment groups. Overall, the mean left ventricular ejection fraction was 32 ± 13% in the ICD group and 31 ± 13% in the drug group. Relatively equal percentages in the ICD limb (10%) and drug limb (12%) underwent coronary revascularization during hospitalization for the index arrhythmia.

Therapy

AVID can be considered as a study essentially testing the ICD versus amiodarone since 356 patients immediately began empirical amiodarone therapy without subrandomization and, after randomization, an additional 79 patients received amiodarone while 74 patients received sotalol. However, only 13 patients given sotalol (2.6% of all those assigned to antiarrhythmic drug therapy) had adequate suppression of arrhythmia and were receiving sotalol at discharge. The remaining 58 patients assigned to sotalol therapy received amiodarone or another antiarrhythmic drug or were treated with an ICD. Thus, more than 435 patients received amiodarone versus only 13 patients given sotalol.

Eighty-seven percent of patients receiving amiodarone at discharge continued to take the drug at 1 year and 85% at 2 years. The mean daily maintenance dose of amiodarone at 3 months, 1 year, 2 years, and 3 years was 389 ± 112 mg, 331 ± 99 mg, 294 ± 94 mg, and 256 ± 95 mg, respectively. The mean daily dose of sotalol at similar intervals was 258 ± 81 mg, 248 ± 88 mg, 280 ± 121 mg, and 240± 113 mg.

Of 507 patients assigned to the ICD, 93% received a nonthoracotomy device, 5% an epicardial system, and 2% received no device.

Approximately three times as many patients were taking beta-blockers (42.3% vs. 16.5%) in the ICD versus the drug group. In addition, more patients in the ICD limb (46.8% vs. 40.6%) were taking digitalis at discharge than in the drug limb. Except for these differences, there was very little difference in drug at discharge between the two groups (Table 2).

Outcome

There were 80 deaths among patients assigned to the ICD limb versus 122 deaths in the drug limb, so that over a mean follow-up of 18.2 ± 12.2 months, the crude death rates were 15.8 ± 3.2% in the ICD group and 24 ± 3.7% in the antiarrhythmic drug group. As can be seen in Figure 2, there were a greater number of patients surviving who received an ICD compared with those treated with a drug at 1, 2, and 3 years, with differences of about 7% in the first and second years

Table 2 Therapy at Discharge and During Follow-Up[a]

Treatment	At discharge		At 12 mo.		At 24 mo.	
	Defibrillator group ($n = 497$)	Antiarrhythmic drug group ($n = 496$)	Defibrillator group ($n = 338$)	Antiarrhythmic drug group ($n = 306$)	Defibrillator group ($n = 171$)	Antiarrhythmic drug group ($n = 162$)
	percent					
Implantable cardioverter-defibrillator	98.6	1.4	97.9	9.5	95.7	9.8
Amiodarone	1.8	95.8	8.3	84.7	9.3	82.4
Sotalol	0.2	2.8	1.8	5.8	3.1	8.5
Beta-blocker	42.3	16.5	38.1	11.0	39.4	10.1
Calcium-channel blocker	18.4	12.1	22.9	16.6	19.4	14.1
Both beta-blocker and calcium-channel blocker	5.3	2.4	6.8	2.1	5.6	0.7
Digitalis	46.8	40.6	45.8	37.9	44.4	32.3
Diuretic agent	48.2	50.7	56.0	59.3	56.9	56.4
Other antiarrhythmic drug	4.2	1.2	7.1	3.8	10.0	4.0
Angiotensin converting enzyme inhibitor	68.8	68.2	68.4	65.5	68.1	63.1
Nitrate	36.4	37.0	29.1	27.9	28.1	29.5
Other antihypertensive agent	7.6	8.8	9.0	9.4	10.0	6.1
Lipid-lowering agent	13.2	11.5	19.5	17.2	23.1	19.5
Aspirin	60.7	59.2	55.4	55.4	62.5	56.4
Warfarin	21.9	34.8	24.8	35.4	22.5	30.2

[a] Patients who died while in the hospital after the index event ($n = 19$) are excluded, as are patients still in the hospital at the termination of the study ($n = 4$).

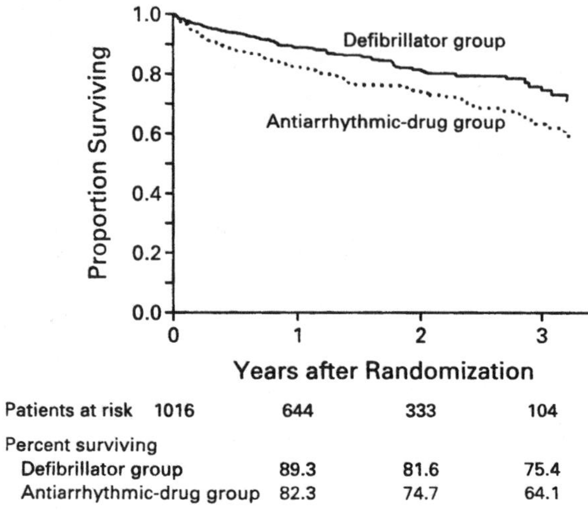

Patients at risk	1016	644	333	104
Percent surviving				
Defibrillator group		89.3	81.6	75.4
Antiarrhythmic-drug group	82.3	74.7	64.1	

Figure 2 Overall survival unadjusted for baseline characteristics. Survival was better among patients treated with the ICD [$p < 0.02$, adjusted for repeated analyses ($n = 6$)].

and 11% at year 3. Thus, over a mean follow-up of 18.2 ± 12.2 months, the crude death rates (95% confidence limits) were $15.8 \pm 3.2\%$ in the ICD group and $24 \pm 3.7\%$ in the drug limb. Patients treated with the ICD had better survival throughout the course of the study (Wilcoxon statistic, 3.32; $p < 0.02$, adjusted for sequential monitoring). While the accuracy of data at 3 years can be questioned because of the few patients followed beyond 2 years (at the time the study was terminated prematurely), calculated survival figures represented decrease in death rates (95% confidence limits) of $39 \pm 20\%$, $27 \pm 21\%$, and $31 \pm 21\%$ at 1, 2, and 3 years, respectively. The average unadjusted length of additional life associated with ICD therapy was 2.7 months at 3 years.

None of the prespecified subgroups differed significantly from the entire population for death from any cause in the ICD limb as compared with the drug limb (Fig. 3). Thus, the hazard ratios for death according to age, left ventricular ejection fraction, cardiac diagnosis, and qualifying arrhythmia were not significantly different for any of these subgroups. Unfortunately, the early termination of the study diminished its power to detect differences between these groups. Those patients with higher ejection fractions tended to show less improvement with the ICD compared to amiodarone, but the wide confidence intervals prevented statistical significance.

Multivariate analysis showed that the beneficial effect of the ICD remained even after adjusting for age, use of beta-blockers during follow-up, presence or absence of heart failure, and ejection fraction at baseline. Revascularization after

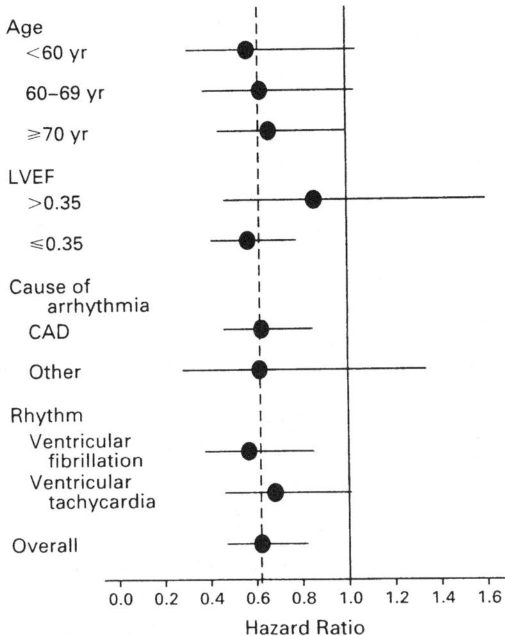

Figure 3 Hazard ratios (and 95% confidence limits) for death from any cause in the ICD group as compared with the antiarrhythmic drug group in prespecified subgroup analyses in the univariate model. No subgroup differed significantly from the entire population. The solid vertical line represents the equal effectiveness of the two treatments so that points to the left indicate better survival in the ICD group and points to the right better survival in the antiarrhythmic drug group. The dotted vertical line represents the results for the entire study, with a hazard ratio of 0.62.

the index arrhythmia did not alter survival differences either. Using the Cox model to adjust for baseline differences in the presence or absence of heart failure, ejection fraction, and history with respect to atrial fibrillation slightly altered the reduction in mortality attributable to the ICD to 37 ± 22%, 24 ± 22%, and 29 ± 23% at 1, 2 and 3 years, respectively. Even after adjusting for the use of beta-blockers, these estimates were unchanged from the unadjusted values.

Therapy from the ICD was more common in patients who entered the study with VT than those who had VF as the index arrhythmia. For patients with ventricular tachycardia, 36% had received treatment from the ICD at 3 months, 68% at 1 year, 81% at 2 years, and 85% at 3 years. Comparable numbers of patients who entered with VF were 15%, 39%, 53%, and 69%, respectively. More therapy was delivered by the ICD to VT patients than VF patients ($p < 0.001$).

Rehospitalization was sooner in patients with an ICD than those treated

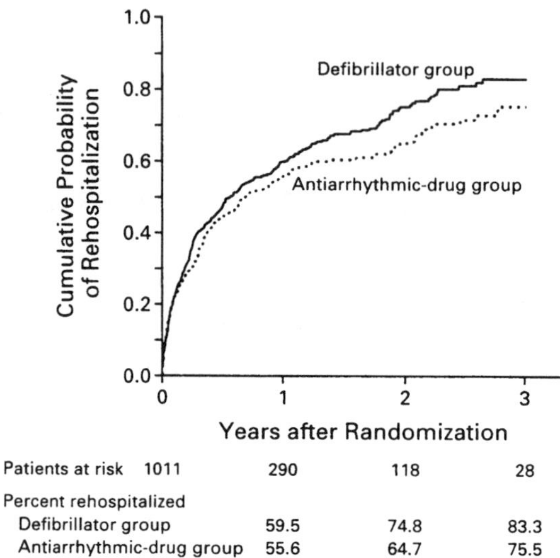

Patients at risk	1011	290	118	28
Percent rehospitalized				
Defibrillator group		59.5	74.8	83.3
Antiarrhythmic-drug group		55.6	64.7	75.5

Figure 4 Time to first rehospitalization. Data on patients who died were censored. Patients with ICDs were rehospitalized sooner than patients treated with antiarrhythmic drugs ($p = 004$). The number of patients at risk at baseline is 1011, because five patients were still hospitalized for the index arrhythmia at the time the study was stopped.

with drugs, so that by 1 year, 60% of the ICD group had been rehospitalized, compared with 56% in the drug group ($p = 0.04$) (Fig. 4). The crossover rate was higher among those initially assigned to therapy with an ICD ($p < 0.001$), with approximately 20% overall of patients crossing over or adding the other therapy by 24 months (Fig. 5).

Complications of Therapy

Thyroid dysfunction requiring replacement medication was prescribed for 10% of the patients treated with amiodarone by 1 year and 16% by 2 years. Pulmonary toxicity was suspected in 3% of amiodarone-treated patients at 1 year and 5% at 2 years, with one patient dying from pulmonary toxicity. Nonfatal torsade de pointes VT was observed once in a patient treated with amiodarone.

In the ICD population, 12 patients (2.4%) died within 30 days of the initiation of therapy (or by the time of possible discharge, if that occurred earlier), as compared with 18 patients (3.5%) in the drug group ($p = 0.27$). Bleeding requiring reoperation or transfusion occurred in 6 patients in the ICD group and serious hematomas in 13. Infection occurred in 10 patients, pneumothorax in 8, and cardiac perforation in 1. Early lead dislodgement or migration of leads occurred in

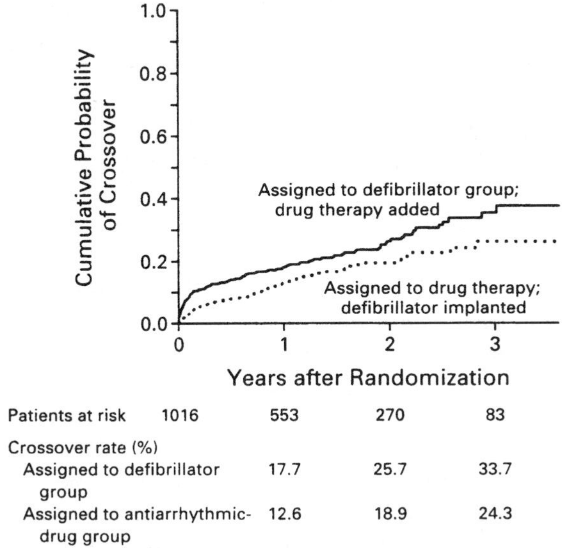

Patients at risk	1016	553	270	83
Crossover rate (%)				
Assigned to defibrillator group		17.7	25.7	33.7
Assigned to antiarrhythmic-drug group		12.6	18.9	24.3

Figure 5 Time to crossover in the two groups. Antiarrhythmic drug therapy was added to ICD therapy more commonly than vice-versa ($p < 0.001$).

three patients. Five patients had unsuccessful nonthoracotomy ICD implantation attempts because of high defibrillation threshold in four and cardiac perforation in one. Three of these five patients subsequently underwent successful ICD implantation.

DISCUSSION

Major Findings

The results from this study definitively show that the ICD improves survival as compared with antiarrhythmic drug therapy in patients who were resuscitated from VF or who had sustained symptomatic VT with hemodynamic compromise.

The baseline clinical characteristics of the ICD and drug limb groups were similar except for minor exceptions noted above. Importantly, the rates of crossover from the ICD to the drug group (25.7%) or from the drug to the ICD limb (18.9%) at 2 years were relatively low and did not compromise the power of the study. Most crossovers occurred because the arrhythmia recurred, rather than because of intolerance to the drugs or devices. More crossovers occurred in the ICD group because of the perceived need to suppress the ventricular arrhythmia with an antiarrhythmic drug to reduce the frequency of shocks received by the patients.

As mentioned earlier, AVID had a registry that demonstrated that the clinical characteristics of the patients who underwent randomization were similar to those in the nonrandomized population. Therefore, the patients randomized in AVID are representative of the general population of patients who are resuscitated from these ventricular arrhythmias so that the conclusions based on the randomized patients can be generalized to this population in general.

Criticisms

Despite the fact that AVID was well conceived and effectively carried out, like any clinical study, it can be criticized. Beta-blockers were used less often in the antiarrhythmic drug group than in the ICD group, as was the case in the Multicenter Automatic Defibrillator Implantation Trial (MADIT) (6). It is likely that many physicians were reluctant to administer a beta-blocker to patients already receiving amiodarone because of resultant bradyarrhythmias, while this was not a problem in the ICD population, who also had backup VVI pacing through the ICD if necessary. In addition, more beta-blockers may have been used in the ICD limb to help control the ventricular response during atrial fibrillation and prevent inappropriate ICD discharge. Interestingly, recent meta-analysis data suggest that beta-blockers added to amiodarone may be more effective in improving survival than either drug alone (7), while information from the Cardiac Arrest Study Hamburg (CASH) indicates that survival was the same in patients treated with amiodarone or beta-blockers (8). Adjustment for this imbalance in beta-blocker use in the Cox regression analysis slightly reduced the estimated benefit of ICD therapy on survival from an unadjusted hazard ratio for the ICD group as compared with the antiarrhythmic drug group of 0.62. Adjusted hazard ratio was 0.67.

In addition, despite randomization, one could argue that the antiarrhythmic drug group was slightly sicker in that the mean left ventricular ejection fraction was nonsignificantly lower in the drug group compared with the ICD group. The entire difference occurred in those who had VF as the index arrhythmia, with the ejection fraction slightly higher in the ICD limb. Further, the incidence of heart failure was slightly greater in the antiarrhythmic drug group. However, stratified regression analysis suggests that these minor imbalances in baseline characteristics explained only about 8% of the observed difference in survival. Thus, the improved survival provided by the ICD remains clear.

Previous Publications

Three other studies of ICDs bear directly on the results from the AVID trial. MADIT (6), in only 196 patients, demonstrated a 56% reduction in mortality in patients treated with an ICD compared with conventional therapy (mostly amiodarone) in patients with prior T-wave myocardial infarction, nonsustained VT, ejection fraction $\leq$ 35%, and inducible VT not suppressed by IV procainamide. MADIT demonstrated the benefits of prophylactic implantation of an ICD in a high-risk population.

CASH (8) was similar to AVID in that patients surviving sudden cardiac death due to VT/VF were randomized to an ICD or drug therapy that included amiodarone, metoprolol, or propafenone. The propafenone limb was stopped at 11 months due to excess mortality. The reported results indicate a 39% reduction in mortality at 1 year in the ICD limb compared with the amiodarone/metoprolol group. Finally, the Canadian Implantable Defibrillator Study (CIDS) (9) was virtually identical to AVID with the exception that they also included patients who had unexplained syncope with later documented ventricular tachycardia exceeding 10 s or inducible sustained VT at electrophysiology study. They studied 650 patients and demonstrated a 20% reduction in mortality in the ICD limb, but this did not reach statistical significance ($p = 0.07$).

Importantly, results from CASH (8) and CIDS (9) are totally concordant with AVID and a meta-analysis using patients in all three studies will be forthcoming.

Study Limitations

Dosing with amiodarone, even after 25 years of use in the United States, is still controversial. Various loading regimens and maintenance doses have been proposed, and its use, empirically as well as following definite endpoints such as electrophysiological testing, has its advocates. The CASCADE (10) trial established the effectiveness of amiodarone used empirically and consequently that was the approach taken for the AVID study. We reasoned that, considering the population, a placebo arm was unethical and therefore we compared one treatment strategy against another. An argument could be made that the antiarrhythmic drugs increased mortality in that limb, making the ICD group appear to have a lower mortality. However, the CAMIAT (11) and EMIAT (12) studies both established that amiodarone did not increase mortality compared with a placebo group and therefore that argument is not likely.

CONCLUSIONS

In summary, data from AVID support the conclusion that the ICD should be the initial treatment of choice for patients who fit the AVID inclusion criteria. Although the absolute magnitude of the benefit associated with the ICD remains unknown, the greater efficacy of this device relative to antiarrhythmic drug therapy is strongly supported by the outcome of this study.

ACKNOWLEDGMENTS

This work was supported in part by the Herman C. Krannert Fund and by a contract N01-HC-25117 with the National Heart, Lung, and Blood Institute of the National Institutes of Health.

REFERENCES

1. Zipes DP, Roberts D. Results of the international study of the implantable pacemaker cardioverter-defibrillator, a comparison of epicardial and endocardial lead systems. Circulation 1995;92:59–65.
2. The Antiarrhythmics Versus Implantable Defibrillators (AVID) Investigators. A comparison of antiarrhythmic drug therapy with implantable defibrillators in patients resuscitated from near-fatal ventricular arrhythmias. N Engl J Med 1997;337:1576–1583.
3. Antiarrhythmics versus Implantable Defibrillators (AVID)—rationale, design, and methods. Am J Cardiol 1995;75:470–475.
4. Kim SG, Fogoros RN, Furman S, Connolly ST, Kuck KH, Moss A. NASPE Policy Statement. Standardized reporting of ICD patient outcome: the report of a North American Society of Pacing and Electrophysiology Policy Conference, February 9-10, 1993. PACE 1993;16:1–5.
5. The Antiarrhythmics Versus Implantable Defibrillators (AVID) trial executive committee. Are implantable cardioverter-defibrillators or drugs more effective in prolonging life? Am J Cardiol 1997;79:661–663.
6. Moss AJ, Hall WJ, Cannom DS, et al. Improved survival with an implanted defibrillator in patients with coronary artery disease at high risk for ventricular arrhythmias. N Engl J Med 1996;335:1933–1940.
7. Amiodarone Trials Metaanalysis Investigators. Effectiveness of prophylactic amiodarone on mortality after acute myocardial infarction and in congestive heart failure: metaanalysis of individual data from 6500 patients in randomized trials. Lancet 1987;350:1417–1474.
8. Kuck KH. Cardiac Arrest Study Hamburg (CASH). Presented at the 47th Annual Scientific Session of the American College of Cardiology.
9. Connolly S. Canadian Implantable Defibrillator Study (CIDS). Presented at the 47th Annual Scientific Session of the American College of Cardiology.
10. The CASCADE Investigators. Randomized antiarrhythmic drug therapy in survivors of cardiac arrest (the CASCADE Study). Am J Cardiol 1993;72:280–287.
11. Cairns JA, Connolly SJ, Roberts R, Gent M. Randomised trial of outcome after myocardial infarction in patients with frequent or repetitive ventricular premature depolarisations: CAMIAT. Lancet 1997;349:675–682.
12. Julian DG, Camm AJ, Frangin G, et al. Randomized trial of effect on amiodarone on mortality in patients with left-ventricular dysfunction after recent myocardial infarction: EMIAT. Lancet 1997;349:667–674.

Bramah N. Singh

*UCLA School of Medicine and West Los Angeles Veterans
Affairs Medical Center, Los Angeles, California*

There is little doubt that over the last decade there has been a revolution in the treatment of cardiac arrhythmias, although a great deal still remains to be done, especially in the preventive arena. With the possible exception of atrial fibrillation, there are relatively few supraventricular arrhythmias that have not been amenable, to varying extents, to the use of radiofrequency catheter ablation. Cure has been possible in many such tachyarrhythmias.

With the advent of implantable devices, the therapeutic excitement is no less in the case of life-threatening ventricular arrhythmias. However, note a critical distinction. On the one hand, in the case of supraventricular tachyarrhythmias, the purpose of suppressing or eliminating the cause of arrhythmias for the most part is to alleviate symptoms. On the other hand, in the case of life-threatening ventricular arrhythmias, the larger purpose of therapy is to prevent sudden arrhythmic death from ventricular fibrillation and tachycardia and thereby prolong survival. Until very recently, this has been an uncertain, if not elusive, goal.

The earliest attempt at prolonging survival by reducing arrhythmic deaths was via the suppression of manifest ventricular arrhythmias. Because the presence of such arrhythmias in the setting of cardiac disease was considered a marker of sudden death, the suppression of these arrhythmias was believed to lead to a reduction in sudden death. The outcome of the Cardiac Arrhythmia Suppression Trial (CAST) clearly laid to rest such a hypothesis (1). The dissociation between the suppression of ventricular arrhythmias in the postmyocardial infarction patients and patient mortality cast serious doubt on the validity of arrhythmia suppression as an approach to mortality reduction in patients with significant cardiac disease. It was assumed that certain drugs, namely, the class Ic agents, which had the highest propensity to reduce simple and complex premature ventricular contractions (PVCs), also appeared to have the greatest and perhaps the most serious proarrhythmic reactions, sometimes culminating in death, especially in patients with significant cardiac disease.

Against this background, the automatic implantable cardioverter-defibrillator (ICD) was developed in the 1980s (2). It had an almost immediate appeal and clinical impact because the device predictably did precisely what it was designed to do, that is, to cardiovert ventricular tachycardia (VT) and defibrillate ventricular fibrillation (VF). In subsequent generations of the device, additional features have been added, such as antitachycardia pacing to terminate VT and various pacing modes to pace the ventricle in the event of life-threatening slow ventricular rhythms.

Clinically, however, the single most important function of the ICD is to prevent sudden arrhythmic death and therefore to prolong survival. Since the mode of arrhythmic deaths in patients with organic or electrical cardiac disease is ultimately due to VT deteriorating into ventricular fibrillation (VF) in most cases (3), and ICD is expected to terminate the majority of spontaneously occurring VT/VF in a repeated fashion, and if the arrhythmia does not change characteristic and deteriorate into electrical storm, survival may be prolonged. Nonetheless, such a consideration conceals the assumption that in all such cases the myocardial substrate is mechanically adequate and cardiocirculatory function will be restored rapidly in the wake of cardioversion or defibrillation when an ''electrical accident'' in the form of VT/VF supervenes. That this does not occur in every case is well known, as is the observation that the ICD has the ability to reduce or essentially eliminate cases of sudden death with only a modest impact on overall total mortality. Clearly, other factors are at play.

The extreme example may be the case of sudden arrhythmic death in patients with advanced class IV congestive heart failure, in whom the defibrillator is unlikely to prolong survival despite its having the capability for terminating sudden episodes of VT/VF in this setting. At the other extreme might be the subsets of patients with left ventricular ejection fractions exceeding 40% to levels that are close to normal and who are subject to repeated bouts of ventricular tachycardia. It is not that such subsets of patients might not benefit from the use of the ICDs for preventing sudden death; in this setting, the benefit is likely to be so small compared to drug therapy that it might be difficult to clearly quantify such benefit in a direct comparison with the effects of the best medical therapy. In between the two extremes are likely to be patients who might meaningfully benefit from the use of the ICD for preventing sudden death with a consequent increase in survival. Clearly, the therapeutic challenge is to precisely define the magnitude of the benefit on total mortality in this group of patients by further adequately controlled trials. This was the clear objective of the AVID (Antiarrhythmics Versus Implantable Defibrillators) trial (4). The AVID investigators found that: ''The defibrillator was superior to antiarrhythmic drug therapy in prolonging survival among patients resuscitated after symptomatic, sustained ventricular tachycardia or ventricular fibrillation causing hemodynamic compromise.'' They recommended that ''it should be offered as first-line therapy to such patients'' (4).

How closely should this advice be followed in every case of VT and VF that present to the cardiologist? There is little doubt that the impact of AVID on clinical practice has been profound. So it should be. It is the first ICD trial of its kind in which the patient population to be enrolled was prospectively defined and characterized; the sample size was appropriately calculated on the basis of available data, and the feasibility of the study was examined in a preliminary pilot study of 200 patients. The drug limb of the study was correctly selected on the evidence available before the initiation of the study. The guidelines for the premature termination were also prospectively defined. Therefore, the outcome data are sound from the point of view of clinical decision making, but clearly they are not flawless in terms of universal applicability on a global scale.

The AVID investigators appreciate the limitations of their study. However, they have not as yet clearly indicated in which subsets of patients with VT or VF the ICD might reasonably not be the first-line therapy. Furthermore, they perhaps could have emphasized that device therapy and drug therapy should be viewed as a continuum, and that for the purposes of device therapy, beta-blockade might be viewed as an integral adjunctive antiarrhythmic therapy that should be offered to all patients with ICDs if there are no specific contraindications.

There are other issues that may merit further scrutiny and considerations, and which may be relevant to the selection of patients for device therapy. It is noted that in AVID (4), at the end of the first year of follow-up, when there were 644 patients at risk, the device reduced the number of total deaths by 39% when compared to the total death rate in the antiarrhythmic drug limb. The difference was highly statistically significant. However, it should be emphasized that the percentage reduction in total mortality after second and third years of therapy was significantly less and few patients had been followed for more than 2 years. It should also be remembered that the average unadjusted length of additional life associated with device therapy was 2.7 months at 3 years. Thus, the overall absolute survival benefit is modest rather than striking, tempered further by the data that patients treated with the ICD needed to be rehospitalized significantly more frequently. Moreover, patients on the device crossed over significantly more frequently to drug therapy than the converse to reduce the number of shocks that were not tolerated by the patient, to treat other arrhythmias not favorably affected by the device, or to slow the arrhythmia rate to enable antitachycardia pacing for termination. While these and other features of device function that may have an impact on the quality of life of the patient, as well as cost of therapy, do not minimize the ICD's demonstrated impact on mortality, they do, however, emphasize two significant issues. First, it is clear that it is imperative to consider that device therapy and drug therapy for VT/VF are complementary rather than competitive. Second, a clearer delineation is needed of the subsets of patients in whom it might still be the best therapeutic option to use the best medical regimen which might prevent the recurrence of sudden death and life-threatening ventricular tachycardia. In these respects the data reported from the AVID trial may provide some further directions and approaches.

It is noted that the mean age of the patients in AVID in both treatment limbs was 65 years. Although there was no significant difference among the groups under 60 years of age, those between 60 and 69 years of age, and those equal to or over 70 years of age, it is not clear how many patients had been enrolled in the study who were over 80 years of age. It is known that life expectancy falls as a function of age and it might be extremely difficult to show benefit in octogenarians who may otherwise be candidates for device therapy if they were to develop VT/VF. Neither AVID nor other reported studies have specifically addressed this issue in the elderly.

Finally, a potentially important observation that may be revisited is the question of the impact of ventricular function on hazard ratio in terms of responses to device and drug therapy. The AVID data bear on this critical point. The mean left ventricular ejection fraction (LVEF) for the AVID patients was 0.32 ± 0.13 for the device limb and 0.31 ± 0.13 in the drug therapy limb. There appeared to be a major difference in outcome in the group that had a LVEF < 0.35 (favoring device), whereas the difference between device therapy and drug therapy was almost negligible in patients with LVEF > 0.35. The numbers of patients in the latter group may have been small, but the data provide the clue that in patients with relatively better preserved LVEF, a stratified randomized trial might show no significant benefit of ICD for survival in patients with VT/VF compared to drug therapy. Such patients may be optimally treated with the best antiarrhythmic drug regimen which may now need to be considered as a combination of beta-blockade and amiodarone as suggested by the data from the EMIAT and CAMIAT trials (5,6). The possibility should be tested that, in this particular subset of patients, the combined regimen of beta-blockade and amiodarone might be at least as effective as the ICD. It should be noted that the patients with lower LVEF appeared to derive greater benefit from ICD therapy compared to those with a higher LVEF. This suggests that the impact of ICD therapy in patients with congestive cardiac failure should be evaluated further in patients with varying grades of decompensation, again possibly in combination with amiodarone and beta-blockers, which have a demonstrated favorable impact on mortality in this subset of patients.

In sum, AVID has been a landmark trial in which the effects on mortality of the perceived best antiarrhythmic therapy and implantable device were compared in patients resuscitated from ventricular fibrillation and other life-threatening ventricular tachyarrhythmias. The clinical context of the trial was such that the impact of neither form of therapy on mortality could be quantified in absolute terms as a control therapy (placebo equivalent) limb was clearly unethical. Similarly, the trial could not be undertaken on the basis of ''pure'' drug treatment and ''sole'' device therapy. On the basis of intention-to-treat analysis of data, device therapy had a significantly greater impact on mortality reduction than did therapy with the drug amiodarone. The outcome data have raised a number of issues of clinical importance that may require consideration in future controlled clinical trials. Perhaps the most significant is whether in patients with relatively well-preserved LVEF there might be little difference between the effects of device as compared to therapy, which now must be considered to be a combination of beta-blockade and amiodarone in regimens best tolerated by the patient. However, the possibility that sotalol, administered empirically or as a guided therapy, might be equally effective in this context cannot be excluded on the basis of the AVID data since relatively few patients were enrolled on this agent. Finally, to date, the impact of device therapy has been such that electrophysiologically guided therapy for VT/VF is unlikely to reemerge as a realistic therapeutic modality. Rather, drug and device therapy in combination are likely to develop *pari passu* as the best therapeutic options for reducing mortality in patients at high risk for death from ventricular tachycardia and fibrillation.

REFERENCES

1. The Cardiac Arrhythmia Suppression Trial (CAST) Investigators. Preliminary report: effect of encainide and flecainide on mortality in randomized trial of arrhythmia suppression after myocardial infarction. N Engl J Med 1989;321:406–412.
2. Mirowfski M, Reid PR, Mower MM, et al. Termination of malignant ventricular arrhythmias with an implanted automatic defibrillator in human beings. N Engl J Med 1980;303:322–324.
3. Bayes de Luna A, Coumel P, Leclerq JF. Ambulatory sudden death: Mechanisms of production on the basis of data from 157 cases. Am Heart J 1989;117:151–160.
4. The Antiarrhythmics Versus Implantable Defibrillators (AVID) Investigators. A comparison of antiarrhythmic-drug therapy with implantable defibrillators in patients resuscitated from near-fatal ventricular arrhythmias. N Engl J Med 1997;337:1576–1583.
5. Julian DG, Camm SAJ, Frangin, et al. Randomized trial of amiodarone on mortality in patients with left ventricular dysfunction after recent myocardial infarction: EMIAT. Lancet 1997;349:667–674.
6. Cairns JA, Connolly SJ, Roberts R, Gent M. Randomized trial of outcome after myocardial infarction in patients with frequent repetitive ventricular depolarizations: CAMIAT. Lancet 1997;349:675–682.

10

The CABG Patch Trial: Prophylactic Use of Implanted Cardiac Defibrillators in High-Risk CABG Surgery Patients

J. Thomas Bigger, Jr., and Daniel M. Bloomfield
*Columbia University and Columbia–Presbyterian
Medical Center, New York, New York*

The CABG Patch Trial tested the hypothesis that implantation of an ICD in high-risk patients who were having CABG surgery would improve survival (1). In September 1990, The CABG Patch Trial started a pilot study in five North American clinical centers under the sponsorship of Guidant/CPI. In January 1992, enrollment was extended to 13 hospitals in North America and Europe and, in March 1993, The CABG Patch Trial entered a cooperative agreement with the National Heart, Lung, and Blood Institute (NHLBI) and enrollment was extended to 37 clinical centers. The full-scale trial, cosponsored by NHLBI and Guidant/CPI, enrolled patients with coronary heart disease who were having elective CABG surgery, were <80 years of age, had a LVEF <0.36, and had an abnormal signal-averaged ECG. Patients who signed a consent form were randomized to ICD therapy or to a control group that received no therapy in addition to their routine CABG surgery. The last of 900 patients was randomized on February 5, 1996. Joint sponsorship by NHLBI and Guidant/CPI made possible a full-scale trial to obtain controlled data for a possible new indication for ICD therapy.

PRIMARY PREVENTION OF SUDDEN CARDIAC DEATH

The poor salvage rate for out-of-hospital cardiac arrest provides a strong rationale for primary prevention of sudden cardiac death. Each year, more than 400,000 cardiac arrests occur in the United States, almost one per minute (2,3). A similar number occur annually in western Europe. Only about 2% of cardiac arrest victims are resuscitated and leave the hospital alive (4,5). Survivors of cardiac arrest treated with implantable cardiac defibrillators (ICDs) have improved survival (6). However, the impact of this approach is small because so few patients survive a cardiac arrest to take advantage of modern treatment. About 25% of sudden cardiac deaths are due to ischemia in previously asymptomatic patients (7–10). These deaths can only be addressed by aggressive treatment of risk factors for coronary heart disease. About 75% of sudden cardiac deaths occur in patients with previously recognized heart disease who are available for screening, risk stratification, and prophylaxis (11,12). If the patients with heart disease who will experience cardiac arrest can be identified, preventive measures should have a substantially larger impact on the sudden cardiac death problem than is currently achieved with the salvage and treat strategy. ICD therapy is an attractive candidate for prophylaxis of high-risk patients.

In the early 1990s, two studies began to evaluate prophylactic use of ICD therapy: The Multicenter Automatic Defibrillator Implantation Trial (MADIT) (13,14) and The CABG Patch Trial (1). This chapter describes the interim results of The CABG Patch Trial.

The Rationale for Prophylactic ICD Treatment of High-Risk CABG Surgery Patients

The planning effort for The CABG Patch Trial began in 1988, long before the Endotak lead was approved by the Food and Drug Administration (August 27, 1993). The planning group realized that there were serious scientific problems with conducting a randomized controlled trial of ICD prophylaxis using transthoracic implantation of epicardial patch defibrillating leads. They anticipated that diagnostic coronary angiography and revascularization procedures would be more likely in patients randomized to receive ICD therapy via thoracotomy and unequal surgical revascularization in the two randomized groups would confound the assessment of ICD efficacy (i.e., benefit due to ICD therapy could not be distinguished from benefit due to revascularization). To avoid confounding by revascularization, patients who were having CABG surgery and were thought to be at high risk for arrhythmic death were selected for study.

High Long-Term Mortality Rates After CABG Surgery

After CABG surgery, mortality rates are high for patients with poor left ventricular function. The 231 patients in the Coronary Artery Surgery Study (CASS) registry with LVEF <0.36 who had CABG surgery between 1975 and 1979 had an average LVEF of 0.30 and a 3-year cumulative mortality rate of 23% (15).

Hochberg et al. (16) reported the surgical mortality and long-term survival of 466 patients with LVEF <0.40 undergoing CABG surgery between 1976 and 1982. All of the patients had previous myocardial infarction and 36% had congestive heart failure. Patients with LVEF of 0.20–0.39 ($n = 425$) had a surgical mortality of 11% and a 3-year mortality rate of 40%. The group with LVEF 0.10–0.19 ($n = 41$) had a surgical mortality of 27% and a 3-year mortality rate of 85%.

The University of Toronto analyzed the relationship between operative death and preoperative LVEF for 12,471 patients who had CABG surgery between January 1982 and December 1990 (17). The 9445 patients with LVEF >0.40 had an operative mortality rate of 2.3%; the 2539 patients with LVEF between 0.20 and 0.40 had an operative mortality rate of 4.8%; and the 487 patients with LVEF <0.20 had an operative mortality rate of 9.8%. No information was provided on long-term mortality rates.

These studies provided the rationale for the use of LVEF in the CABG Patch trial (i.e., requiring a LVEF <0.36 for eligibility and stratifying randomization at a LVEF of 0.20).

Arrhythmic Death and Hospitalization for Arrhythmic Events After CABG Surgery

There is not much information on the causes of death during long-term follow-up after CABG surgery. Holmes reported the mortality experience during 5 years of follow-up in 11,843 medically treated patients and 8103 surgically treated patients in the CASS registry (18,19). After CABG surgery, sudden cardiac death represented a significantly lower fraction of deaths than in medically treated patients, but substantial numbers of sudden deaths occurred in the surgical cohort (19). In surgically treated patients, death was sudden in 204 patients (25%), not sudden but cardiac in 390 (47%), and not cardiac in 230 (28%) (18). CASS found no baseline variables that predicted sudden death better than nonsudden cardiac death after CABG surgery. In a small study, Bolooki reported 35% of all deaths after CABG surgery were sudden during 50 months of follow-up (20). Tresch et al. reported the long-term follow-up of 49 patients who had CABG surgery after cardiac arrest (21). The mean LVEF for the group was 45%. Seven (16%) of the 45 patients discharged alive died during an average follow-up of 55 months. Five of the seven deaths (71%) were due to recurrent ventricular fibrillation and two were due to congestive heart failure.

A CASS registry study reported that rehospitalization for arrhythmias occurred in 21.2% of the surgical group and in 17.9% of the medical group, suggesting that CABG surgery does not substantially reduce arrhythmic risk (15).

The literature indicates that operative mortality for CABG surgery in patients with LVEF <0.36 ranges from 4% to 24%; 3-year all-cause mortality after

CABG surgery in patients with LVEF <0.36 ranges from 24% to 50%; and the percentage of all deaths after CABG surgery that are sudden ranges from 25% to 50%.

The CABG Surgery Survey

Because there was so much variability among the reports in the literature and because most of the relevant studies were 10 to 20 years old, The CABG Patch Trial planning group surveyed seven of their institutions to determine the percentage of patients who had CABG surgery during 1986 who were <80 years of age and had LVEF <0.36 to determine the survival experience of this high-risk subset. A total of 3217 CABG operations were done in the seven hospitals in 1986 and 17% were <80 years of age and had LVEF <0.36 (1). The surgical mortality rate for patients with LVEF <0.36 was 11.6% and the 2-year actuarial mortality rate was 28%. Follow-up after 2 years was too infrequent to permit an estimate of 3-year mortality. A number of arrhythmic deaths and nonfatal cardiac arrests were reported in patients with LVEF <0.36, but the data on mechanism of death were too incomplete to estimate a rate for arrhythmic death.

The CABG Patch Trial Pilot Study

A 1-year pilot study was undertaken between September 1, 1990 and August 31, 1991 to obtain information needed to plan a full-scale trial (1). The major objectives of the pilot study were to determine: (1) whether the signal-averaged ECG was a worthwhile arrhythmia qualifier; (2) the percentage of CABG surgery patients who were fully eligible for the trial; (3) the percentage of fully eligible patients who would consent to the study; and (4) the percentage of enrolled patients who could be randomized.

Because the ICD only prevents arrhythmic deaths, the investigators wanted a marker to identify patients at high risk for arrhythmic events during follow-up. Three tests were considered: (1) signal-averaged ECG; (2) ventricular arrhythmias in 24-h Holter ECG recordings; and (3) electrophysiological testing. Most patients were admitted much less than 24 h before their CABG surgery, making 24-h ECG recordings or electrophysiological studies much less feasible than the signal-averaged ECG, a noninvasive test that can be completed in less than 30 min. Early or late after myocardial infarction, the signal-averaged ECG identifies patients at high risk for sudden cardiac death or nonfatal cardiac arrest better than spontaneous ventricular arrhythmias detected by Holter recordings; the overall relative risk for an abnormal signal-averaged ECG is 6 to 8 (22–24) compared with a relative risk of 2 to 4 for arrhythmias detected by Holter recordings (25–27). There were relatively few data comparing the predictive accuracy of the signal-averaged ECG and electrophysiological testing. The signal-averaged ECG was chosen based on its feasibility and its high predictive value for arrhythmic events.

During the 1-year pilot study, 2508 patients were screened and 18% of them were less than 80 years of age and had a LVEF <0.36 (1). Overall, 3.3% of the screened patients were fully eligible and 68% of the eligible patients signed a consent form. Of those who signed a consent form, 80% were randomized. About 65% of the otherwise eligible patients had an abnormal signal-averaged ECG and the relative risk of patients with abnormal signal-averaged ECG for death or cardiac arrest was about 3.0 (1,28).

Sample Size and Power for the Full-Scale CABG Patch Trial

The CABG Patch Trial was designed as a fixed-sample size, randomized, clinical trial with group sequential monitoring for safety (1). Qualified patients were randomized 50:50 to ICD therapy or to no therapy. Randomization was stratified by clinical center and LVEF ≤0.20 versus 0.21 to 0.35. The average follow-up was expected to be about 40 months. The primary endpoint for the study was all-cause mortality. The primary hypothesis was tested using the intention-to-treat principle; data were analyzed using the Cox regression model; the significance of differences between groups was tested with the long rank test. The alpha error was set at 0.05 (two-tailed) and the power at about 0.85. For the sample size calculation, the 40-month mortality rate was expected to be 36.5% and ICD treatment was assumed to reduce mortality by 26%. The drop-in rate was expected to be 11% and the dropout rate was expected to be 6%. Using these parameters, the sample size required for the trial was calculated to be about 800 patients, 400 in each group. In October 1994, the Data and Safety Monitoring Board (DSMB) recommended that the sample size be increased to 900 patients and calendar time of follow-up be increased to correct for a lower than expected mortality rate in the control group and a shortening of follow-up time caused by a June 1994 subpoena from the Office of the Inspector General. A quantitative comparison of the options considered by the DSMB to deal with the power problems was published recently (29).

Phases of The CABG Patch Trial

The CABG Patch Trial recruitment was conducted in three phases: pilot, bridging, and full scale. Five clinical centers recruited during the pilot phase (August 14, 1990 to August 31, 1991) to determine the feasibility of recruiting high-risk CABG surgery patients and to evaluate the performance of the signal-averaged ECG for increasing the mortality rate. Ten clinical centers recruited during the bridging phase (September 1, 1991 to March 12, 1993), which spanned the time between the end of the pilot phase and the beginning of the full-scale, NHLBI-sponsored trial. Thirty-seven centers in the United States and Germany recruited during the full-scale trial (March 12, 1993 to February 5, 1996).

Patients who were fully eligible and signed consent forms proceeded to CABG surgery. After the bypass grafts were done, the surgeon made the judgment whether the patient was stable enough to implant an ICD. If so, the patient was randomized and the ICD system implanted and tested in the operating room, usually while patients were on partial cardiopulmonary bypass after coronary grafts were completed. More than 90% of patients who signed a consent form and remained eligible were randomized. Also, about 350 patients were enrolled in the substudy to determine the value of the signal-averaged ECG for predicting death or nonfatal arrhythmic events after CABG surgery (1).

Baseline Studies

Patients with coronary artery disease scheduled for elective CABG surgery were screened at The CABG Patch Trial clinical centers. All patients had coronary angiography and measurement of LVEF within a year, 84% within 30 days of the CABG surgery, and 72% of patients were screened within 24 h of CABG surgery. Most qualifying ejection fraction determinations were made on the basis of a preoperative left ventriculogram (77%), with small percentages qualified on the basis of a radionuclide study (12%) or a quantitative echocardiogram (10%). The LVEF was one of the tests used to identify those at higher risk of dying after CABG surgery.

To obtain a sample with higher risk of arrhythmic deaths and sustained arrhythmic events, we used the signal-averaged ECG to exclude low-risk patients from the trial. Any of the following criteria qualified patients for the study: (1) a filtered QRS duration of $\geq$114 ms; (2) a root-mean-square voltage <20 μV in the terminal 40 ms of the filtered QRS duration; or (3) duration of the terminal filtered QRS complex of >38 ms after the QRS voltage falls below 40 μV (1). Requiring only one abnormality to qualify high-risk patients made more patients eligible than conventional criteria would have.

Because of the exceptionally short interval from the time of screening to surgery, qualification for patient inclusion in the trial was determined at the clinical centers, with subsequent quality control review for the two primary qualifying laboratory tests, left ventricular ejection fraction and signal-averaged electrocardiogram. Quality control review of ventriculographic ejection fraction found no evidence of any investigator bias to include ineligible patients in the trial (discussed in detail in Ref. 30). All signal-averaged ECGs were reread by the Core Laboratory in Philadelphia and 100% satisfied the criteria to qualify for the trial.

Rationale for Policy on Antiarrhythmic Drugs

Aside from beta-blockers (32–35), no antiarrhythmic drug therapy had proven efficacy at the time The CABG Patch Trial was recruiting. On the contrary, clinical trials available when The CABG Patch Trial started suggested that antiarrhythmic drugs with class I action had a substantial harmful effect (36–44) and that drugs with class III action might have some benefit (44). Several trials of amiodarone therapy reported results long after The CABG Patch Trial was started that showed ~10% reduction in mortality rate for prophylaxis after myocardial infarction or in heart failure patients with arrhythmias (45–47). These previous studies indicate that a substantial difference in antiarrhythmic drug use in the two arms of the trial could confound the primary results. Accordingly, The CABG Patch Trial adopted a policy of no treatment of unsustained VT with either class I or class III antiarrhythmic drugs.

Lack of treatment in the control group is an important difference between The CABG Patch Trial and other recently published ICD trials. The AVID study specifically compared ICD therapy to antiarrhythmic drug therapy (the majority of medically treated patients received empiric amiodarone) (6). The MADIT trial compared ICD therapy to conventional therapy: 74% of patients randomized to conventional therapy in MADIT were taking amiodarone and 10% were taking class I antiarrhythmic drugs 1 month after randomization (14).

Patient Screening and Randomization

During recruitment, 71,855 patients were screened, 1422 eligible patients were identified, 1055 were enrolled (signed consent forms), and 900 patients were randomized. The accrual of patients during the course of the trial is shown in Figure 1.

Of the 71,855 patients in the registry, 73% were male, the age was 65 ± 10 years, and the left ventricular ejection fraction averaged 0.51 ± 0.15. Of all screened patients, 74% were excluded because they had a left ventricular ejection fraction greater than 0.35, and 5% of the patients were excluded on the basis of age ≥80. As expected, only 20% of all screened patients were eligible by both age and ejection fraction criteria. About half of otherwise eligible patients had a normal signal-averaged ECG (30,31).

Baseline Characteristics

Demographic and Clinical History

The demographic characteristics and baseline medical history for patients randomized in The CABG Patch Trial are shown in Table 1 and discussed in greater detail in Ref. 30. A total of 446 patients were randomized to the ICD group and 454 to the control group. For the 900 randomized patients, the mean age was 63 years and 85% were male; 46% were over the age of 65 years. There were no significant differences between the two groups for any medical history or baseline variables. The majority of patients had a history of hypertension (55%), smoking

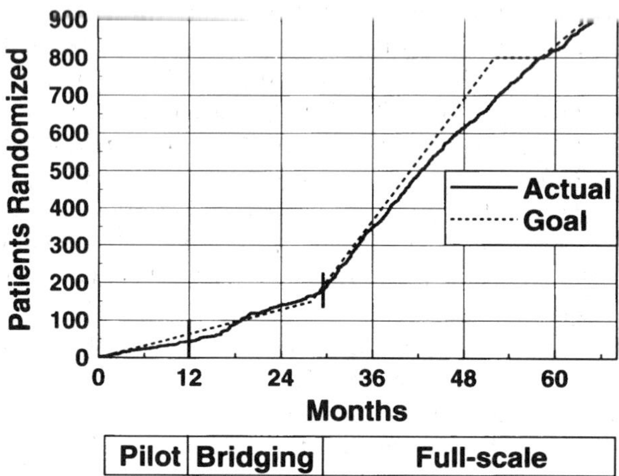

Figure 1 Recruitment for The CABG Patch Trial. The first patient was randomized on August 14, 1990 and the last on February 5, 1996, 67 months after randomization began. In each phase of the trial—pilot, bridging, and full-scale—the number of clinical centers increased and the rate of randomization showed a corresponding increase. (From Ref. 30.)

(78%), and hypercholesterolemia (54%). Forty-eight percent had received specific treatment for heart failure, 37% had been hospitalized for heart failure, and 24% were in NYHA functional class III or IV. Fifty-five percent of the patients had three-vessel coronary artery disease.

Ejection Fraction

The mean ejection fraction for both patient groups was 0.27 ± 0.06, 16% of patients had a left ventricular ejection fraction ≤ 0.20 (the stratifying value for randomization). Figure 2 shows the distribution of ejection fraction by treatment group for the 900 randomized patients.

Electrocardiographic Characteristics

Overall, 73% of the patients had a QRS duration >100 ms on their baseline 12-lead ECG and 39% had a QRS duration ≥ 120 ms. The rhythm was sinus in 92% of the patients, atrial fibrillation in 2.9%, and paced in 1.2%. A nonspecific intraventricular conduction defect with a QRS duration ≥ 120 ms was present in 18% of patients, complete right bundle branch block in 9%, and left bundle branch block in 11%. ECG evidence for a myocardial infarction was present in 63% of patients and the ECG was indeterminate in an additional 16%. The signal-averaged ECG showed a prolonged QRS duration (≥ 114 ms) in 85% of patients,

Table 1 Baseline Characteristics by Treatment Group

	ICD (*n* = 446)	No ICD (*n* = 454)
Age (years)	64 ± 9[a]	63 ± 9
Sex (men/women)	386/60	373/81
Cardiovascular history (%)		
Cigarette smoking (any time)	79	76
Angina pectoris	76	76
Myocardial infarction	83	82
≥2 prior myocardial infarctions	30	33
Heart failure	51	49
Treatment for heart failure	49	47
NYHA functional class II–IV	44	43
Treatment for hypertension	54	52
Diabetes mellitus	36	40
Diabetes treated with insulin	17	20
Treatment for ventricular arrhythmias	7	7
PTCA or atherectomy	11	11
CABG surgery	12	10
Electronic cardiac pacemaker	2	2
Physical findings (%)		
Heart rate (beats/min)	79 ± 15	79 ± 14
Systolic blood pressure (mmHg)	126 ± 19	123 ± 19
Pulmonary rales	20	25
S3 gallop	14	11
LV Function		
LV ejection fraction (mean ± SD)	0.27 ± 0.06	0.27 ± 0.06
LV end diastolic pressure (mmHg)	21 ± 10	22 ± 10
Electrocardiographic findings (%)		
QRS duration > 100 ms	71	74
Left bundle branch block	10	12
Q-wave myocardial infarction	52	53
Coronary angiography (%)		
One-vessel disease	8	9
Two-vessel disease	36	36
Three-vessel disease	55	55
Medications at baseline (%)		
Oral antiarrhythmics	8	8
Digitalis	37	35
Diuretics	51	48
Converting enzyme inhibitors	50	55
Antihypertensives	42	44
Nitrates	61	61
Beta-blockers	30	30
Calcium channel blockers	37	32
Antiplatelet drugs	59	63
Oral anticoagulants	5	5
Lipid-lowering drugs	18	15

Abbreviations: CABG = coronary artery bypass graft; ECG = electrocardiogram; ICD = implantable cardiac defibrillator; LV = left ventricular; NYHA = New York Heart Association; and PTCA = percutaneous transluminal coronary angioplasty.

[a] Plus–minus values are means ± standard deviations. There was no significant difference between the two groups for any of the variables listed in this table.

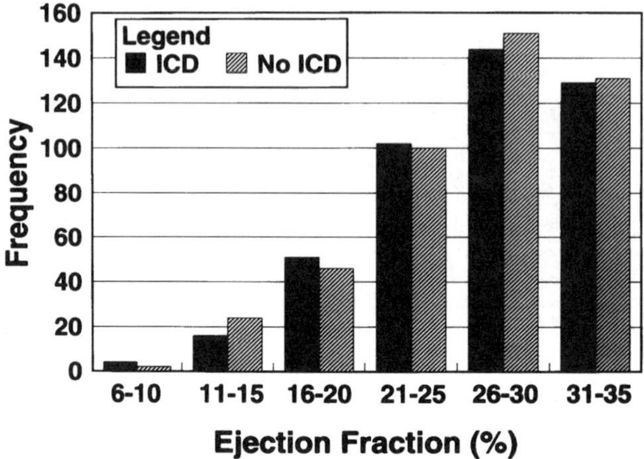

Figure 2   The distribution of the qualifying left ventricular ejection fractions of patients randomized in The CABG Patch Trial. Solid bars indicate patients randomized to the ICD group and hatched bars indicate patients randomized to the control group. Sixteen percent of the patients had a left ventricular ejection fraction ≤ 0.20, the value used to stratify patients for randomization; 55% had a left ventricular ejection fraction in the 0.21–0.30 range, and 29% had a left ventricular ejection fraction in the 0.31–<0.36 range.

a root-mean-square voltage of the terminal 40 ms of $<20\ \mu V$ in 71%, and a low-amplitude signal duration >38 ms in 67%. There were 249 patients who had a baseline Holter ECG recording with ≥ 12 h of analyzable ECG data. Of these, 65% of 116 ICD patients and 62% of 133 control patients had ≥ 10 VPC/h and 39% of the ICD patients and 33% of the control patients had unsustained ventricular tachycardia.

Medications

Drugs taken during the 3 months before admission for CABG surgery are also listed in Table 1. Reflecting the serious medical condition of these patients, a majority were taking nitrates and at least one-third were taking antihypertensive drugs, digitalis, diuretics, converting enzyme inhibitors, or antiplatelet drugs.

Results of Surgery

Extent of Revascularization

The mean number of distal anastomoses was 3.6 ± 1.1. Internal mammary artery grafts were used in 62% of the patients. The surgeons assessed the completeness of revascularization by coronary artery territory; in the left anterior descending artery distribution, revascularization was judged to be complete in more than 80% of the cases, in the circumflex territory, revascularization was judged to be complete in 70% of the cases, and in the right coronary artery territory, revascularization was judged to be complete in 68% of the cases.

ICDs

Most (88%) of the devices implanted in the patients assigned to ICD were CPI Models 1550, 1555, and 1600, which are simple shock-only ICDs without pacing capability or electrogram storage. Forty-one patients got newer ICD models that are capable of bradycardia pacing and electrogram storage. Twelve patients who were randomized to ICD therapy did not receive ICDs because of hemodynamic instability or death that occurred in the operating room after randomization.

Complications of Surgery

At the trial's inception, investigators were concerned that ICD therapy could increase surgical mortality, shock, bleeding, CHF, arrhythmias, or deep sternal wound infections (48). Cardiopulmonary bypass time averaged 108 min in the control group and 127 min in the ICD group. There was no statistically significant difference between groups suggesting a difference in intraoperative hemodynamic instability, including the incidence of inotropic drug administration or mechanical circulatory assistance. Of the potential complications of ICD implantation outlined by the investigators, only deep sternal wound infections occurred more frequently in the ICD group compared with controls (2.2% vs. 0.4%; $p <$ 0.05).

The change in LVEF as a function of signal-averaged ECG status was studied at one trial center. A 56% average increase in LVEF was found for patients who were excluded from the trial only by a normal signal-averaged ECG compared with a 19% increase in LVEF for patients with an abnormal signal-averaged ECG (49).

Adherence to Protocol

Crossovers

During follow-up, 70 crossovers occurred: 18 patients in the control group had an ICD implanted during the course of the trial. As mentioned above, 12 patients assigned to ICD therapy never had an ICD implanted because of death or hemodynamic instability in the operating room, and 40 had their ICD removed, primarily because of infection ($n = 19$), because the ICD reached end of service and no replacement was done ($n = 5$), or because the patient requested removal ($n =$

5). The small crossover rate during 4 years of follow-up in the trial is illustrated in Figure 3. The upper curve represents the proportion of patients randomized to ICD therapy who had an ICD capable of delivering therapy, whereas the lower curve represents the proportion of patients randomized to the control group who had an ICD capable of delivering therapy. The difference between these two curves represents the treatment gradient between the two groups in the trial. At 42 months, the cumulative rate of crossover to the control group was 10% and the cumulative rate of crossover to the ICD group was less than 5%.

Cardiac Drugs

Figure 4 illustrates the use of antiarrhythmic drugs and beta-blockers over the course of the trial. There was an increase in the use of antiarrhythmic drugs from immediately preoperatively to hospital discharge due to treatment of postoperative atrial fibrillation. This increase in antiarrhythmic drugs after discharge was similar in the control and ICD groups, and decreased substantially by the 3-month follow-up visit in both groups. Throughout the trial, approximately 15% of patients in both groups were treated with antiarrhythmic drugs, mostly for the treat-

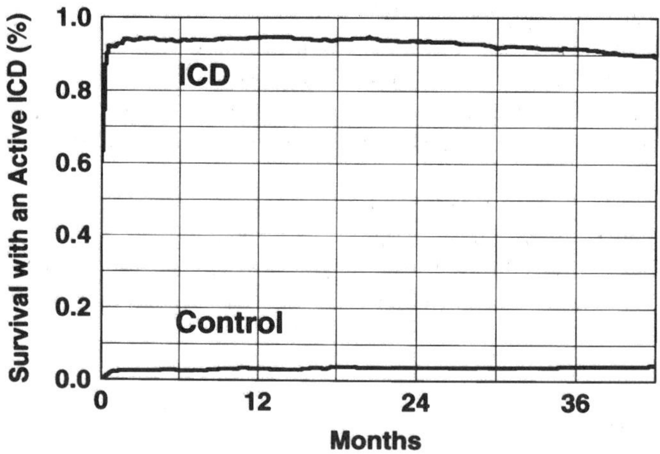

Figure 3   Adherence to treatment assigned at randomization. The upper curve shows the proportion of patients who were assigned to ICD therapy, were alive, and had an ICD capable of antiarrhythmic therapy over the first 48 months of the trial. At 42 months, 90% had a working ICD. The lower curve shows the proportion of patients who were assigned to the control group, were alive, and had an ICD capable of antiarrhythmic therapy over the first 48 months of the trial. At 42 months, only 5% of the control group had crossed over to ICD therapy. Adherence to the original treatment assignment was remarkably good.

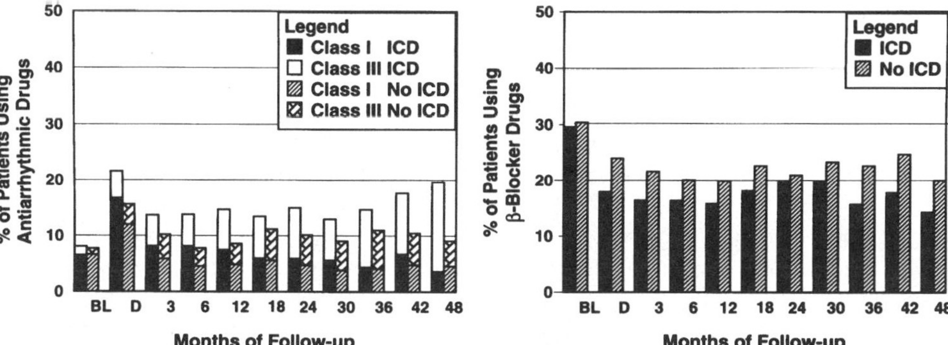

Figure 4 Antiarrhythmic drug and beta-blocker use in The CABG Patch Trial. (Left panel) The overall incidence of class I or class III antiarrhythmic drugs was less than 20% (the trial's goal) at any time during 48 months of follow-up except at the time of discharge, when treatment and prophylaxis for atrial fibrillation were at their peak. There was no significant difference between the two groups with respect to antiarrhythmic drug use. (Right panel) The overall use of beta-blocking drugs was about 20% and remarkably constant over 48 months of follow-up. There was a trend for beta-blockers to be used more in the control group, but the difference was not statistically significant.

ment of atrial fibrillation (31). There was no statistically significant difference in antiarrhythmic drug use in the two groups over the entire trial.

Also, there was similar use of beta-blockers in both groups in the trial. This is another important contrast to both the AVID study and the MADIT trial, where there was a substantial inequity in the use of beta-blockers favoring the ICD group (6,14). In the MADIT trial, 5% of patients randomized to conventional therapy compared with 27% of patients randomized to ICD were taking beta-blockers at the time of the last recorded contact with the patient (14). In the AVID study, 10% of patients randomized to antiarrhythmic (amiodarone or dl-sotalol) therapy also were taking a beta-blocker compared with 39% of patients randomized to ICD therapy (6).

Effects of Treatment on Survival

The primary endpoint for The CABG Patch Trial was death of any cause. On April 2, 1997, the Data and Safety Monitoring Board took the last of four interim looks at the mortality data with 76% of the anticipated mortality information available. The fourth interim analysis showed no difference between the ICD and control groups and a negligible chance that a difference would ever be found. Accordingly, the Board recommended that data on the primary endpoint be reported as of April 30, 1997, while the trial continued to pursue its secondary objectives. On April 10, 1997, the Director of the National Heart, Lung, and Blood Institute accepted the Board's recommendation.

When the interim results were reported in November 1997, the average follow-up was 32 months. During an average follow-up of 32 $\pm$ 16 months, there were 101 deaths in the ICD group (71 from cardiac causes) and 95 in the control group (72 from cardiac causes) (31). Of these, there were 44 deaths in the first 30 days after randomization, 24 in the ICD group, and 20 in the control group ($p = 0.60$). The Kaplan–Meier cumulative mortality curves for the two treatment groups shows that the ICD group mortality rate was almost identical to that found in the control group (Fig. 5). The hazard ratio from a Cox regression analysis that compared the risk of death per unit of time in the ICD group with the control group was 1.07 (95% CI, 0.81 to 1.42). The hazard ratio and 95% CI derived from a Cox regression was similar for the period beginning 30 days after randomization (''postsurgical'' survival, hazard ratio 1.03, 95% CI, 0.75 to 1.41).

Cause-specific death was classified by an external Events Committee using the modified Hinkle–Thaler definitions (50,51). Of the 198 deaths that were known to have occurred as of April 30, 1997 (2 deaths were added between

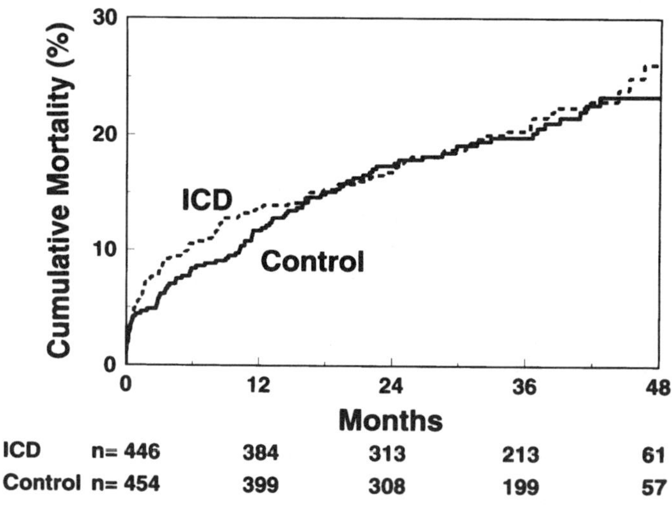

Figure 5 The probability of dying according to assigned treatment. By April 30, 1997, 95 deaths had occurred in the control group and 101 deaths had occurred in the implanted defibrillator group. By 4 years of follow-up, the actuarial (Kaplan–Meier) mortality rate was 24% in the control group and 27% in the group assigned to implanted defibrillator therapy ($p = 0.64$). (From Ref. 31.)

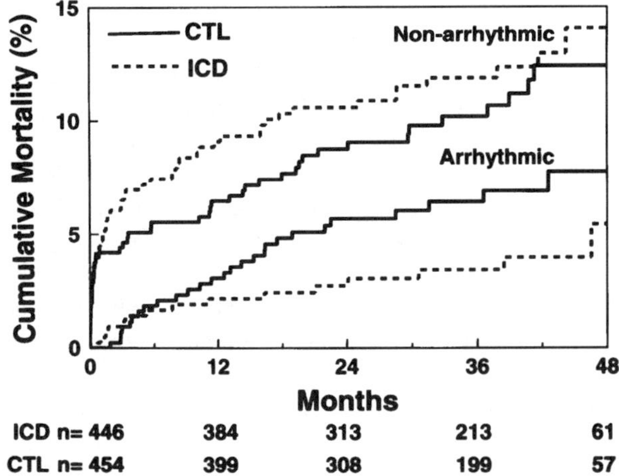

Figure 6 The probability of dying arrhythmic deaths and nonarrhythmic deaths stratified by treatment group. There was a substantial decrease in arrhythmic death and a modest increase in nonarrhythmic cardiac death when the ICD group was compared with the control group. (From Ref. 51.)

version 1 and version 2 of the database), 73% occurred in hospital or in the emergency room (52). Eighty-two percent of the 96 control group deaths were cardiac, 29% were arrhythmic, and 48% were nonarrhythmic cardiac deaths (52). The 42-month cumulative arrhythmic death rate was 6.9% in the control group compared with 4.0% in the ICD group (a 42% decrease; $p = 0.057$) (Fig. 6). The 42-month cumulative nonarrhythmic cardiac death rate was 12.4% in the control group compared with 13.0% in the ICD group ($p = 0.275$), a 5% increase. The results were compared to those found in MADIT. The percent of patients in the control group that died arrhythmic deaths and the percent reduction in arrhythmic deaths were quite similar for the two studies (52). In MADIT, nonarrhythmic cardiac deaths and noncardiac deaths were reduced about as much as arrhythmic deaths; nonarrhythmic cardiac deaths and noncardiac deaths were not reduced in The CABG Patch Trial (52).

A Search for Statistical Interactions with Ten Prespecified Covariates

The CABG Patch Trial specified 10 covariates of interest before the study began: age, gender, heart failure, New York Heart Association (NYHA) functional class, diabetes mellitus, left ventricular ejection fraction, QRS duration >100 ms, angiotensin converting enzyme inhibitors, β-adrenergic blocking drugs, and class I or class III antiarrhythmic drugs (31). There was no statistically significant interaction between any of these 10 covariates and treatment effect, and the hazard ratio and 95% CI derived from a Cox model after adjustment for the 10 prespecified covariates were similar to those obtained without adjustment.

One example of the lack of interaction between a covariate and the treatment is illustrated in Figure 7. In this example, the presence of congestive heart failure (indicated by the heavy lines) is clearly associated with an increased mortality compared with those patients who did not have congestive heart failure (indicated by the thin lines). However, the mortality of patients in the ICD group (solid lines) and the control group (dashed lines) was similar whether or not congestive heart failure was present.

Comparisons of the mortality rates for patients in the ICD group and control group stratified by the presence or absence of the covariate are listed in Table 2. The hazard ratios and the 95% CI describe the difference in mortality rates

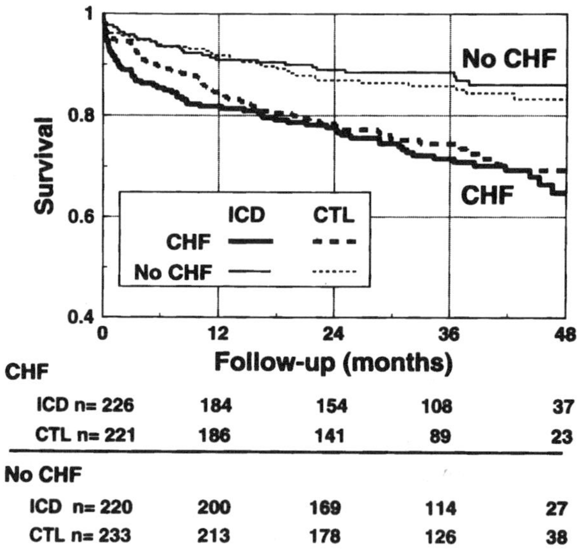

CHF				
ICD n= 226	184	154	108	37
CTL n= 221	186	141	89	23
No CHF				
ICD n= 220	200	169	114	27
CTL n= 233	213	178	126	38

Figure 7 The probability of survival comparing patients with and without congestive heart failure at baseline stratified by treatment group. Heavy lines represent patients with congestive heart failure at baseline and thin lines represent patients without congestive heart failure at baseline. Solid lines are used to indicate patients randomized to ICD therapy and dashed lines are used to indicate patients randomized to control. The presence of congestive heart failure at baseline is associated with a significantly worse survival regardless of treatment group (ICD or control).

Table 2　Lack of Statistical Interactions Between Ten Prespecified Covariates and Treatment: Hazard Ratios at 4 Years for the ICD Group Compared with the Control Group

Variable	n	4-Year mortality (%) ICD	Control	4-Year hazard ratio	95% CI
Age					
≥65	449	36.8	29.6	1.20	0.84, 1.70
<65	451	17.2	18.8	0.82	0.50, 1.32
Gender					
Male	759	26.5	25.0	1.01	0.74, 1.36
Female	141	29.9	20.6	1.19	0.54, 2.62
CHF					
Yes	448	35.9	31.2	1.11	0.78, 1.58
No	452	16.8	18.0	0.86	0.53, 1.41
NYHA class					
No CHF/I	510	18.0	19.1	0.87	0.56, 1.36
II, III, IV	390	37.5	31.7	1.16	0.80, 1.68
Diabetes					
Yes	344	29.7	23.6	1.21	0.76, 1.92
No	556	25.7	24.6	0.95	0.66, 1.36
LVEF					
>20	757	25.9	22.4	1.08	0.78, 1.48
≤20	143	32.8	33.5	0.88	0.47, 1.67
QRS duration					
>100 ms	653	29.1	26.2	1.08	0.78, 1.49
≤100 ms	247	22.3	18.5	0.97	0.53, 1.78
Converting enzyme inhibitors					
Yes	473	22.8	20.1	0.97	0.62, 1.51
No	427	31.7	28.4	1.10	0.76, 1.60
Beta-blocker drugs					
Yes	183	17.9	15.1	0.87	0.37, 2.00
No	717	29.0	26.9	1.02	0.76, 1.39
Antiarrhythmic drugs					
Yes	160	27.1	32.3	0.93	0.50, 1.73
No	740	26.7	22.7	1.05	0.76, 1.45

Abbreviations: CHF = congestive heart failure; NYHA class = New York Heart Association Functional Class; LVEF = left ventricular ejection fraction.

attributed to treatment with an ICD in patients with and without each covariate. The odds ratios are close to 1 (and all of the 95% CI include one), indicating the absence of any interaction between these covariates and treatment effect.

ICD Discharges

Despite the lack of a survival benefit associated with ICD therapy, 57% of the patients randomized to ICD therapy had a shock within the first 2 years after implantation (31). The cumulative probability of the first ICD discharge in the group assigned to ICD therapy is shown in Figure 8. In most patients the rhythm that resulted in shock delivery could not be ascertained. However, in the final phase of enrollment, 41 patients randomized to ICD therapy at the time of surgery received devices capable of storing intracardiac electrograms. In this subgroup, ICDs were programmed for committed, single-zone, shock-only therapy (criterion for tachyarrhythmia detection, 175 bpm) to emulate device programming in the overall trial.

Thirteen of the 41 patients (32%) with stored-electrogram ICDs received at least one ICD shock during the first 18 months of follow-up (53). Either stored electrograms or telemetry monitoring strips documented the first shock in 12 of these patients. The remaining patient received a shock 3.5 months after surgery, but died before electrograms were retrieved. Shocks were delivered for sustained ventricular arrhythmias in only 4 of 12 patients (33%): uniform VT within a

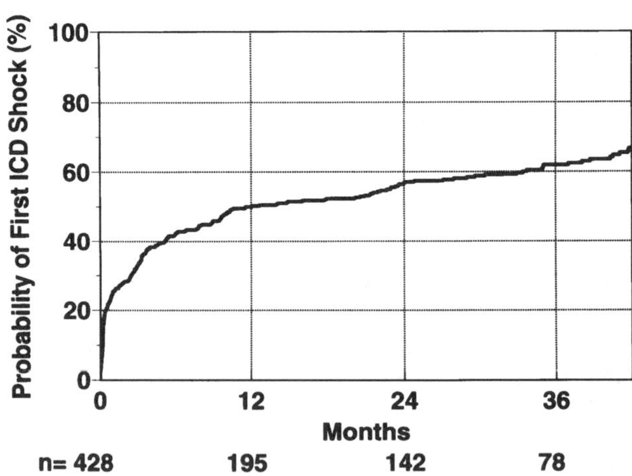

Figure 8   The probability for the discharge of a first shock from implanted cardiac defibrillators. At 1 year, the actuarial incidence was 50% and, at 2 years, the incidence was 57%. (From Ref. 31.)

week of CABG surgery in three patients, and multiform VT in one patient 72 days after surgery. In two patients, an ICD shock was delivered after the spontaneous termination of unsustained VT. The remaining six patients had ICD shocks for supraventricular rhythms: two of these occurred within a week, three occurred at about 2 months, and one occurred 5 months after surgery. The data from this substudy of The CABG Patch Trial demonstrates that ICD shocks were common (32%), but the majority of these (67%) were for unsustained VT or supraventricular rhythms. Only a few patients received shocks for sustained ventricular arrhythmias; only one patient received a shock after hospital discharge (53).

What Did We Learn from The CABG Patch Trial?

The CABG Patch Trial showed that ICD prophylaxis did not improve survival of high-risk patients having CABG surgery. These results indicate that not all high-risk groups of coronary heart disease patients will benefit from ICD therapy. In the past, we assumed that when high-risk groups of coronary heart disease patients were identified, that they would benefit from ICD therapy. Taken together, the results of The CABG Patch Trial and those of MADIT indicate that this assumption is wrong. Table 3 shows that many characteristics of patients in The CABG Patch Trial and those in MADIT are almost identical: age, gender, etiologic heart disease, prevalence and severity of heart failure, number with multiple previous myocardial infarcts, and average LVEF. Despite the similarity in the MADIT patients and The CABG Patch Trial patients, ICD therapy had no benefit whatsoever in The CABG Patch Trial while ICD therapy halved the mortality rate in MADIT.

Why Was There No Benefit from ICD Therapy in The CABG Patch Trial?

Although the patients recruited for The CABG Patch Trial were very similar to those recruited for MADIT (see Table 3), the benefit of ICD therapy was nil in The CABG Patch Trial, but large in MADIT. The two characteristics that differ substantially between these two primary prevention trials are inducible VT and revascularization with CABG surgery. One of these two differences is likely to explain the difference in ICD benefit in the two trials.

A Low Prevalence of Inducible Sustained VT

A likely explanation for the difference in ICD benefit between MADIT and The CABG Patch Trial is that a small proportion of patients randomized in The CABG Patch Trial had inducible sustained VT, as contrasted with MADIT, in which all patients had inducible sustained VT. The electrophysiology substudy of The

Table 3 Comparison of Patients in The MADIT and CABG Patch Trials

	MADIT (n = 196)	The CABG Patch Trial (n = 900)
Similarities		
Age <80 years	100	100
Age in years (mean ± SD)	63 ± 9	64 ± 9
Male	92	84
Coronary heart disease	100	100
LV ejection fraction < 0.36	100	100
LV ejection fraction (mean ± SD)	0.26 ± 0.07	0.27 ± 0.06
History of myocardial infarction	100	85
History of ≥2 myocardial infarctions	31	31
History of heart failure	51	50
Differences		
CABG surgery	45	100
Coronary angioplasty/atherectomy	22	11
Unsustained ventricular tachycardia	100	30
Positive signal-averaged ECG (fQRS)	57	100
Positive signal-averaged ECG (fQRS or LP)	70	100
Positive electrophysiological study	100	?

Abbreviations: ECG = electrocardiogram; fQRS = filtered QRS; LP = late potential; LV = left ventricular; SD = standard deviation.
Except where indicated, the numbers in the table indicate percentages.

CABG Patch Trial (in progress at the time of this publication) will allow us to estimate the proportion of patients with inducible ventricular tachycardia in all 454 control subjects randomized in The CABG Patch Trial.

The estimation of the prevalence of inducible ventricular tachycardia in all 454 control subjects randomized in The CABG Patch Trial is based on a ''mixture model'' (discussed in detail in Ref. 54). A simplification of the mixture model is provided in Table 4. This model utilizes two numbers to estimate the prevalence of inducible ventricular tachycardia in all 454 control subjects randomized in The CABG Patch Trial: (1) the observed prevalence of inducible ventricular tachycardia among all surviving control subjects ([c/(c + d)] in Table 4) and (2) an estimation of the relative risk of death for patients with inducible ventricular tachycardia compared to patients without inducible ventricular tachycardia (in Table 4, the relative risk is equivalent to [a/(a + c)]/[b/(b + d)]). MADIT estimated the relative risk of patients with inducible VT to be more than 4; patients with inducible sustained VT had a mortality rate of 39% versus 8% for patients who were not inducible (55). For our estimates, we assumed a relative risk of 3 to obtain a conservative estimate.

Table 4 Mixture Model for Calculating
the Prevalence of Inducible Ventricular
Tachycardia in All Randomized Control
Patients

	Inducible VT		
	Yes	No	Totals
Dead	a[a]	b[a]	m
Alive	c[b]	d[b]	n
Totals	a + c	b + d	N
	Inducible VT		
	Yes	No	Totals
Dead	36[a]	64[a]	100
Alive	35[b]	315[b]	350
Totals	71	379	450

Abbreviation: VT = ventricular tachycardia.

[a] These values will be measured in the electro-physiology substudy of The CABG Patch Trial.

[b] These values can be calculated based on an assumption of the relative risk of death for patients with inducible ventricular tachycardia compared to patients without inducible ventricular tachycardia (the relative risk is equivalent to [a/(a + c)]/[b/(b + d)]). The lower table provides these calculations assuming an observed prevalence of inducible ventricular tachycardia of 10% and a relative risk of 3. See text for further explanation.

The lower portion of Table 4 provides these calculations. If the observed prevalence of inducible VT among all surviving control subjects is 10% (i.e., 35 of 350 subjects enrolled in the electrophysiology substudy), and we assume a relative risk of 3, this model estimates a 15.8% prevalence (71/450) of inducible VT in all control subjects randomized in The CABG Patch Trial. If the observed prevalence of inducible VT among all surviving control subjects is 15% (i.e., 53 of 350), and we assume the same relative risk of 3, this model estimates a 22% prevalence of inducible ventricular tachycardia for all control subjects at the time of randomization in The CABG Patch Trial (54).

If a low fraction of inducible patients is found in the electrophysiology substudy of The CABG Patch Trial, it will indicate that electrophysiological testing should play a dominant role in identifying patients who will benefit from prophylactic ICD therapy.

Alternatively, if the proportion of patients with inducible VT is large (e.g., >0.30) in The CABG Patch Trial, then it can be concluded that CABG surgery uncoupled inducible VT from spontaneous arrhythmic events during follow-up.

The latter finding will indicate that CABG surgery should play a more important role in the primary prevention of sudden cardiac death.

Future efforts to extend ICD prophylaxis must assess each risk group in a controlled study. While new prophylaxis studies are going on, we should make every effort to salvage more patients with cardiac arrest (e.g., more people trained for effective bystander CPR, wider deployment of automatic external defibrillators, and improvements in pharmacological therapy of patients who have recurrences of VF at the scene of the cardiac arrest) (56–58). For patients who survive a cardiac arrest, ICD therapy plays the leading role (6).

REFERENCES

1. The CABG Patch Trial Investigators and Coordinators. The CABG Patch Trial. Prog Cardiovasc Dis 1993;36:97–114.
2. National Center for Health Statistics: Advance report, final mortality statistics, 1981. DHHS Pub. No. (PHS)84-1120. Monthly Vital Stat 33(suppl 3):4–5.
3. Weaver WD, Cobb LA, Hallstrom AP, Fahrenbruch C, Copass MK, Ray R. Factors influencing survival after out-of-hospital cardiac arrest. J Am Coll Cardiol 1986;7:752–757.
4. Becker LB, Ostrander MP, Barrett J, Kondos GT. Outcome of cardiopulmonary resuscitation in a large metropolitan area: where are the survivors? Ann Emerg Med 1991;20:355–361.
5. Lombardi G, Gallagher EJ, Gennis P. Outcome of out-of-hospital cardiac arrest in New York City. J Am Med Assoc 1994;271:678–683.
6. The Antiarrhythmics Versus Implanted Defibrillators (AVID) Trial Investigators. A comparison of antiarrhythmic drug therapy with implantable defibrillators in patients resuscitated from near-fatal ventricular arrhythmias. N Engl J Med 1997;337:1576–1583.
7. Davies MJ, Thomas A. Thrombosis and acute coronary artery lesions in sudden cardiac ischemic death. N Engl J Med 1984;310:1137–1140.
8. Marshall JC, Waxman HL, Sauerwein A, Gilchrist I, Kurnik PB. Frequency of low-grade residual coronary stenosis after thrombolysis during acute myocardial infarction. Am J Cardiol 1990;66:773–778.
9. Fuster V, Badimon L, Badimon JJ, Chesebro JH. The pathogenesis of coronary artery disease and the acute coronary syndromes. N Engl J Med 1992;326:242–250, 310–318.
10. Spaulding CM, Joly LM, Rosenberg A, Monchi M, Weber SN, Dhainaut JFA, Carli P. Immediate coronary angiography in survivors of out-of-hospital cardiac arrest. N Engl J Med 1997;336:1629–1633.
11. Gordon T, Kannel WB. Premature mortality from coronary heart disease. The Framingham Study. J Am Med Assoc 1971;215:1617–1625.
12. Lown B. Sudden cardiac death: the major challenge confronting contemporary cardiology. Am J Cardiol 1979;43:313–328.

13. MADIT Executive Committee. Multicenter Automatic Defibrillator Implantation Trial (MADIT): design and clinical protocol. PACE 1991;14:920–927.

14. Moss AJ, Hall WJ, Cannom DS, Daubert, JP, Higgins SL, Klein H, Levine JH, Saksena S, Waldo AL, Wilber DJ, Brown MW and Heo M for the MADIT Investigators. Improved survival with an implantable defibrillator in coronary patients at high risk for ventricular arrhythmias. N Engl J Med 1996;335:1933–1940.

15. Alderman EL, Fisher LD, Litwin P, Kaiser GC, Myers WO, Maynard C, Levine F, Schloss M. Results of coronary artery surgery in patients with poor left ventricular function (CASS). Circulation 1983;68:785–795.

16. Hochberg MS, Parsonnet V, Gielchinsky I, Hussain SM. Coronary artery bypass grafting in patients with ejection fractions below forty percent. Early and late results in 466 patients. J Thorac Cardiovasc Surg 1983;86:519–527.

17. Christakis GT, Weisel RD, Fremes SE, Ivanov J, David TE, Goldman BS, Salerno TA, Cardiovascular Surgeons of the University of Toronto. Coronary artery bypass grafting in patients with poor left ventricular function. J Thorac Cardiovasc Surg 1992;103:1083–1092.

18. Holmes DR, David K, Gersh BJ, Mock MB, Pettinger MB and CASS participants. Risk factor profiles of patients with sudden cardiac death and death from other cardiac causes: a report from the Coronary Artery Surgery Study (CASS). J Am Coll Cardiol 1989;13:524–530.

19. Holmes DR, Jr, Davis KB, Mock MB, Fisher LD, Gersh BJ, Killip T, III, Pettinger MB, and participants in the Coronary Artery Surgery Study. The effect of medical and surgical treatment on subsequent sudden cardiac death in patients with coronary artery disease: a report from the Coronary Artery Surgery Study. Circulation 1986; 73:1254–1263.

20. Bolooki H. Discussion of CABG in patients with ejection fractions below forty percent. J Thorac Cardiovasc Surg 1983;86:526.

21. Tresch DD, Wetherbee JN, Siegel R, Troup PJ, Keelan MH, Olinger JN, Brooks HL. Long-term follow-up of survivors of prehospital sudden cardiac death treated with coronary bypass surgery. Am Heart J 1985;110:1139–1145.

22. Cripps TR, Bennett ED, Camm AJ, Ward DE. High gain signal averaged electrocardiogram combined with 24-hour monitoring in patients early after myocardial infarction for bedside prediction of arrhythmic events. Br Heart J 1988;60:181–187.

23. Steinberg JS, Regan A, Sciacca RR, Bigger JT, Jr, Fleiss JL. Predicting arrhythmic events after myocardial infarction: results of a prospective study and a meta-analysis using the signal-averaged electrocardiogram. Am J Cardiol 1992;69:13–21.

24. El-Sherif N, Denes P, Katz R, Capone R, Mitchell LB, Carlson M, Reynolds-Haertle R, for the Cardiac Arrhythmia Suppression Trial/Signal-Averaged Electrocardiogram (CAST/SAECG) Substudy Investigators. Definition of the best prediction criteria of the time domain signal-averaged electrocardiogram for serious arrhythmic events in the postinfarction period. J Am Coll Cardiol 1995;25:908–914.

25. Bigger JT, Jr, Fleiss JL, Kleiger R, Miller JP, Rolnitzky LM, and The Multicenter Post-Infarction Research Group. The relationships among ventricular arrhythmias, left ventricular dysfunction and mortality in the 2 years after myocardial infarction. Circulation 1984;69:250–258.

26. Mukharji J, Rude RE, Poole KE, Gustafson N, Thomas LJ, Jr, Strauss HW, Jaffe AS, Muller JE, Roberts R, Raabe DS, Jr, Croft CH, Passamani E, Braunwald E, Willerson JT, the MILIS Study Group. Risk factors for sudden death after acute myocardial infarction: two-year follow-up. Am J Cardiol 1984;54:31–36.

27. Nicod P, Gilpin E, Dittrich H, Henning H, Ross J, Jr. Prognostic significance of complex ventricular arrhythmia for cardiac death during the first year after myocardial infarction. J Electrophysiol 1987;1:93–102.

28. Gottlieb CD, Bigger JT, Jr, Steinman RC, Rolnitzky LM for The CABG Patch Trial Investigators. Signal averaged ECG predicts death after CABG surgery. Circulation 1995;92:I–406.

29. Bigger JT, Jr, Parides MK, Levin B, Meier P, Rolnitzky LM, Egan D. Changes in sample size and length of follow-up to maintain power in The CABG Patch Trial. Controlled Clin Trials 1998;19:1–14.

30. Curtis AB, Cannom DS, Bigger JT, Jr, DiMarco JP, Estes NAM, III, Steinman RC, Parides MK, for The CABG Patch Trial Investigators. Baseline characteristics of Patients in The Coronary Artery Bypass Graft (CABG) Patch trial. Am Heart J 1997; 134:787–799.

31. Bigger JT, Jr for The Coronary Artery Bypass Graft (CABG) Patch Trial Investigators. Prophylactic use of implanted cardiac defibrillators in patients at high risk for ventricular arrhythmias after coronary artery bypass graft surgery. N Engl J Med 1997;337:1569–1575.

32. Hjalmarson A, Elmfeldt D, Herlitz J, Holmberg S, Malek I, Nyberg G, Ryden L, Swedberg K, Vedin A, Waagstein F, Waldenstrom A, Waldenstrom J, Wedel H, Wilhelmsen L, Wilhelmsson C. Effect on mortality of metoprolol in acute myocardial infarction. A double-blind randomized trial. Lancet 1981;iv:823–827.

33. Norwegian Multicenter Study Group. Timolol-induced reduction in mortality and reinfarction in patients surviving acute myocardial infarction. N Engl J Med 1981; 304:801–807.

34. Beta-blocker Heart Attack Trial Research Group. A randomized trial of propranolol in patients with acute myocardial infarction. Mortality results. J Am Med Assoc 1982;247:1707–1714.

35. Yusuf S, Peto R, Lewis J, Collins R, Sleight P. Beta blockade during and after myocardial infarction: an overview of the randomized trials. Prog Cardiovasc Dis 1985;27:335–371.

36. The Cardiac Arrhythmia Suppression Trial (CAST) Investigators. Effect of encainide and flecainide on mortality in a randomized trial of arrhythmia suppression after myocardial infarction. N Engl J Med 1989;321:406–412.

37. The Cardiac Arrhythmia Suppression Trial II Investigators. Effect of the antiarrhythmic agent moricizine on survival after myocardial infarction. N Engl J Med 1992; 327:227–233.

38. May GS, Eberlein KA, Furberg CD, Passamani ER, DeMets DL. Secondary prevention after myocardial infarction: a review of long-term trials. Prog Cardiovasc Dis 1982;24:331–352.

39. Furberg CD. Effect of antiarrhythmic drugs on mortality after myocardial infarction. Am J Cardiol 1983;52:32C–36C.

40. Hine L, Laird N, Hewitt P, Chalmers T. Meta-analysis of empiric chronic antiarrhythmic therapy after myocardial infarction. J Am Med Assoc 1989;262:3037–3040.

41. Coplen SE, Antman EM, Berlin JA, Hewitt P, Chalmers TC. Efficacy and safety of quinidine therapy for maintenance of sinus rhythm after cardioversion. A meta-analysis of randomized control trials. Circulation 1990;82:1106–1116.

42. Morganroth J, Goin JE. Clinical investigation: quinidine-related mortality in the short-to-medium-term treatment of ventricular arrhythmias: a meta-analysis. Circulation 1991;84:1977–1983.

43. Yusuf S, Teo KK. Approaches to prevention of sudden death: need for fundamental reevaluation. J Cardiovasc Electrophysiol 1991;2:S233–S239.

44. Teo KK, Yusuf S, Furberg CD. Effects of prophylactic antiarrhythmic drug therapy in acute myocardial infarction. An overview of results from randomized controlled trials. J Am Med Assoc 1993;270:1589–1595.

45. Zarembski DF, Nolan PE, Slack MK, Caruso AC. Empiric long-term amiodarone prophylaxis following myocardial infarction: a meta-analysis. Arch Intern Med 1993;153:2661–2667.

46. Sim I, McDonald KM, Lavori PW, Norbutas CM, Hlatky MA. Quantitative overview of randomized trials of amiodarone to prevent sudden cardiac death. Circulation 1997;96:2823–2829.

47. Amiodarone Trials Meta-Analysis Investigators. Effect of prophylactic amiodarone on mortality after acute myocardial infarction and in congestive heart failure; meta-analysis of individual data from 6500 patients in randomised trials. Lancet 1997; 350:1417–1424.

48. Spotnitz HM, Herre JM, Raza ST, Hammon JW, Jr, Baker LD, Fitzgerald DM, Kron IL, Bigger JT, Jr, for The CABG Patch Trial Investigators. Effect of ICD implantation on surgical morbidity in The CABG Patch Trial. Circulation 1998;98(suppl II): II-77–II-80.

49. Cook JR, Flack JE, Gregory CA, Deaton DW, Rousou JA, Engelman RM, for The CABG Patch Trial. A preoperative signal-averaged electrocardiogram predicts the change in left ventricular ejection fraction after CABG surgery in patients with preoperative left ventricular dysfunction. Am J Cardiol 1998;82:285–289.

50. Hinkle LE, Jr, Thaler HT. Clinical classification of cardiac deaths. Circulation 1982; 65:457–464.

51. Epstein AE, Carlson MD, Fogoros RN, Higgins SL, Venditti FJ, Jr. Classification of death in antiarrhythmia trials. J Am Coll Cardiol 1996;27:433–442.

52. Bigger JT Jr, Whang W, Rottman JN, Kleiger RE, Gottlieb CD, Namerow PB, Steinman RC, Estes NAM. Mechanisms of death in The CABG Patch Trial: A randomized trial of prophylactic use of implantable cardiac defibrillators in patients at high risk of death after coronary artery bypass graft surgery. Circulation 1999;99: 1416–1421.

53. Bloomfield D, Block M, Windle J, Cook J, Wilber D, for The CABG Patch Trial Investigators and Coordinators. Stored electrogram analysis of shocks in The CABG Patch Trial: A potential explanation for the limited survival benefit of implantable cardiac defibrillators. PACE 1998;21(Part II):818 (abstr).

54. Rottman JN, Levin B, Paik MC, Tsai W-Y, Bigger JT, Jr, for The CABG Patch

Investigators. Using missing data techniques to explore the lack of effect: illustration with The CABG Patch Trial. Stat Med 1999;18:1943–1959.

55. Daubert JP, Higgins SL, Zareba W, Wilber DJ. Comparative survival of MADIT-eligible but noninducible patients. J Am Coll Cardiol 1997;29(suppl A):78A.

56. Weisfeldt ML, Kerber RE, McGoldrick RP, Moss AJ, Nichol G, Ornato JP, Palmer DG Riegel B, Smith CS, Jr. American Heart Association report on the Public Access Defibrillation Conference, December 8–10, 1994. Circulation 1995;92:2740–2747.

57. Cummins RO, Ornato JP, Thies WH, Pepe PE. Improvement in survival from sudden cardiac arrest: the ''chain of survival'' concept. Circulation 1991;83:1832–1847.

58. Kerber RE, Becker LB, Bourland JD, Cummins RO, Hallstrom AP, Michos MB, Thies WH, White RD, Zuckerman BD. Automatic external defibrillators for public access defibrillation: recommendations for specifying and reporting arrhythmia analysis algorithm performance, incorporating new waveforms, and enhancing safety. Circulation 1997;95:1677–1682.

Peter J. Zimetbaum and Mark E. Josephson
Beth Israel Deaconess Medical Center, Boston, Massachusetts

The CABG Patch Trial was initiated in 1993 to determine whether prophylactic implantation of an ICD would prevent sudden cardiac death and improve overall survival in high-risk patients (1). High-risk patients were defined as individuals with coronary artery disease requiring surgery, depressed left ventricular function (<36%), and a positive, signal-averaged ECG (SAECG). There were a total of 37 participating centers that screened 1422 patients and enrolled 1055. Nine hundred of these subjects were randomized, with 446 receiving ICDs and 454 in the non-ICD or control group. A total of 70 patients crossed over from one arm to the other. Eighteen patients in the control arm ultimately received an ICD. Twelve patients in the ICD arm never received a device secondary to intraoperative developments that precluded implantation. Forty patients with an ICD had them removed, 19 secondary to infection, 10 because of patient preference either before or at the end of battery life, and 11 for uncertain reasons. There was an average of 32 ± 16 months of follow-up with no significant difference in total or cardiovascular mortality between the two study arms.

BACKGROUND

Analysis of the clinical relevance of The CABG Patch Trial requires a brief review of the greater problem of the primary prevention of sudden cardiac death in patients with coronary artery disease. It is well recognized that the most important risk factor for sudden death is impaired ventricular function (2,3). Left ventricular function is believed to serve as a substrate for ventricular arrhythmias that may become manifest when exposed to a trigger. The presence of ventricular dysfunction by itself does not identify high-risk patients accurately enough. It is likely that the highest risk patients are those whose LV myocardium is both mechanically and electrically abnormal. Studies of the risk of sudden death have attempted to identify markers of this abnormal electrical substrate that will identify patients at highest absolute risk for sudden death. Such potential markers include late potentials documented by signal-averaged ECG, nonsustained VT (NSVT), inducible ventricular arrhythmias at electrophysiology study, abnormal heart rate variability, and abnormal baroreceptor sensitivity (4–6). The prevention of sudden death in patients with abnormal substrate requires the prevention of triggers or the prompt termination of ventricular arrhythmias once they have developed. The CABG Patch Trial sought to identify a group of patients with impaired LV function and electrical substrate identified by a positive, signal-averaged ECG. The potential arrhythmic trigger and/or substrate in these patients was coronary ischemia that was then modified by revascularization. The ICD allowed a method of termination of ventricular arrhythmias that might occur despite prior modification of the trigger (revascularization).

STRENGTHS/WEAKNESSES

The CABG Patch Trial was a well-run investigation that addressed an important facet of the problem of primary prevention of sudden cardiac death. It chose a well-defined group of patients at potentially high risk for sudden death based on depressed left ventricular function and an arrhythmic substrate. The arrhythmic substrate is implied by a positive SAECG and coronary artery disease. One can assume that most patients had depressed left ventricular function secondary to prior infarction—therefore, defining a possible substrate identified by the positive SAECG. The SAECG was chosen as an easy, noninvasive marker of substrate. Although the theoretical grounds for utilizing SAECG can be questioned (see below), this technology is widely available and easily applied. The 18% mortality at 2 years and 24% mortality observed at 42 months is higher than expected for surgical patients with depressed LV function and validates the SAECG as a marker of increased risk. This study also successfully identified a control group (not receiving antiarrhythmic medication) to compare with patients receiving an ICD. Finally, and perhaps most important, this study is unique amongst primary and secondary prevention studies of sudden death in that it addresses the issue of ischemia as a trigger for sudden death by attempting to completely revascularize all patients.

Many of the important weaknesses of The CABG Patch Trial resulted from the evolution in ICD technology that occurred during the course of the study. Specifically, the ICDs implanted in the study were epicardial committed devices without stored electrograms. The time added to bypass surgery as well as the increased risk of infection associated with implantation resulted in the removal of a significant proportion of the devices in this study. It is likely that many of these complications would have been avoided in the succeeding era of nonthoracotomy ICDs.

The initial CABG Patch report did not specify the percentage of cardiac deaths that were arrhythmic (1). It is possible that the defibrillator group had fewer arrhythmic deaths but more mortality related to procedural complications. Finally, though not apparently statistically significant, the defibrillator group had fewer patients on beta-blockers and more on type 1 antiarrhythmic agents and diuretics. We now recognize that class 1 antiarrhythmic agents and beta-blockers have a significant impact on mortality in patients with coronary artery disease and depressed left ventricular function (7,8). Furthermore, diuretics may be associated with metabolic abnormalities and an increased risk of sudden death (9).

Another important issue is the choice of a positive SAECG as a marker of high risk. Although the positive SAECG may have accounted for the increased mortality in this group of patients compared with the standard mortality for this surgical group, a number of potential problems are possible with the use of this marker. Specifically, it is important to know the timing of the documentation of late potentials. It is well recognized that the frequency of late potentials is greatest in the perimyocardial infarction period and may disappear during the following weeks or months as will the incremental risk of ventricular arrhythmias associated with the positive SAECG (10). It is quite possible that many of the patients enrolled in The CABG Patch Trial had had recent myocardial infarctions or ischemic episodes associated with the recording of a positive SAECG. In many instances, the surgery was probably performed weeks to months later and the late potentials and, therefore, the potential increased risk of sudden death had disappeared. For those patients in whom the positive SAECG was unassociated with recent infarction or ischemia, the question remains as to the effect of myocardial revascularization on late potentials. One study evaluating the effect of CABG on the SAECG noted post-CABG normalization of the pre-CABG positive SAECG in 29% of patients (11). It would have been useful for the CABG Patch investigators to have performed post-CABG SAECGs to make sure that the marker was stable and equally distributed between groups.

Finally, an important potential limitation of this study was the statistical power to detect a difference in mortality between the two groups. As will be discussed below, the 24-month total mortality was 18%. However, 5% of this mortality occurred in the early postoperative period leaving a post-30-day mortality of 13%. The overall mortality rates were less than anticipated and efforts were required to improve power by extending follow-up and slightly increasing the sample size (12).

WHAT HAS THE CABG PATCH TRIAL TAUGHT US?

The CABG Patch Trial was a study evaluating the preventative value of ICD implantation in patients with depressed LV function, electrically abnormal substrate, and active ischemic heart disease undergoing revascularization. The central questions of this study were: (1) if a positive SAECG (preoperatively) further identifies a fixed substrate and risk of postoperative events, does a prophylactic ICD save lives? and (2) What is the effect of surgical revascularization in patients with severe left ventricular dysfunction and such a substrate?

The findings of The CABG Patch Trial are best interpreted when compared with the results of other studies of primary and secondary prevention of sudden death. The 13% 2-year mortality (excluding 30-day post-op mortality) is higher than that seen in comparable patients in other surgical studies and suggests that the SAECG increased the risk of death. However, the causes of death are not reported and one cannot assume that they were arrhythmic. Furthermore, the overall mortality was not significantly impacted upon by the presence of an ICD. This would suggest that nonarrhythmic causes of death were dominant. The MADIT study evaluated the benefit of ICDs in patients with depressed LV function, NSVT, and inducible ventricular tachycardia (13). In both the MADIT and CABG Patch studies the device discharge rate approached 60% at 2 years of follow-up. However, the ICD only improved mortality in MADIT. It is likely that the older generation of devices in CABG Patch delivered many of the shocks for atrial arrhythmias or NSVT (secondary to the committed nature of these older devices) rather than more lethal ventricular arrhythmias. It is possible that part of the excess mortality in the CABG Patch patients was due to the relatively high prevalence (70%) of class 2 or 3 heart failure in this population. Other studies (14,15) assessing methods of primary prevention in patients with congestive heart failure have shown this group of patients to be amongst the highest risk groups for sudden death and total mortality (see Table 1).

Other important risk groups for sudden death include patients who are post-MI, particularly with depressed left ventricular function (see Table 1). The Beta Blocker Heart Attack Trial (BHAT) treated patients between 9 and 21 days following a heart attack with propranolol or placebo (17). The control group demonstrated a total mortality at 2 years of follow-up of 9.8% versus 7.2% in the beta-blocker group. The EMIAT trial evaluated the benefit of empiric amiodarone in postmyocardial infarction patients with depressed left ventricular function (18). There was no difference in outcome between the studied groups and the 2-year mortality was 14%. This compares with a 2-year mortality of 32% in the MADIT study, where depressed LV function, NSVT, and EPS-induced ventricular arrhythmias were required. In conclusion, the answer to the first question is that the SAECG probably identified a slight increase in risk above that imposed by coronary artery disease and depressed LV function. However, the prevalence of

Table 1 Two-Year Mortality in Studies of Primary and Secondary
Prevention of Sudden Death

Study (Ref.)	Patient characteristics	Two-year mortality
BHAT (17)	Post-MI	9.8%
EMIAT (18)	LVEF 30%, post-MI	14%
CABG Patch (1)	Ischemic heart disease + SAECG LVEF 36%	18%
AVID (16)	Sudden death, LVEF 32%	24%
MADIT (13)	LVEF 26%, NSVT, inducible VT	32%
CHF-STAT (14)	LVEF <40%, CHF Frequent VPDs	34%

congestive heart failure in this population may have accounted for the excess
mortality. Nonetheless, we cannot recommend ICD placement in comparable patients in our practice.

The second question regarding the value of revascularization in preventing
sudden death has been neglected by most primary and secondary prevention trials
of sudden death. An example is the CASCADE study, which evaluated the benefit
of empiric amiodarone in survivors of sudden death with depressed LV function
and congestive heart failure (19). Nearly 44% of the population in this study were
revascularized at or following randomization; however, no subgroup analysis is
available. The Coronary Artery Surgery Study (CASS) was not specifically a
study of primary prevention of sudden death but did document a reduction in
sudden death and total mortality in patients with multivessel CAD and depressed
LV function who underwent surgical revascularization compared with medical
management (20). This benefit was particularly pronounced if there was also
congestive heart failure (21). The CABG Patch Trial is the first prospective primary prevention study that controls this variable by selecting a homogeneous
group of patients all undergoing revascularization. The relatively low observed
total mortality compared with other trials of patients with comparable risk factors,
including CHF, suggests that revascularization conferred some benefit. It would
now be useful to test the value of ICDs in higher risk groups of patients (e.g.,
NSVT, inducible ventricular arrhythmias) with coronary artery disease undergoing CABG.

In conclusion, The CABG Patch Trial has demonstrated that ICDs are not
routinely indicated in patients with depressed left ventricular function and a positive SAECG who are undergoing CABG. It does suggest that revascularization
is an important method for the primary prevention of sudden death.

REFERENCES

1. Bigger JT. Prophylactic use of implanted cardiac defibrillators in patients at high risk for ventricular arrhythmias after coronary-artery bypass graft surgery. N Engl J Med 1997;337:1569–1575.

2. Bigger JT, Fleiss JL, Kleiger RE, Miller JP. Multicenter Post-Infarction Research Group. The relationships among ventricular arrhythmias, left ventricular dysfunction, and mortality in the 2 years after myocardial infarction. Circulation 1984;69: 250–258.

3. Mukharji J, Rude RE, Poole WK. The MILIS Study Group. Risk factors for sudden death after acute myocardial infarction: Two year follow-up. Am J Cardiol 1984; 54:31–36.

4. Buxton AE. Patients with nonsustained ventricular tachycardia. In: Akhtar M, Myerberg RJ, Ruskin JN. Sudden Cardiac Death: Prevalence, Mechanisms and Approaches to Diagnosis and Management. Baltimore: Williams and Wilkins, 1994: 486–496.

5. Wellens HJJ. Sudden death late after a myocardial infarction: Substrate and risk stratification. In: Akhtar M, Myerberg RJ, Ruskin JN. Sudden Cardiac Death: Prevalence, Mechanisms and Approaches to Diagnosis and Management. Baltimore: Williams and Wilkins, 1994:147–154.

6. Farrell TG et al. Risk stratification for arrhythmic events in postinfarction patients based on heart rate variability, ambulatory electrocardiographic variables and the signal-averaged electrocardiogram. J Am Coll Cardiol 1991;18:687.

7. Widerhorn J, Rahimtoola SH. Results of large-scale studies with β-adrenergic-blocking drugs and other non-antiarrhythmic agents for the prevention of sudden cardiac death. In: Akhtar M, Myerberg RJ, Ruskin JN. Sudden Cardiac Death: Prevalence, Mechanisms and Approaches to Diagnosis and Management. Baltimore: Williams and Wilkins, 1994:419–439.

8. Echt DS, Liebson PR, Mitchell LB. Mortality and morbidity in patients receiving encainide, flecainide, or placebo: The Cardiac Arrhythmia Suppression Trial. N Engl J Med 1991;324:781–788.

9. Siscovick DS, Raghunathan TE, Psaty BM, Kuepsell TD. Diuretic therapy and hypertension and the risk of primary cardiac arrest. N Engl J Med 1994;330(6):1852–1857.

10. El-Sheriff N, Ursell SN, Bekheit S. Prognostic significance of the signal-averaged ECG depends on the time of recording in the postinfarction period. Am Heart J 1989;118:256–264.

11. Borbola J, Serry C, Goldin M, Denes P. Short-term effect of coronary artery bypass grafting on the signal-averaged electrocardiogram. Am J Cardiol 1988;61:1001–1005.

12. Bigger JT, Parides MK, Rolnitzky LM, Meier P, Levin B, Egan DA. Changes in sample size and length of follow-up to maintain power in The Coronary Artery Bypass Graft (CABG) Trial. Controlled Clin Trials 1998;19:1–14.

13. Moss AJ, Hall WJ, Cannom DS, et al. Improved survival with an implanted defibrillator in patients with coronary artery disease at high risk for ventricular arrhythmia. N Engl J Med 1996;335:1933–1940.

14. Singh S, Fletcher RD, Fisher SG, Singh B. Amiodarone in patients with congestive heart failure and asymptomatic ventricular arrhythmia. N Engl J Med 1995:33:77–82.

15. Kober L, Torp-Pedersen C, Carlsen JE, Bagger H. A clinical trial of the angiotensin-converting-enzyme inhibitor Trandolapril in patients with left ventricular dysfunction after myocardial infarction. N Engl J Med 1995;333:1670–1676.

16. The Antiarrhythmics Versus Implantable Defibrillators (AVID) Investigators. A comparison of antiarrhythmic drug therapy with implantable defibrillators in patients resuscitated from near-fatal ventricular arrhythmias. N Engl J Med 1997;337:1576–1583.

17. Beta-blocker heart attack trial research group: A randomized trial of propranolol in patients with myocardial infarction: 1. Mortality results. JAMA 1982;247:1707–1717.

18. Julian DG, Camm AJ, Frangin G, Janse MJ. Randomised trial of effect of amiodarone on mortality in patients with left ventricular dysfunction after recent myocardial infarction: EMIAT. Lancet 1997;349:667–674.

19. The CASCADE investigators. Randomized antiarrhythmic drug therapy in survivors of cardiac arrest (The Cascade Study). Am J Cardiol 1993;72:280–287.

20. Passamani E, David KB, Gillespie MJ. A randomized trial of coronary artery bypass surgery: Survival of patients with a low ejection fraction. N Engl J Med 1985;312:1665–1671.

21. Holmes DR, Davis KB, Mock MB, Fisher LD. The effect of medical and surgical treatment on subsequent sudden cardiac death in patients with coronary artery disease: a report from the Coronary Artery Surgery Study. N Engl J Med 1986;73:1254–1263.

11

The European Myocardial Infarct Amiodarone Trial (EMIAT)

Yee Guan Yap and A. John Camm
St. George's Hospital Medical School, London, England

INTRODUCTION

The major cause of death in the first year after acute myocardial infarction (AMI) is sudden death, usually due to ventricular arrhythmias (1,2). Recognition of the relatively high rate of arrhythmic death has prompted the search for an effective antiarrhythmic drug that will prevent arrhythmias following an AMI. Apart from beta-blockers (3–5), angiotensin converting enzyme inhibitors (6), and aspirin (7), no other agents have been shown conclusively to reduce mortality. To date, there is little evidence that antiarrhythmic agents can reduce arrhythmic death. Amiodarone, however, is a unique antiarrhythmic agent that has proven to be effective in the treatment of sustained, life-threatening ventricular arrhythmias (8,9). Amiodarone is a coronary vasodilator, an anti-ischemic drug, and an anti-fibrillatory agent. Amiodarone is a complex molecule in that it uniquely possesses pharmacological properties from all four antiarrhythmic classes (10).

Class I: Sodium channel blockade that blocks or depresses ventricular conduction, resulting in suppression or slowing of ventricular tachycardia as well as suppression of ventricular premature depolarization.

Class II: Sympatholytic effects may lead to sinus node and atrioventricular node suppression and may also exert some protection against sudden death following acute myocardial infarction when there is sympathetic autonomic predominance.

Class III: Prolongation of action potential duration by amiodarone can prevent both reentrant atrial and ventricular arrhythmias.

225

Class IV: Calcium channel antagonism action that inhibits atrioventricular node conduction and may also reduce arrhythmogenesis (e.g., torsades de pointes) caused by early after-depolarization.

Several previous studies showed that amiodarone has a favorable effect in reducing mortality of high-risk patients, although the number of patients studied was too small to draw a definite conclusion. The Polish Amiodarone Study demonstrated that amiodarone significantly reduced cardiac mortality among survivors of MI who were not eligible for beta-blockers (11). In the Basel Antiarrhythmic Study of Infarct Survival (BASIS), amiodarone significantly reduced mortality in the first year after MI in patients with frequent or repetitive ventricular premature complexes (12). Similarly, the Canadian Amiodarone Myocardial Infarction Arrhythmia Trial (CAMIAT) pilot study showed that amiodarone substantially suppressed ventricular ectopic activity with little toxicity and was associated with a favorable trend toward a reduction in all-cause mortality (13). In the meta-analysis on placebo-controlled trials published by Teo et al. (14), amiodarone substantially improved survival in patients after myocardial infarction or with heart failure. These results formed the background against which both EMIAT and CAMIAT were designed. The EMIAT investigators decided to conduct a large trial of amiodarone in survivors of MI who were at increased risk of death.

HYPOTHESIS

EMIAT was a randomized placebo-controlled, double-blind trial. The aim of EMIAT was to assess whether amiodarone reduced all-cause mortality (primary endpoint), cardiac mortality, arrhythmic death, and arrhythmic death plus resuscitated cardiac arrests (secondary endpoints) in survivors of myocardial infarction with a left ventricular ejection fraction (LVEF) ≤40% (15,16).

RATIONALE AND METHODS

All patients with acute myocardial infarction admitted to coronary care units were screened. Eligible patients were those aged between 18 and 75 years who had a LVEF on multiple-gated nuclear angiography (MUGA) of ≤40%, performed between 5 and 21 days following AMI (Fig. 1). Some of the eligible patients had an initial echocardiographic ejection fraction assessed prior to the MUGA scan and those with echocardiographic left ventricular ejection fraction ≥50% were excluded from further enrolment into the trial. Patients with contraindications to amiodarone, those requiring active antiarrhythmic therapy, patients with

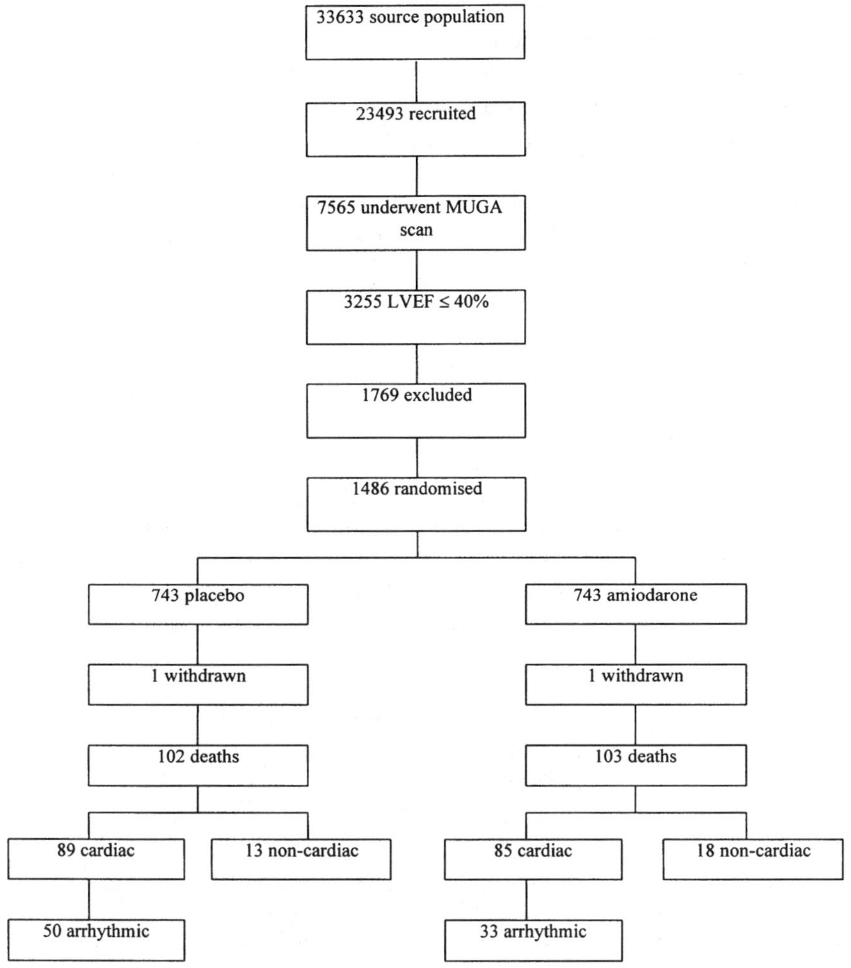

Figure 1 Trial profile. (Adapted from Ref. 16.)

severe angina or left ventricular failure, and patients likely to undergo imminent cardiac surgery were also excluded. Patients were randomized to treatment with amiodarone 800 mg/day, or matching placebo for 14 days, followed by amiodarone 400 mg/day for 14 weeks and 200 mg/day for the remainder of the study. A total of 1486 patients were recruited, 743 for each arm. The median follow-up was 21 months. The sample size calculations were based on a 15% 2-year mortality rate in the placebo group, with type I and type II error rates of 0.05

and 0.20, respectively. The calculation indicated that 1500 patients should be enrolled. The primary analyses were by intention to treat, although on-treatment (efficacy) analysis of outcome events in eligible patients while on study medication or within 3 months of early permanent discontinuation of treatment was also performed. At baseline (day of enrollment), continuous and categorical variables were compared by t test and χ^2 test, respectively. Survival curves according to treatment group were calculated by the Kaplan–Meier method and compared by the log-rank test. The risk ratio and 95% CI values were calculated by Cox's proportional hazards model.

RESULTS

The results showed that in an intention-to-treat analysis, at 24 months, the primary endpoint of all-cause mortality did not differ between the two groups (103 vs. 102 deaths; $p = 0.96$), nor did the cardiac mortality (85 vs. 89 deaths; $p = 0.67$) (Table 1 and Fig. 2) (16). However, in the amiodarone group, there was a 35% reduction in the risk of arrhythmic deaths (33 vs. 50 deaths, 95% CI 0.42-1.00; $p = 0.05$) (16). A similar risk reduction of 32% was obtained after the inclusion of resuscitated cardiac arrest to the arrhythmic deaths (42 vs. 61 deaths, 95% CI 0.46-1.00; $p = 0.05$). However, there was an excess of 13 cardiac but nonarrhythmic deaths (which could have resulted from chance or, at least in part, from the imbalance in baseline characteristics and treatments between the groups) and five noncardiac deaths (three pulmonary fibrosis), which offset this reduction in the arrhythmic deaths in the amiodarone group (Tables 2 and 3). EMIAT also demonstrated that, at 3 months, amiodarone treatment was associated with a significant reduction of arrhythmic death (with or without resuscitated cardiac arrest) compared with placebo (on-treatment analysis) (Table 4). Amiodarone significantly delayed the time to death for both all-cause mortality and arrhythmic death by more than 7 months in patients with LVEF=31–40% (Fig. 3). However, the

Table 1 Two-Year Mortality (Intention to Treat)

	Placebo	Amiodarone	RR	CI (95%)	p-Value
ACM	101	102	0.99	0.75–1.31	0.952
TCM	88	84	0.94	0.69–1.26	0.667
AD	50	33	0.65	0.42–1.01	0.05
AD + CAr	61	42	0.68	0.46–1.00	0.05

ACM = all-cause mortality; TCM = total cardiac mortality; AD = arrhythmic death; AD + CAr = arrhythmic death + resuscitated cardiac arrest.

Two-year Mortality (Intention to Treat)

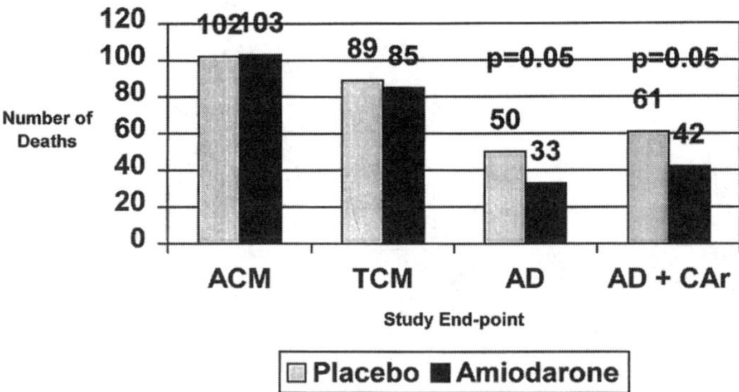

Figure 2 Endpoints analysis by treatment groups. Note that there is no difference in all-cause mortality and total cardiac mortality between the treatment groups. ACM = all-cause mortality. TCM = total cardiac mortality; AD = arrhythmic death; CAr = cardiac arrest.

survival benefit on all-cause mortality disappeared at 24 months. EMIAT also showed that there was an important synergistic interaction between amiodarone and beta-blockers in the reduction of mortality (Table 5). There were fewer cardiac deaths among amiodarone-treated patients who were receiving concomitant beta-blockers than among those who were not. Similarly, of those patients who

Table 2 Nonarrhythmic Cardiac Deaths

	Placebo (no.)	Amiodarone (no.)
Progressive LVF	25	26
Cardiogenic shock	2	4
Reinfarction	3	10
Surgery	3	3
EMD	2	0
Other	1	3
Unknown	3	6
Total	39	52

LVF = left ventricular failure; EMD = electromechanical dissociation.

Table 3 Unbalanced Baseline Parameters

Risk factors	Placebo (%)	Amiodarone (%)	p-Value
Previous MI	26	32	0.014
Angina history	33	36	0.208
Hypertension	30	35	0.119
NYHA (II/III)	50	55	0.087
Dyslipidemia	28	32	0.125
LVEF < 30%	46	48	0.074

received beta-blockers, there was a substantial reduction in the cardiac and arrhythmic mortality among those who were also given amiodarone.

DISCUSSION

EMIAT showed that amiodarone was associated with a significant reduction in the 2-year arrhythmic deaths and resuscitated cardiac arrests in patients with depressed left ventricular function after myocardial infarction. Such antiarrhythmic effect of amiodarone on arrhythmic death and resuscitated cardiac arrest was evident at 3 months after discontinuation of the treatment. However, there was neither a significant nor corresponding reduction in all-cause or total cardiac mortality at 2 years due to an increase in noncardiac, or cardiac but nonarrhythmic, mortality. The reduction in arrhythmic deaths and resuscitated cardiac arrests in EMIAT is offset by other forms of cardiac death (e.g., pump failure or reinfarction) and noncardiac death attributed to amiodarone toxicity. Thus, the risk in patients with LVEF $\leq$40% consists of both arrhythmic and nonarrhythmic deaths and despite the increased duration of life associated with amiodarone treat-

Table 4 On-Treatment Analysis (3 Months Rule)

	Placebo	Amiodarone	%RRR	p-Value
ACM	90	84	0	0.95
TCM	80	70	6	0.71
AD	45	23	44	0.018
AD + CAr	59	30	45	0.006

ACM = all-cause mortality; TCM = total cardiac mortality; AD = arrhythmic death; AD + CAr = arrhythmic death + resuscitated cardiac arrest.

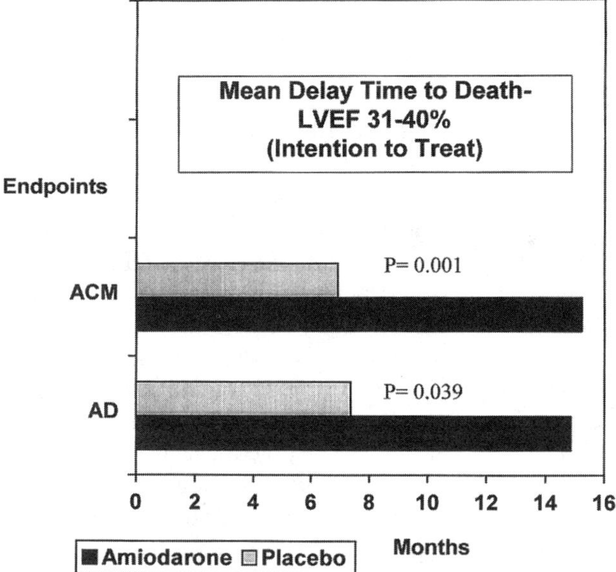

Figure 3 Mean delay time to death for both all-cause mortality and arrhythmic death in patients with LVEF 31–40%. Note that amiodarone significantly increased the duration of life for both all-cause mortality and arrhythmic death by more than 7 months. ACM = all-cause mortality; AD = arrhythmic death.

Table 5 Effect of Beta-Blocker on Total Cardiac Mortality

Beta-blocker	Amiodarone ($n = 743$)	Placebo ($n = 743$)	p-Value
Yes	15/325	28/333	0.005
($n = 658$)	(4.6%)	(8.4%)	
No	70/418	61/410	N.S.
($n = 828$)	(16.7)	(14.9%)	

Interaction between beta-blocker and total cardiac mortality: $p = 0.057$.

ment compared with placebo therapy, some of the patients probably died eventually from heart failure after having an arrhythmic death prevented by amiodarone. Based on the results of EMIAT alone, it is not clear whether the beneficial effect of amiodarone on arrhythmic death might translate into a beneficial effect on all-cause mortality. Hence, the evidence from EMIAT alone does not support the routine use of amiodarone in survivors of MI with depressed left ventricular function. However, the reduction in the risk of arrhythmic death suggests that, on balance, amiodarone is not proarrhythmic and affords protection from arrhythmic death in high-risk survivors of myocardial infarction. An additional benefit may be conferred by concomitant beta-blocker treatment. This is in contrast to the increase in arrhythmic death associated with prophylactic use of other class III agents such as d-sotalol (17) in post-MI patients with reduced LVEF.

Unlike other studies, such as the CAST (18) or CAMIAT (19), in which the mortality among placebo-group patients was lower than expected, EMIAT used a low LVEF ($\leq$ 40%) as the main inclusion criterion and achieved the anticipated number of trial endpoints. EMIAT also showed that many arrhythmic deaths occurred in patients who did not have frequent or complex ventricular premature complexes at baseline. An explanation may be that reducing arrhythmic deaths with amiodarone in patients with poor LVEF makes them "available" to die eventually from pump failure, whereas in patients with frequent or complex ventricular premature complexes but moderate LVEF, prophylactic treatment with amiodarone will prevent arrhythmic deaths but will not necessarily be followed by deaths due to pump failure. EMIAT represented one of the largest trials to date examining the prophylactic use of amiodarone in patients following acute myocardial infarction. However, despite relatively large numbers, EMIAT was underpowered to detect what turned out to be a modest reduction in the total mortality. The definitive indications of amiodarone require further clinical trials and/or meta-analysis with other placebo-controlled amiodarone survival studies.

To improve the selection of high-risk subgroups of patients who might benefit from prophylactic amiodarone treatment for future clinical trial, the EMIAT investigators recently performed a retrospective analysis on the baseline factors of the patients (20). The results showed that in a univariate analysis, all-cause mortality is reduced by amiodarone in patients with a LVEF <30%, with arrhythmia on the initial Holter, in patients on concomitant beta-blocker treatment, and in those with an increased initial heart rate. On the other hand, a trend toward an increase in all-cause mortality was noted in patients with a LVEF 30–40%, without arrhythmia on Holter, off beta-blockers, and with a low baseline heart rate. Such effects are additive in multivariate analysis. Thus, the results from the EMIAT substudy may help design future prospective trials in which amiodarone can be tested in patients with a recent MI, reduced LVEF, a high initial heart rate, and who are on beta-blocking drugs.

There have been two large meta-analyses examining the prophylactic use of amiodarone published since the publication of EMIAT (21,22). In the meta-analysis by the Amiodarone Trials Meta-Analysis Investigators (21), patient data from 13 randomized controlled trials of the prophylactic use of amiodarone in patients with recent MI (eight trials including CAMIAT and EMIAT) or congestive cardiac failure (CHF) (five trials) were pooled. Nine trials were double-blind, placebo-controlled and four compared amiodarone with usual care. A total of 6553 patients were randomized (78% post-MI and 22% with CHF). The results showed that sudden death or arrhythmic death in patients after a recent MI or patients with CHF was reduced by 29%, with this translating into an overall reduction of 13% in all-cause mortality when amiodarone was used prophylactically. The effect on nonarrhythmic death was neutral. There was no difference in the treatment effect between post-MI and CHF studies. Similarly, in a separate meta-analysis by Sim et al. (22), 15 randomized trials (5864 patients) were pooled and the effect of amiodarone on mortality was assessed. The result showed that amiodarone significantly reduced the total mortality by 19%, cardiac mortality by 23%, and sudden death by 30%. The mortality reductions were similar between trials enrolling patients after MI, with left ventricular dysfunction, and after cardiac arrest.

In conclusion, the results from these meta-analyses appear to strengthen the role of amiodarone as a prophylactic agent in suppressing arrhythmic deaths, as well as reducing all-cause mortality, which EMIAT was underpowered to detect in high-risk post-MI patients (i.e., those with poor LVEF or frequent ventricular premature complexes). Although amiodarone is not recommended for systematic prophylactic use in survivors of AMI, these findings appear to support early amiodarone treatment in high-risk patients with poor LVEF or ventricular arrhythmias after infarction. Use of low-dose amiodarone will prevent one death for every 43 postmyocardial infarction patients treated for 2 years (21).

REFERENCES

1. Rosenthal ME, Oseran DS, Gang E, Peter T. Sudden cardiac death following acute myocardial infarction. Am Heart J 1985;109:865–875.
2. Bigger JT, Jr, Heller CA, Wenger TL, et al. Risk stratification after acute myocardial infarction. Am J Cardiol 1978;42:202–210.
3. Beta-blocker Heart Attack Trial Research Group. A randomised trial of propranolol in patients with acute myocardial infarction. JAMA 1982;247:1701–1714.
4. The Norwegian Multicentre Study Group. Timolol-induced reduction in mortality and reinfarction in patients surviving acute myocardial infarction. Lancet 1979;11: 865–872.
5. Hjalmarson A, Elmfeldt D, Herlitz J, et al. Effect on mortality of metoprolol in acute myocardial infarction. A double-blind randomised trial. Lancet 1981;1:823–827.

6. Kober L, Torp-Pedersen C, Carlsen JE, Bagger H, Eliasen P, Lyngborg K, Videbaek J, Cole D, Auclert L, Pauly N, Aliot E, Persson S, Camm AJ, for the TRAndolapril Cardiac Evaluation (TRACE) Study Group. New Engl J Med 1995;333(25):1670–1676.

7. Second International Study of Infarct Survival Collaborative Group. Randomised trial of intravenous streptokinase, oral aspirin, both, or neither among 17,187 cases of suspected acute myocardial infarction: ISIS-2. Lancet 1988;2:349–360.

8. Podrid PJ. Amiodarone: re-evaluation of an old drug. Ann Intern Med 1995;122:689–700.

9. Herre JM, Sauve MJ, Malone P, et al. Long-term results of amiodarone therapy in patients with recurrent sustained ventricular tachycardia or ventricular fibrillation. J Am Coll Cardiol 1989;13:442–449.

10. Nattel S. Comparative mechanisms of action of antiarrhythmic drugs. Am J Cardiol 1993;72:13F–17F.

11. Ceremuzynski L, Leczar E, Krzeminska-Pakula M et al. Effect of amiodarone on mortality after myocardial infarction: a double-blind, placebo-controlled, pilot study. J Am Coll Cardiol 1992;20:1056–1062.

12. Burkart F, Pfisterer M, Kiowski W, Follath F, Burckhardt D. Effect of antiarrhythmic therapy on mortality of survivors of myocardial infarction with asymptomatic complex ventricular arrhythmias: Basel Antiarrhythmic Study of Infarct Survival (BASIS). J Am Coll Cardiol 1990;16:1711–1718.

13. Cairns JA, Connolly SC, Gent M, Roberts RS. Post myocardial infarction mortality in patients with ventricular premature depolarisations: Canadian Amiodarone Myocardial Infarction Arrhythmia Trial Pilot Study. Circulation 1991;84:550–557.

14. Teo KK, Yusuf S, Furberg CD. Effect of antiarrhythmic drug therapy in acute myocardial infarction: an overview of results from randomised controlled trials. JAMA 1993;270:1589–1995.

15. Camm AJ, Julian D, Janse G, Munoz A, Schwartz PJ, Simon P, Fragin G, on behalf of the EMIAT Investigators. The European Myocardial Infarct Amiodarone Trial (EMIAT). Am J Cardiol 1993;72:95F–102F.

16. Julian D, Camm AJ, Frangin G, Janse MJ, Munoz A, Schwartz PJ, Simon P, for the European Myocardial Infarct Amiodarone Trial Investigators. Lancet 1997;349:667–674.

17. Waldo AL, Camm AJ, deRuyter H, Friedman PL, MacNeil DJ, Pauls JF, Pitt B, Pratt CM, Schwartz PJ, Veitri EP, for the SWORD investigators. Effect of dsotalol on mortality in patients with left ventricular dysfunction after recent and remote myocardial infarction. Lancet 1996;348:7–12.

18. Echt DS, Liebson PR, Mitchell LB, Peters RW, Obias-Manno D, Barker AH, et al. Mortality and morbidity in patients receiving encanide, flecanide or placebo. The Cardiac Arrhythmia Suppression Trial. N Engl J Med 1991;324:781–787.

19. Cairns JA, Connolly SJ, Roberts R, Gent M for the Canadian Amiodarone Myocardial Infarction Arrhythmia Trial Investigators. Randomised trial of outcome after myocardial infarction in patients with frequent or repetitive ventricular premature depolarisarions: CAMIAT. Lancet 1997;349:675–682.

20. Janse MJ, Malik M, Camm AJ, Julian DG, Frangin GA, Schwartz PJ, on behalf of the CAMIAT Investigators. Eur Heart J 1998;19:85–95.

21. Amiodarone Trials Meta-Analysis Investigators. Effect of prophylactic amiodarone on mortality after acute myocardial infarction and in congestive heart failure: meta-analysis of individual data from 6500 patients in randomised trials. Lancet 1997; 350:1417–1424.

22. Sim I, McDonald KM, Lavori PW, Norbutas CM, Hlatky MA. Quantitative overview of randomised trials of amiodarone to prevent sudden cardiac death. Circulation 1997;96:2823–2829.

Andrew E. Epstein

The University of Alabama at Birmingham, Birmingham, Alabama

The European Myocardial Infarct Amiodarone Trial (EMIAT) was a primary prevention study designed to determine whether amiodarone reduces the mortality of patients at high risk for death after myocardial infarction (1). Unlike most other trials evaluating amiodarone, EMIAT studied patients with impaired left ventricular function (left ejection fraction ≤ 0.40) irrespective of ambient ventricular arrhythmias. This double-blind, placebo-controlled trial showed that all-cause and cardiac mortality were no different in the amiodarone-treated and placebo-treated patient groups. However, in the amiodarone group, a 35% reduction in the risk for antiarrhythmic death was observed. Unfortunately, this was offset by a 33% increase in nonarrhythmic death leading to negation of any benefit for overall survival.

STRENGTHS OF EMIAT

Studies such as EMIAT, with an apparently negative conclusion, are sometimes viewed as being unimportant. On the contrary, EMIAT is important. Sudden cardiac death remains a serious public health problem, especially in survivors of myocardial infarction (2). Those with left ventricular dysfunction and ambient ventricular ectopy identify individuals at particularly high risk. Thus, primary prevention interventions with antiarrhythmic drugs and devices to prevent fatal arrhythmia occurrence have been studied. The Cardiac Arrhythmia Suppression Trial (CAST) (3) and the Survival With ORal d-Sotalol (SWORD) trial (4) found antiarrhythmic drug prophylaxis to prevent sudden cardiac death disappointing. However, a meta-analysis by Teo et al. raised the possible utility of amiodarone for this purpose (5). The EMIAT results are consistent with this hypothesis. In

EMIAT, amiodarone was a safe drug in patients with ischemic heart disease. It decreased the rate of arrhythmic death and resuscitated cardiac arrest and did not increase total mortality. Although the Multicenter Automatic Defibrillator Implantation Trial (MADIT) showed that implantable defibrillators could decrease all-cause and arrhythmic mortality in high-risk patients following myocardial infarction (6), patients in MADIT were highly selected, and the implantable defibrillator is not universally available.

EMIAT has several important strengths: first, high-risk patients were enrolled irrespective of ambient ventricular arrhythmias. This is a distinctly different population from those enrolled in previously reported primary prevention trials to improve survival following myocardial infarction. It was eminently reasonable to enroll such patients since left ventricular dysfunction is such a powerful predictor of mortality. A second strength of EMIAT is the inclusion of a registry that details the source population, the patients recruited, the individuals who underwent assessment of left ventricular function, reasons for exclusion, and, finally, the 1486 patients randomized in the trial. These data provide assurance that the patients included in EMIAT were representative of our clinical practices. Of the 3255 patients with qualifying left ventricular ejection fractions (≤ 0.40), 1769 were excluded (54%), a not unusual proportion in the conduct of clinical trials. Furthermore, the reasons for exclusion were reasonable, including lack of patient consent (409), imminent cardiac surgery (286 patients), other serious illnesses presumed to limit longevity (205 patients), important congestive heart failure (179 patients), amiodarone treatment within the previous 6 months (142 patients), antiarrhythmic treatment that was deemed essential (142 patients), and other contraindications (406 patients). Indeed, the rate of exclusion for lack of physician or patient consent is lower than those excluded in other trials where registries are detailed [35% in CAST (7) and 26% in the Antiarrhythmics Versus Implantable Defibrillators (AVID) trial (8)].

A third strength of EMIAT is that amiodarone given in the doses used in the trial (800 mg for 14 days, 400 mg for 14 weeks, and then 200 mg a day until end of the study) can be given on an entirely outpatient basis. Although the authors suggest that high dosing may have accounted for the increased early mortality, the doses, in fact, were not as large as those used for sustained, life-threatening ventricular arrhythmias. In the recently launched Atrial Fibrillation Follow-Up Investigation of Rhythm Management (AFFIRM) study (9), doses such as these are often given on an outpatient basis for patients with atrial fibrillation. It is further gratifying to recognize that there was no torsades de pointes ventricular tachycardia observed in EMIAT, and even if there was proarrhythmia due to amiodarone, any such events did not outweigh amiodarone's antiarrhythmic benefit since the risk of arrhythmic death was decreased in the trial.

The final strength of the study is that not only intention-to-treat but also on-treatment analyses were performed. Indeed, the benefit of amiodarone to decrease arrhythmic death was even more evident in patients receiving the drug than when analyzed on an intention-to-treat basis. Nevertheless, by reporting overall mortality, problems of event classification are circumvented (10).

LIMITATIONS OF EMIAT

Despite its strengths, EMIAT, as is the case for all studies of this type, was not perfect. In EMIAT, 284 (38.5%) of the amiodarone-treated patients discontinued their study medication compared to 158 (21.4%) of placebo-treated patients. The most common reasons for discontinuance were noncompliance (placebo-treated patients 7.8%, amiodarone-treated patients 9.4%) and endocrine disorders (1.6% placebo-treated patients, 5.9% amiodarone-treated patients). Although this high dropout rate limits the interpretation of both the intention-to-treat and on-treatment analyses, one must recognize that in a trial of prophylactic treatment of patients without arrhythmic events, the impetus for continuing a drug with important adverse effects is probably less than in a secondary prevention trial when the patients have already manifested a life-threatening problem. Thus, the high dropout rate is easily understandable from the clinician's point of view.

Some may view the classification of cardiac deaths as sudden, nonsudden, or unwitnessed as being artificial. However, there is, unfortunately, no other mechanism than the use of ''validation'' committees to adjudicate events in clinical trials. Although some may argue that the classification system is imperfect, most would agree that the use of event committees is probably more desirable than having the responsibility for assigning cause of death rest with individual investigators (11).

Finally, it must be recognized that the use of the most effective drugs available to decrease overall mortality in patients with myocardial infarction were not optimally employed. Beta-blockers and ACE inhibitors were used in only 45% and 44%, respectively, and 58% and 59%, respectively, of the placebo-treated and amiodarone-treated patients. Despite the imperfect application of these life-saving therapies, it still must be recognized that their use exceeds the administration witnessed in other important antiarrhythmic trials such as CAST (3), MADIT (6), and AVID (12). The relevance of the suboptimal application of known beneficial therapies is discussed below.

QUESTIONS RAISED BY EMIAT

Although EMIAT did not show that amiodarone enhances overall survival in patients who survive myocardial infarction, it does raise several important questions that are left unanswered. First, the roles of concomitant therapies, such as beta-blockers and ACE inhibitors, are still open to question. A subanalysis showed a distinct benefit of beta-blockers to patients in the trial (1). There were fewer nonsudden and arrhythmic cardiac deaths among amiodarone-treated patients who were receiving beta-blockers than among those who were not. Thus, EMIAT raises the question whether agents that are known to improve overall survival (such as beta-blockers and ACE inhibitors) can be combined with drugs that decrease arrhythmic death to synergistically decrease both nonsudden and sudden cardiac death. There is, in fact, an emerging literature on the role of beta-blockade to decrease mortality in patients with heart failure and left ventricular dysfunction (13). Would it not be interesting if beta-blockers (to decrease death due to heart failure) combined with amiodarone (to decrease death due to arrhythmias) together improved overall survival with less sudden and nonsudden cardiac death?

EMIAT differed from other primary prevention trials using antiarrhythmic drugs in that the presence of ambient ventricular ectopy was not a criterion for inclusion. However, ambulatory electrocardiograms were obtained on most patients (1367 of whom 191 died). Interestingly, the mortality rate was higher in those with arrhythmias [112/548 (20%)] compared to those without ambient ventricular arrhythmias [79/819 (10%)]. Thus, one ''sub-subset'' of myocardial infarction survivors who may receive a special benefit from combined antiarrhythmic/antiischemic/heart failure therapy may be those with both left ventricular dysfunction and nonsustained ventricular arrhythmias.

IMPLICATIONS FOR FURTHER RESEARCH

The major challenge for further research is the identification of subsets of patients who may benefit from specific antiarrhythmic therapies. Myerburg et al. called attention to the fact that the majority of sudden deaths occur in patients without prior identifiable heart disease (2). Thus, although certain groups may be identified as being at high risk, they, in fact, contribute only a minority of the events of arrhythmic death from the larger population of patients who have no apparently predisposing factors. This concept has been extended by Wilber et al. who showed that postinfarction patients with left ventricular dysfunction, nonsustained ventricular tachycardia, and inducible sustained ventricular tachycardia, although at high risk, contribute only a trivial, minority of sudden deaths in the population at risk for the event (14). Thus, the major challenge for further research as identified by EMIAT is the identification of patients who may most benefit from prophylactic antiarrhythmic therapy.

IMPLICATIONS FOR THE PRACTICE OF MEDICINE

The authors of EMIAT clearly state that ''Our findings do not support the systematic prophylactic use of amiodarone in patients with poor left ventricular function after myocardial infarction, irrespective of the presence of symptomless ventricular ectopy activity.'' This is a responsible conclusion in view of the adverse drug reactions that can be caused by amiodarone and the lack of improvement in overall survival in their trial. However, EMIAT also showed that amiodarone can be administered safely to patients with left ventricular dysfunction at risk for cardiac death. Torsades de pointes ventricular tachycardia proarrhythmia was not observed.

One explanation for the failure of amiodarone to reduce nonarrhythmic death is that nonarrhythmic death increased because arrhythmic death was prevented. The reasons for the relatively high dropout rate of patients receiving amiodarone is probably due to reasons detailed above, specifically that the enthusiasm for continuing a drug with systemic adverse drug reactions that are potentially fatal or morbid was not felt to be justified in a primary prevention clinical trial. The effect of patient drop-out (and crossover) in clinical trials is to decrease to power of studies to establish a difference in treatments when one in fact exists. Thus, the utility of amiodarone prophylaxis in patients with cardiovascular disease has probably not been resolved by EMIAT. Indeed, the results of trials examining the use of amiodarone to extend life and prevent sudden, arrhythmic cardiac death have been inconsistent. Using a variety of analytic methods, grouped data (that include the results of EMIAT) suggest that amiodarone may reduce overall and sudden death mortality by up to 19% (15,16).

A final message from EMIAT is that patients at risk for cardiac death should not be deprived of therapies unequivocally known to be life-saving. Specifically, beta-blockers, ACE inhibitors, and aspirin are not being prescribed optimally. It is well known that the patients at greatest risk derive the greatest benefit, and that these are the patients who are probably being systematically excluded from receiving the therapy that may be the most beneficial. If the general care of patients with cardiovascular disease were enhanced, other potentially life-saving therapies could be used to give an even greater ''extra edge'' to these patients.

REFERENCES

1. Julian DG, Camm AJ, Frangin G, Janse MJ, Munoz A, Schwartz PJ, Simon P, for the European Myocardial Infarct Amiodarone Trial Investigators. Randomised trial of effect of amiodarone on mortality in patients with left-ventricular dysfunction after recent myocardial infarction: EMIAT. Lancet 1997;349:667–674.
2. Myerburg RJ, Kessler KM, Castellanos A. Epidemiology of sudden cardiac death: Emerging strategies for risk assessment and control. In: Dunbar SB, Ellenbogen KA, Epstein AE, eds. Sudden Cardiac Death: Past, Present, and Future. Mt. Kisco: Futura Publishing Company, Inc, 1997:29–51.

3. Epstein AE, Hallstrom AP, Rogers WJ, Liebson PR, Seals AA, Anderson JL, Cohen JD, Capone RJ, Wyse DG, for the CAST Investigators. Mortality following ventricular arrhythmia suppression by encainide, flecainide, and moricizine after myocardial infarction: The original design concept of the Cardiac Arrhythmia Suppression Trial (CAST). JAMA 1993;270:2451–2455.

4. Waldo AL, Camm AJ, deRuyter H, Friedman PL, MacNeil DJ, Pauls JF, Pitt B, Pratt CM, Schwartz PJ, Veltri EP, for the SWORD Investigators. Effect of d-sotalol on mortality in patients with left ventricular dysfunction after recent and remote myocardial infarction. Lancet 1996;348:7–12.

5. Teo KK, Yusuf S, Furberg CD. Effects of prophylactic antiarrhythmic drug therapy in acute myocardial infarction: An overview of results from randomized controlled trials. JAMA 1993;270:1589–1595.

6. Moss AJ, Hall WJ, Cannom DS, Daubert JP, Higgins SL, Klein H, Levine JH, Saksena S, Waldo AL, Wilber D, Brown MW, Heo M, for the Multicenter Automatic Defibrillator Implantation Trial Investigators. Improved survival with an implanted defibrillator in patients with coronary disease at high risk for ventricular arrhythmia. N Engl J Med 1996;335:1933–1940.

7. Gorkin L, Schron EB, Handshaw K, Shea S, Kinney MR, Branyon M, Campion J, Bigger JT, Sylvia SC, Duggan J, Stylianou M, Lancaster S, Ahern KD, Follick MJ. Clinical trial enrollers vs. nonenrollers: The Cardiac Arrhythmia Suppression Trial (CAST) Recruitment and Enrollment Assessment in Clinical Trials (REACT) Project. Controlled Clin Trials 1996;17:46–59.

8. Curtis AB, Hallstrom AP, Klein RC, Nath S, Pinski SL, Epstein AE, Wyse DG, Cannom DS, Renfroe E, and the AVID Investigators. Influence of patient characteristics in the selection of patients for defibrillator implantation (The AVID Registry). Am J Cardiol 1997;79:1185–1189.

9. The Planning and Steering Committees of the AFFIRM Study for the NHLBI AFFIRM Investigators. Atrial Fibrillation Follow-up Investigation of Rhythm Management—The AFFIRM Study design. Am J Cardiol 1997;79:1198–1202.

10. Kim SG, Fogoros RN, Furman S, Connolly S, Kuck KH, Moss AJ, for the Participants of the Policy Conference. Standardized reporting of ICD patient outcome: The report of a North American Society of Pacing and Electrophysiology Policy Conference, February 9–10, 1993. PACE 1993;16:1358–1362.

11. Epstein AE, Carlson MD, Fogoros RN, Higgins SL, Venditti FJ. Classification of death in antiarrhythmia trials. J Am Coll Cardiol 1996;27:433–442.

12. The AVID Investigators (prepared by the AVID Executive Committee: Zipes DP, Wyse DG, Friedman PL, Epstein AE, Hallstrom AP, Greene HL, Schron EB, Domanski M). A comparison of antiarrhythmic drug therapy with implantable defibrillators in patients resuscitated from near-fatal sustained ventricular arrhythmias. N Engl J Med 1997;337:1576–1583.

13. Heidenreich PA, Lee TT, Massie BM. Effect of beta-blockade on mortality in patients with heart failure: A meta-analysis of randomized clinical trials. J Am Coll Cardiol 1997;30:27–34.

14. Wilber DJ, Kall JG, Kopp DE. What can we expect from prophylactic implantable defibrillators? Am J Cardiol 1997;80:20F–27F.

15. Amiodarone Trials Meta-Analysis Investigators. Effect of prophylactic amiodarone on mortality after acute myocardial infarction and in congestive heart failure: Meta-analysis of individual data from 6500 patients in randomised trials. Lancet 1997; 350:1417–1424.
16. Sim I, McDonald KM, Lavori PW, Norbutas CM, Hlatky MA. Quantitative overview of randomized trials of amiodarone to prevent sudden cardiac death. Circulation 1997;96:2823–2829.

12

The Canadian Amiodarone Myocardial Infarction Arrhythmia Trial (CAMIAT)

John A. Cairns

University of British Columbia, Vancouver, British Columbia, Canada

INTRODUCTION

The genesis of CAMIAT (1,2) lay in the recognition in 1983 by a group of Canadian investigators that the presence of ventricular arrhythmias in the post-acute myocardial infarction (AMI) period was predictive of a worse prognosis, that the prevalence was high, and that there was no consensus as to appropriate prophylactic therapy (3–7). The presence of frequent or repetitive ventricular premature depolarizations (VPDs) had been shown to contribute to mortality risk independently of left ventricular dysfunction (6,7). A variety of approaches to the detection of the arrhythmias were followed and the use of antiarrhythmic drugs, particularly those in Vaughan Williams class I, was common. There was no clear evidence for their benefit, although there appeared to be a sound rationale to their use. Several randomized trials of antiarrhythmic drug therapy had been reported prior to 1981, but none demonstrated a benefit (8). There was clearly a need for a well-designed clinical trial to evaluate drug therapy among survivors of AMI with frequent or repetitive VPDs.

At that time, the profile of amiodarone in North America was of a drug that was complex to use, had a high incidence of dangerous side effects, and that should be reserved for patients with life-threatening ventricular arrhythmias who had failed conventional antiarrhythmic drugs. Nevertheless, to the group of Canadian cardiologists, amiodarone appeared to be the most promising drug to test with its apparent efficacy against major ventricular arrhythmias, and its acceptable risk profile during extensive clinical experience. Accordingly, a team of cardiologists and biostatisticians/epidemiologists at McMaster University, in

245

conjunction with colleagues from centers across Canada, undertook to test the following hypothesis: "The administration of amiodarone will reduce 2-year mortality from cardiac arrhythmias among survivors of AMI found, within 45 days of infarction, to have frequent or repetitive VPDs on 24-hour ambulatory electrocardiogram."

PILOT STUDY

In preparation for a large, multicenter clinical trial, we undertook a pilot study, the objectives of which were to evaluate the efficacy of amiodarone for the suppression of VPDs, the toxicity of amiodarone, the rates of outcome events, and the feasibility of the planned multicenter trial (9). Funding was provided by the Medical Research Council of Canada and by Sanofi Pharmaceuticals (New York, New York). The study was conducted during 1986–1988 in the five coronary care units of the university teaching hospitals of Hamilton, Ontario, Canada. There were 77 patients enrolled; each had experienced an AMI within the previous 6 to 45 days and had $\geq$ to 10 VPDs/h, or ≥ 1 run of ventricular tachycardia during 24 h of electrocardiographic (ECG) recording. They were randomized in a double-blind fashion in a 2:1 amiodarone-to-placebo ratio. The loading dose was 10 mg/kg/day for 3 weeks. The maintenance dose was 300 to 400 mg/day with reductions at 4-month intervals in response to VPD suppression, excessive amiodarone plasma levels, or toxicity. VPD suppression on amiodarone at week 1 and week 2 was 63% and 85%, respectively, and on placebo 17% and 27%, respectively.

Apart from elevation of serum thyrotropin and skin reactions, no side effects occurred more frequently with amiodarone. The study drug was stopped for side effects or noncompliance in 35% of amiodarone patients and 34% of placebo patients. The patients were followed for a maximum of 2 years (mean, 20 months). Arrhythmic death or resuscitated ventricular fibrillation occurred in 2 of 48 amiodarone patients (4%) and 4 of 29 placebo patients (14%), whereas the rates of all-cause mortality were 5 of 48 (10%) and 6 of 29 (21%), respectively. We concluded that amiodarone, in moderate loading and maintenance doses with adjustments in response to plasma levels, VPD suppression, and side effects, resulted in effective VPD suppression and acceptable levels of toxicity. The rate of recruitment and the degree of compliance indicated that a multicenter trial should be feasible. Slight modifications were made to the pilot study protocol, including shortening the loading period to 2 weeks, establishing a minimum dose of 200 mg 5 to 7 days/week, simplifying monitoring of holters, chest x-rays, pulmonary function measurements and blood tests, and omitting monitoring of amiodarone blood levels.

METHODS

The main trial was eventually funded jointly by the MRC and Sanofi under the University-Industry Program in 1989, but it was 1990 before the Health Protection Branch (HPB) was satisfied with the protocol and the first patient was randomized in June 1990. The final patient was randomized in November 1994, about 5 months later than originally projected, and follow-up was complete by November 1995. There was concern that the unfavorable results of CAST (10) might diminish enthusiasm for the trial, but the opposite occurred, and when CAST II (11) was published, interest and participation was further stimulated. Evidence for benefit of amiodarone emerging from the BASIS trial (12) and the Polish Arrhythmia trial (13) did not appear to diminish interest in the CAMIAT hypotheses.

Patient Entry

The source population was patients older than 19 years who had survived AMI 6 to 45 days previously. The target population were those with an ambulatory ECG (minimum duration 18 h) showing a mean of 10 VPD/h or more, or at least one run of VT (>3 beats at a rate of 100–120/min or 3–10 beats at a rate of >120/min). Exclusion criteria were contraindications to amiodarone (previous intolerance, sustained heart rate <50/min; first-degree, second-degree, or third-degree heart block, QTc >480 ms, moderate or severe peripheral neuropathy, chronic or acute hepatitis, suggestion of interstitial fibrosis on chest radiographs, clinical hypothyroidism or hyperthyroidism or current therapy for these conditions, asthma, women of child-bearing potential); perceived requirement for antiarrhythmic therapy (run of VT >120/min, length >10 beats, arrhythmia which in the opinion of the attending physician required antiarrhythmic drug therapy other than beta-blocker or digoxin, requirement for tricyclic antidepressant, phenytoin, or sotalol); concurrent disease (class 4 congestive heart failure or angina, severe hypotension, uncorrected hypokalemia, or noncardiac illness likely to shorten survival to less than 2 years); and geographical or social factors that made study participation impractical.

A nurse practitioner visited the coronary care units of the participating hospitals regularly and documented every case of myocardial infarction according to study criteria. All patients with AMI were assessed for the presence of any cause for exclusion. Eligible patients were monitored by 24-h ambulatory ECG, which had to be done within 6 to 45 days of onset of AMI. Patients with 10 or more VPDs/h or at least one run of VT according to the hospital's interpretation of the 24-h ECG recording, were asked to give their informed consent to take part in the study. Most monitor tapes were also interpreted at the central facility,

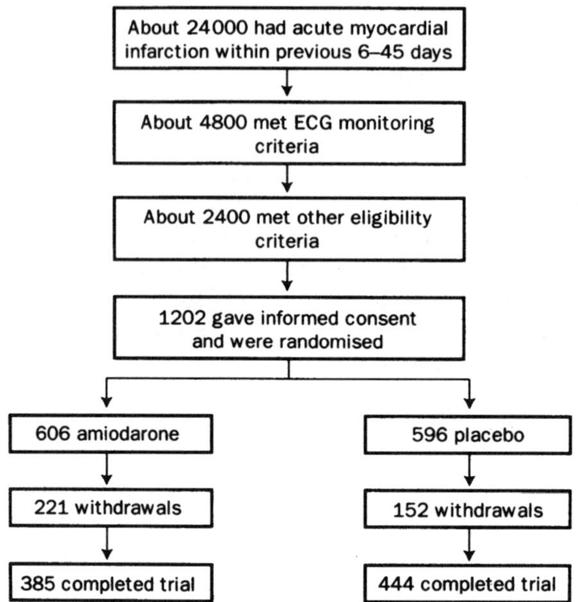

Figure 1   Patient flow diagram. (Reprinted from Ref. 1, with permission.)

but 5% of the recordings were in real-time format and interpreted only at the local hospital.

The flow diagram of patients screened, entry, and follow-up is depicted in Figure 1. Following consent, patients were assigned a study identification number and follow-up began. The corresponding, previously randomly ordered treatment pack was opened and drug loading was begun. The complete randomization code was available only to the Chair of the External Safety and Efficacy Monitoring Committee. Hence, patients, treating physicians, steering committee, external safety and efficacy monitoring committee, the coordination and methods center, and Sanofi Winthrop were unaware of therapeutic allocation. In an emergency, the randomization code could be broken by opening a sealed drug identification label stored on site or by contacting the 24-h telephone response line.

Treatment and Follow-Up

Patients received a loading dose of 10 mg/kg amiodarone or placebo in two divided daily doses for 2 weeks, when the dose was reduced to 400 mg/day. Patients who weighed less than 60 kg or who were older than 75 years received

300 mg/day. Holter monitors were repeated at 4 and 8 months, and if VPDs were suppressed, the dose of amiodarone was reduced to 300 or 200 mg/day, then 200 mg 7 or 5 days/week. Arrhythmia suppression was defined as the absence of ventricular tachycardia and a reduction in the rate of VPDs relative to the rate recorded on ambulatory ECG at baseline (i.e., a reduction to 10% or less for a baseline rate of 240–720 VPDs per 24 h, and a reduction to 20% or less for a baseline rate of more than 720 VPDs/24 h.

Patients were assessed by a nurse practitioner in consultation with a physician at baseline, week 2, month 4, and then every 4 months for up to 24 months. In addition, intermediate follow-up was done by telephone every 2 months. Planned follow-up was for 2 years, except for patients who entered the study during the final year of enrollment, who were followed up for 1 to 2 years. A schedule defined the timing of chest x-rays and measurement of thyrotropin, AST, and alkaline phosphatase. Hypothyroidism was defined as a thyrotropin concentration of >10 mU/L or a perceived need to prescribe thyroxin. The nurses followed protocols for the management of known toxic effects of amiodarone. Proarrhythmia was defined as the occurrence of a run of VT of >20 beats in duration at a rate >120/min, or as an increase in the number of episodes of VT/24 h on ambulatory electrocardiography (from June 1990 to January 1993: more than a tenfold increase from baseline number of episodes; from January 1993 to November 1995: for a baseline number of episodes of 1–10 per 24 h, 11–50 per 24 h, or >50 per 24 h, an increase of >30-fold, >20-fold, or >10-fold, respectively). Canadian Health Protection Branch regulations required withdrawal of the patient from treatment for the occurrence of proarrhythmia or resuscitated VF.

Outcome Events

Resuscitated ventricular fibrillation—loss of consciousness and pulse, VF documented on ECG monitor, direct current counter shock administered, patient establishes spontaneous cardiac output (no longer dependent on external massage), and survives for at least 7 days.

Arrhythmic death—death from rapid VT or VF, patient expected to survive at least 4 months had this rhythm not occurred. Loss of cardiac output and pulse is sudden and precedes collapse of the circulation (defined as a state of very low cardiac output, poor peripheral perfusion, systolic blood pressure <80 mmHg, or dependence on intravenous inotropic support) or severe pulmonary edema, characterized by severe respiratory distress of sudden onset without evidence of noncardiac cause. The patient is not already in shock or pulmonary edema at the time of onset of the arrhythmia.

Other cardiac death—patient develops collapse of the circulation or is in shock or severe pulmonary edema before loss of cardiac output and fatal

arrhythmia. Special categories included monitored patients who had profound bradycardia or asystole, or a rhythm generally compatible with
normal cardiac output, and, therefore, probably electromechanical dissociation, immediately before abrupt circulatory collapse.
  Noncardiac vascular death—for example, ruptured aortic aneurysm, other
    hemorrhage, cerebral vascular accident, pulmonary embolus.
  Nonvascular death—for example, trauma, infection, malignant disease.

  The outcome events reported by the clinical investigators were all reviewed
by an External Validation Committee, the members of which were blinded as to
treatment allocation. This committee had final responsibility for the verification
of resuscitated VF and the classification of deaths.
  The primary outcome was the composite of resuscitated VF or arrhythmic
death among patients who had not been permanently discontinued from amiodarone for 3 months or more. The secondary outcomes were arrhythmic death,
cardiac death, and all-cause mortality. No patient who had an outcome event
could be deemed retrospectively to have previously stopped study medication,
and once a patient had stopped study medication for more than 3 months, it
could not be restarted. All outcomes were also analyzed by the intention-to-treat
principle.

Statistics

We anticipated a 2-year all-cause mortality rate of 15%, with 50% of deaths from
arrhythmia. We expected that amiodarone would reduce the arrhythmic deaths
by 50% (from 7.5% to 3.75%), but would have no effect on nonarrhythmic deaths
(25% reduction of total mortality from 15% to 11.25%). With a beta error of 0.2
and a one-sided alpha of 0.05, we estimated that 1200 patients were required to
detect 50% reduction of arrhythmic death. We expected that the composite outcome of resuscitated ventricular fibrillation or arrhythmic death would provide
increased statistical power for the detection of benefit from amiodarone. The
sample size was not large enough to detect the anticipated 25% reduction in all-
cause mortality with any reasonable power. Several studies had suggested a benefit of amiodarone over placebo, and the aim of our study was to show such a
benefit. We established asymmetric stopping guidelines for the External Safety
and Efficacy Monitoring Committee, so the trial would have been stopped at any
one of three formal, interim analyses during the trial at about 25%, 50%, and
75% of the accumulated years at risk. The trial was to have been stopped early
if the efficacy analysis for the primary outcome showed a p value of less than
0.001, or if the 95% Cl ruled out a relative risk reduction of more than 20% in

favor of amiodarone. We, therefore, used a one-sided test of significance to test the differences in outcome events between the amiodarone and placebo groups.

RESULTS

Patient Population

We enrolled 1202 patients (606 in the amiodarone group, 596 in the placebo group) and followed them for a minimum of 1 year and a maximum of 2 years [mean 1.79 years (SD 0.44)]. No patient was lost to follow-up. The baseline ambulatory ECG showed that 20% of patients had only VT, 60.4% had only a mean of $\geq$ to 10 VPD/h, and 18.6% met both these criteria. Eleven (1%) enrolled patients did not meet the arrhythmia criteria, but were retained in the trial. The amiodarone and placebo groups were well matched in terms of baseline characteristics and use of concomitant medications at the time of enrollment. Aspirin (83%), beta-blockers (60%), and ACE inhibitors (32%) were commonly used, and 47% and 50% had received thrombolytic therapy.

The mean VPD frequencies on baseline ambulatory ECG monitoring were for amiodarone 100/h and for placebo 104/h, and median frequencies were, respectively, 30/h and 34/h.

Compliance and Side Effects

The mean loading doses of study drug were 776 mg/day for amiodarone and 771 mg/day for placebo. By month 4, the mean daily doses had fallen to 308 mg and 351 mg, respectively. By 1 year, they were 208 mg and 294 mg, respectively, and during year 2, they were 211 mg and 301 mg, respectively. By month 4, arrhythmia suppression was detected in 84% of amiodarone group patients and in 35% of placebo patients, and by month 8, in 86% and 39%, respectively.

Adherence to the treatment regimen was assessed by pill count at each 4-monthly follow-up visit and was defined as the percentage of the prescribed dose that had been taken during the preceding 4 months. The mean percentage of the prescribed drug being taken at each follow-up was 75% of the amiodarone group, 78% in the placebo group, and only 6% of patients in each group took less than 50% of the prescribed dose.

Early permanent discontinuation of study drug for reasons other than outcome events occurred in 36.4% of amiodarone patients and 25.5% of placebo patients. The main reason for discontinuation of treatment was the high rate of adverse effects: 26.2% of amiodarone patients and 13.7% of placebo patients, with hypothyroidism, sleep disturbances, bradyarrhythmias, hepatic dysfunction, and pulmonary, neurological, or skin abnormalities more common in amiodarone-

Table 1 Early Permanent Discontinuation of Study Medication for Reasons Other Than Outcome Events

	Amiodarone $n = 606$	Placebo $n = 596$	Excess (amiodarone vs. placebo)		
Adverse experience	159 (26.2)	82 (13.7)	ever	severe	D/C 12.5%
Pulmonary	23 (3.8)	7 (1.2)	6%	1.2%	2.6%
Hepatic	6 (1.0)	2 (0.3)	1%	0	0.7%
Hypothyroid	20 (3.3)	1 (0.2)	15%		3.1%
Hyperthyroid	4 (0.6)	4 (0.7)	3%		0
Neurological	19 (3.1)	5 (0.8)	13%	1.4%	2.3%
Visual	5 (0.8)	0 (0)	3%	0	0.8%
Sleep disturbance	10 (1.7)	2 (0.3)	12%	1.3%	1.4%
Gastrointestinal	13 (2.1)	8 (1.3)	5%	0	0.8%
Skin	12 (1.9)	8 (1.3)	9%	0.3%	0.6%
Proarrhythmia	2 (0.3)	18 (3.0)			−2.7%
Other ventricular tachyarrhythmias	4 (0.7)	12 (2.0)			−1.3%
Bradyarrhythmia	8 (1.3)	5 (0.8)			0.5%
Other	33 (5.4)	10 (1.7)			3.7%
Uncooperative	44 (7.3)	46 (7.7)			−0.4%
Concomitant illness	17 (2.8)	14 (2.3)			0.5%
Other	1 (0.2)	10 (1.7)			−1.5%
Any reason	221 (36.4)	152 (25.5)			10.9%

treated patients than in the placebo group (Table 1). Proarrhythmia or other ventricular tachyarrhythmia led to early discontinuation of study drug in 5% of placebo patients and 1% of the amiodarone patients. No patient died of pulmonary toxic effects. At some point during follow-up, 15% of amiodarone patients and 2.3% of placebo patients had a serum concentration of thyrotropin above 10 mU/L and 3.1% and 0.8%, respectively, had thyrotropin concentrations below 0.1 mU/L. Mean serum concentration of AST decreased after randomization in both treatment groups. Serum concentrations of AST reached a level more than three times the upper limit of normal in 1.8% of amiodarone patients and 0.6% of placebo patients.

Clinical Outcomes

The primary outcome, the composite of resuscitated VF or arrhythmic death by efficacy analysis occurred in 6.0% of placebo patients and 3.3% of amiodarone patients (Kaplan-Meier estimates at 24 months) (relative risk reduction 48.5%,

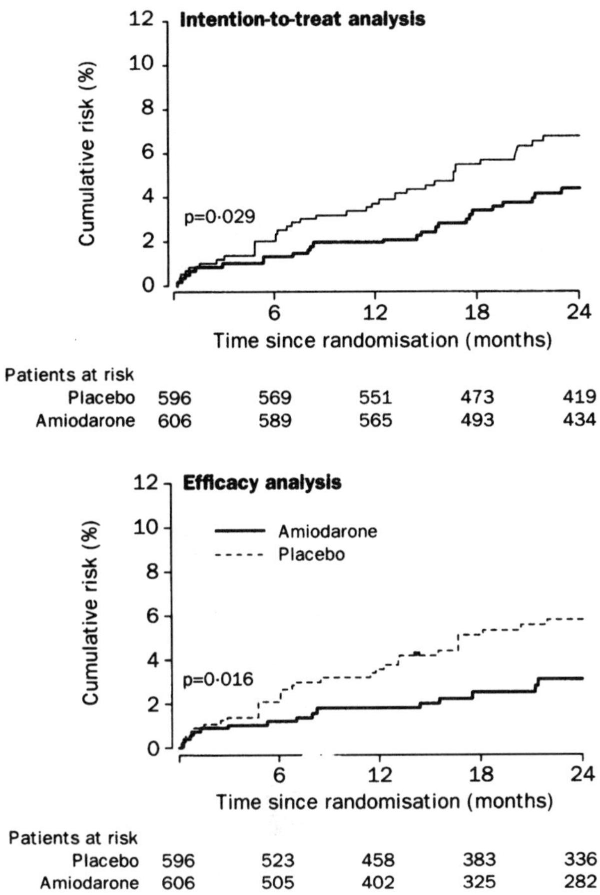

Figure 2 Actuarially determined rates of resuscitated ventricular fibrillation or arrhythmic death. Numbers below graph indicate patients at risk. (Upper graph) Intention-to-treat analysis: placebo 6.9%, amiodarone 4.5%. (Lower graph) Efficacy analysis: placebo 6.0%, amiodarone 3.3%. (Reprinted from Ref. 1, with permission.)

90% CI, 13.5 to 69.3, one-sided $p = 0.016$) and is shown in Figure 2 and Table 2. The table also shows the results of all secondary analyses and the intention-to-treat analyses. The efficacy analysis of arrhythmic death alone yielded a relative risk reduction of 32.6% (one-sided $p = 0.114$), which fell to 27.4% for all cardiac mortality and to 21.2% for all-cause mortality. The intention-to-treat analyses showed a similar pattern of amiodarone effects, but the risk reductions were diluted by outcome events and time beyond the discontinuation of the study

Table 2 Principal and Secondary Outcome Events

	Amiodarone ($n = 606$)			Placebo ($n = 596$)		
	Events (no.)	Follow-up (years)	Rate/year (%)	Events (no.)	Follow-up (years)	Rate/year (%)
Efficacy						
RVF or AD	15	848.6	1.77	31	917.6	3.38
AD	15	848.7	1.77	24	921.9	2.60
Cardiac mortality	30	848.7	3.53	44	921.9	4.77
All-cause mortality	37	848.7	4.36	50	921.9	5.42
Intention-to-treat						
RVF or AD	25	1089.5	2.29	39	1050.8	3.71
AD	24	1090.0	2.20	33	1061.3	3.11
Cardiac mortality	44	1090.0	4.04	55	1061.3	5.18
All-cause mortality	57	1090.0	5.23	68	1061.3	6.41

RVF = resuscitated ventricular fibrillation; AD = arrhythmic death; RRR = relative risk reduction; CI = confidence interval.

medication when patients were unlikely to benefit from active therapy. We found no evidence of rebound after active therapy was stopped. Figure 3 shows the cumulative rates of nonarrhythmic death: 6.2% in the placebo group versus 5.8% in the amiodarone group (two-sided $p = 0.70$).

The rates of resuscitated VF or arrhythmic death were substantially increased among placebo patients with certain baseline risk factors (Table 3). Thus, the risk of this primary outcome was doubled for individuals older than 70 years, or for those with diabetes mellitus, and was more than tripled for those with a history of congestive heart failure or MI before the qualifying event or pulmonary adema with the qualifying event. The relative risk reductions varied somewhat among the baseline risk factors, but there were no statistically significant differences.

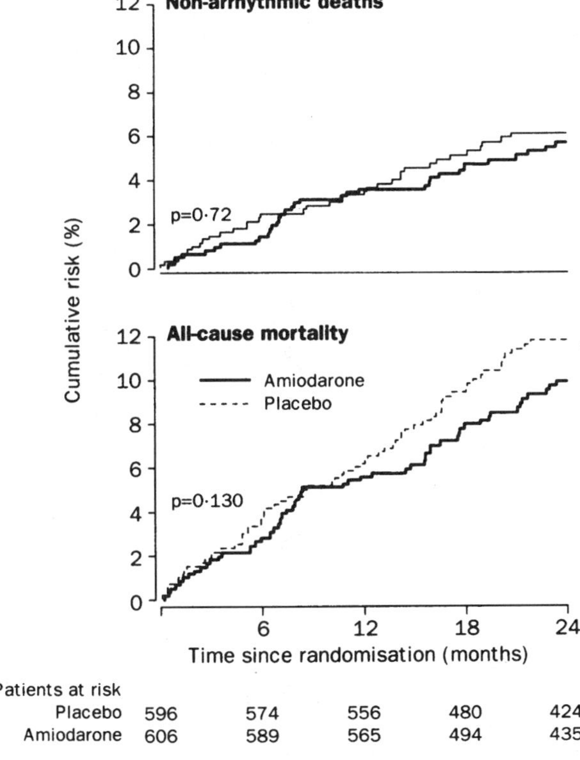

Patients at risk					
Placebo	596	574	556	480	424
Amiodarone	606	589	565	494	435

Figure 3 Actuarially determined rates of death. (Upper graph) Nonarrhythmic deaths: placebo 6.2%, amiodarone 5.8%. (Lower graph) All-cause mortality: placebo 11.8%, amiodarone 9.9%. (Reprinted from Ref. 1, with permission.)

Table 3 Relative and Absolute Risk Reduction

	Amiodarone		Placebo				
Subgroup	Events (no.)	Rate/yr (%)	Events (no.)	Rate/yr (%)	RRR (%)	p-Value (Interaction)	ARR (%)
All	15	1.77	31	3.38	48.5		1.61
Age < 70 year	10	1.57	16	2.56	38.7		0.99
≥ 70 year	5	2.37	15	5.12	53.8	0.65	2.75
Sex male	13	1.82	25	3.28	44.5		1.46
female	2	1.48	6	3.84	61.4	0.68	2.36
Diabetes no	11	1.51	23	2.97	49.2		1.46
yes	4	3.31	8	5.55	40.4	0.81	2.24
Prior MI no	9	1.52	11	1.75	13.2		0.23
yes	6	2.33	20	6.89	66.2	0.14	4.56
Prior CHF no	7	1.01	16	2.21	54.2		1.20
yes	8	5.13	15	7.8	34.0	0.56	2.67
Pulmonary edema no	11	1.52	18	2.32	34.7		0.80
(qualifying MI) yes	4	3.24	13	9.09	64.4	0.37	5.85
VPDs < 20/h	6	1.47	12	2.94	50.0		1.47
≥ 20/h	9	2.07	19	3.73	44.5		1.66
Concomitant drugs							
β-blocker no	13	4.07	15	4.03	−1.0		−0.04
yes	2	0.38	16	2.93	87.1	0.008	2.55
Diltiazem no	14	2.03	28	3.75	46.0		1.72
yes	1	0.63	3	1.75	63.8	0.74	1.12
Digoxin no	8	1.10	24	3.02	63.7		1.92
yes	7	5.85	7	5.68	−2.9	0.12	−0.17
Thrombolytic no	10	2.35	18	4.10	42.7		1.75
yes	5	1.19	13	2.73	56.4	0.64	1.54

RRR = relative risk reduction; ARR = absolute risk reduction; CHF = congestive heart failure.

The use of concomitant medications at baseline also predicted risk of the primary outcome events in the placebo patients (Table 3). The baseline risk of these events increased among those who were not taking beta-blockers or diltiazem, those who had not received thrombolytic therapy, and those who were not taking digoxin. The benefit of amiodarone over placebo was marked among patients who were taking beta-blockers, but was not evident among those who were not, the only statistically significant interaction noted.

CONCLUSIONS

1. Among survivors of AMI with frequent or repetitive VPDs, amiodarone produced a statistically significant reduction of the composite outcome of resuscitated VF or arrhythmic death and favorable trends for the reduction of arrhythmic death, cardiac death, and all-cause mortality among patients who had not been off drug for more than 3 months.

2. More conservative analyses by intention to treat showed a statistically significant reduction of resuscitated VF or arrhythmic death, and favorable trends for the reduction of arrhythmic death, cardiac death, and all-cause mortality.

3. Amiodarone had no effect on nonarrhythmic deaths.

4. Serious side effects of sufficient severity to lead to discontinuation of study drug were uncommon, with absolute excesses of amiodarone over placebo as follows: pulmonary (2.6%), hepatic (0.7%). Absolute excesses of moderate side effects leading to discontinuation of study drug were: hypothyroid (3.1%), hyperthyroid (−0.1%), neurological (2.3%), visual (0.8%), gastrointestinal (0.8%), bradyarrhythmias (0.5%). Proarrhythmia was 10 times as frequent on placebo as on amiodarone. Early drug discontinuation for reasons other than study outcomes was common in both groups with an absolute excess of 10.9% in the amiodarone group.

5. Baseline risk was substantially increased among patients with age greater than 70 years, diabetes, history of congestive heart failure or MI before the qualifying MI, or pulmonary edema during the qualifying MI. Hence, the absolute benefits of amiodarone for the reduction of resuscitated VF or arrhythmic death were increased in these patients.

6. There was a positive, statistically significant interaction between beta blocker therapy and amiodarone assignment.

7. The NNT to prevent one episode of resuscitated VF or arrhythmic death in 1 year is 62, whereas to prevent one death from any cause is 94 (assuming the favorable trend is real). Among patients at increased baseline risk, the NNTs are lower. To prevent one episode of resusci-

tated VF or arrhythmic death, NNTs are as follows: prior MI 22, prior CHF 37, pulmonary edema in conjunction with the present MI 17.

CRITIQUE

Our trial was designed to select patients at increased risk of arrhythmic death and to assess the benefit of amiodarone by its specific reduction of the composite of resuscitated ventricular fibrillation or arrhythmic death. The sample size of 1200 was calculated to give adequate power to detect a substantial reduction in this outcome cluster but would not be large enough to reliably detect a reduction of all-cause mortality. Whereas it is always desirable, if possible, to conduct a trial of sufficient size to detect a reduction in all-cause mortality, we were limited by constraints of resources and available CCU patients in the Canadian clinical trials network.

The relative reduction in the composite outcome of arrhythmic death or resuscitated VF was 48.5%, remarkably close to the 50% predicted in the sample size calculation. Although 46% of the deaths were arrhythmic (close to the predicted 50%), the rate was somewhat less than predicted, the relative risk reduction with amiodarone was 32.6% rather than the predicted 50%, and the benefit was not statistically significant. The mortality benefit of amiodarone occurred as a result of a reduction in arrhythmic deaths. There was no suggestion in any analysis of a compensatory excess of nonarrhythmic deaths in amiodarone-treated patients. Although there was a favorable trend for the reduction of all-cause mortality, this did not reach statistical significance, as we originally anticipated it would not. This was almost certainly due to a lack of sufficient statistical power since the ATMA overview (14) demonstrates a statistically significant 13% reduction in mortality based on 6500 randomized patients in 13 amiodarone trials. CAMIAT confirms that the presence of frequent or repetitive VPDs on ambulatory monitoring following myocardial infarction identifies an appropriate at-risk population in which to test antiarrhythmic therapies, and strongly indicates that these patients may benefit from amiodarone.

We chose to use a one-sided P test of statistical significance because there was evidence in several trials for benefit of amiodarone over placebo, and at the time of initiating the trial, amiodarone was not standard therapy for asymptomatic patients with frequent or repetitive VPDs following myocardial infarction. Our objective was to demonstrate, if possible, that amiodarone was superior to placebo; there was no interest in proving that amiodarone was inferior to placebo. Accordingly, the full 5% type 1 error was focused on demonstrating superiority of amiodarone over placebo rather than a simple difference between amiodarone and placebo. Asymmetrical stopping rules were set up with an intent to stop for early efficacy only if there was a highly statistically significant benefit of amiodarone emerging over placebo, but to stop for futility if there was a trend against amiodarone with a low likelihood of demonstrating at least a 20% benefit in its favor.

Constraints on sample size and resources, and an interest in demonstrating that amiodarone used properly would be more effective than placebo, caused us to choose an efficacy analysis for our principal outcome. This analysis was statistically significant for the principal outcome of resuscitated ventricular fibrillation or arrhythmic death. All outcomes were also analyzed by intention-to-treat, and the outcome of resuscitated ventricular fibrillation or arrhythmic death was again statistically significantly different in favor of amiodarone.

Careful attention was given to the documentation of side effects. The trial demonstrated the power of the double-blind design in determining the true incidence of potentially dangerous or troublesome side effects. The absolute difference between amiodarone and placebo was modest for most side effects and consistent with the rates observed in the ATMA overview. Importantly, proarrhythmia was ten times as common in placebo as in amiodarone; there was no suggestion of causation of proarrhythmia by amiodarone.

There were substantial differences in baseline risks among patients in various categories. The twofold increase in risk for individuals older than 70 years or those with diabetes mellitus, and the threefold increase in risk for those patients with a history of congestive heart failure or myocardial infarction before the qualifying event or pulmonary edema with the qualifying event, allows the selection of particularly high-risk individuals who may enjoy larger absolute benefits of amiodarone. These high-risk groups are observed in the ATMA overview (14) as well.

One of the concerns in designing the trial was that the patient receiving beta-blocker therapy post-myocardial infarction might be exposed to increased risk of dangerous bradyarrhythmias from the addition of amiodarone. Special precautions were introduced to ensure that such patients were carefully followed, and that given the known efficacy of beta-blockers postmyocardial infarction, when patients experienced bradyarrhythmias, amiodarone dosage was to be reduced before the reduction of beta-blocker dosage. There were about 60% of patients receiving beta-blockers at baseline. The surprising observation was a positive interaction between beta-blocker therapy and amiodarone. The relative risk reduction for the composite outcome of resuscitated ventricular fibrillation or arrhythmic death was 87.1% among patients receiving beta-blockers, but was −1.0% for patients not on beta-blockers. This finding was observed in EMIAT (15) and the ATMA overview as well. There is no obvious explanation for this positive interaction, but it is encouraging given the previously demonstrated efficacy and widespread use of beta-blockers in this population.

One of the questions that emerges as a result of the CAMIAT outcomes is, ''Should all patients surviving myocardial infarction undergo ambulatory ECG monitoring?'' It does not seem practical, nor is it likely to be cost effective to arrange for ambulatory monitoring on all survivors of myocardial infarction. Frequent or repetitive VPDs are much more likely to be found among those survivors of AMI with left ventricular dysfunction, age over 65 years, or prior myocardial infarction (16). Ambulatory monitoring of only such patients would be much more cost effective. There is also evidence that shorter periods of ambulatory monitoring, as little as 1 to 6 h, yield most of the information contained in a 24-h recording and accordingly further economies and simplicity might be achieved by such an approach (17). There is persisting uncertainty as to the role of ambulatory monitoring or other measures of electrical instability for practical risk prognostication in survivors of myocardial infarction.

Based upon the results of CAMIAT and in the context of the ATMA overview, the following recommendations for the use of amiodarone postmyocardial infarction appear reasonable.

1. If there is a strong indication for antiarrhythmic drug therapy (sustained VT or resuscitated VF after the first few days of onset), amiodarone is the drug of choice.
2. If there are frequent or repetitive VPDs *plus* LV dysfunction (EF <40% or pulmonary edema during the hospital course), amiodarone is likely to be efficacious.
3. If there are frequent or repetitive VPDs *only*, or LV dysfunction *only*, amiodarone should be considered, but as yet the evidence comes only from the overview, the benefit is relatively modest, and the p value is marginal ($p=0.03$).
4. The benefits of beta-blockers and amiodarone are additive.

ACKNOWLEDGMENTS

This work is supported by The MRC of Canada and Sanofi Winthrop through the University-Industry Programme (Grant U10034).

REFERENCES

1. Cairns JA, Connolly SJ, Roberts RS, Gent M. Canadian Amiodarone Myocardial Infarction Arrhythmia Trial (CAMIAT): rationale and protocol. Am J Cardiol 1993; 72:87F–94F.
2. Cairns JA, Connolly SJ, Roberts R, Gent M, for the Canadian Amiodarone Myocardial Infarction Arrhythmia Trial Investigators. Randomised trial of outcome after myocardial infarction in patients with frequent or repetitive premature depolarisations: CAMIAT. Lancet 1997;349:675–682.
3. Moss AJ, Davis HT, DeCamilla J, Bayer LW. Ventricular ectopic beats and their relation to sudden and non-sudden cardiac death after myocardial infarction. Circulation 1979;60:998–1003.

4. Ruberman W, Weinblatt E, Goldberg JD, Frank CW, Chaudhary BS, Shapiro S. Ventricular premature complexes and sudden death after myocardial infarction. Circulation 1981;64:297–305.

5. The Multicenter Postinfarction Research Group. Risk stratification and survival after myocardial infarction. N Engl J Med 1983;309:331–336.

6. Bigger JT, Fleiss JL, Kleiger R, Miller JP, Rolnitzky LM, the Multicenter Post-Infarction Research Group. The relationships among ventricular arrhythmias, left ventricular dysfunction, and mortality in the 2 years after myocardial infarction. Circulation 1984;69:250–258.

7. Kostis JB, Byington R, Friedman LM, Goldstein S, Furberg C, for the BHAT Study Group. Prognostic significance of ventricular ectopic activity in survivors of acute myocardial infarction. J Am Coll Cardiol 1987;10:231–242.

8. Furberg CD. Effect of antiarrhythmic drugs on mortality after myocardial infarction. Am J Cardiol 1983;52(suppl):32C–36C.

9. Cairns JA, Connolly SJ, Gent M. Roberts R. Post-myocardial infarction mortality in patients with ventricular premature depolarizations. Canadian Amiodarone Myocardial Infarction Arrhythmia Trial Pilot Study. Circulation 1991;84:550–557.

10. The Cardiac Arrhythmia Suppression Trial (CAST) Investigators. Effect of encainide and flecainide on mortality in a randomized trial of arrhythmia suppression after myocardial infarction. N Engl J Med 1989;321:406–412.

11. The Cardiac Arrhythmia Suppression Trial II Investigators. Effect of the antiarrhythmic agent moricizine on survival after myocardial infarction. N Engl J Med 1992; 327:227–233.

12. Burkart F, Pfisterer M, Kiowski W, Follath F, Burckhardt D. Effect of antiarrhythmic therapy on mortality of survivors of myocardial infarction with asymptomatic complex ventricular arrhythmias: Basel Antiarrhythmic Study of Infarct Survival (BASIS). J Am Coll Cardiol 1990;16:1711–1718.

13. Ceremuzynski L, Leczar E, Krzeminska-Pakula M, et al. Effect of amiodarone on mortality after myocardial infarction: a double-blind, placebo-controlled, pilot study. J Am Coll Cardol 1992;20:1056–1062.

14. Amiodarone Trials Meta-Analysis Investigators. Effect of prophylactic amiodarone on mortality after acute myocardial infarction and in congestive heart failure: meta-analysis of individual data from 6,500 patients in randomised trials. Lancet 1997; 350:1417–1424.

15. Julian DG, Camm AJ, Frangin G, Janse MJ, Munoz A, Schwartz PJ, Simon P, EMIAT Investigators. Randomised trial of effect of amiodarone on mortality in patients with left ventricular dysfunction after recent myocardial infarction: EMIAT. Lancet 1997;349:667–674.

16. Connolly SJ, Cairns JA, on behalf of the CAMIAT Pilot Study Group. Prevalence and predictors of ventricular premature complexes in survivors of acute myocardial infarction. Am J Cardiol 1992;69:408–411.

17. Connolly SJ, Cairns JA, on behalf of the CAMIAT Pilot Study Group. Comparison of one-, six- and 24-hour ambulatory electrocardiographic monitoring for ventricular arrhythmia as a predictor of mortality in survivors of acute myocardial infarction. Am J Cardiol 1992;69:308–313.

Jeffrey L. Anderson
University of Utah School of Medicine, Salt Lake City, Utah

SYNOPSIS

The Canadian Amiodarone Myocardial Infarction Arrhythmia Trial (CAMIAT) enrolled patients with a myocardial infarction (MI) occurring within the previous 6 to 45 days who showed >10 ventricular premature complexes (VPCs) per hour on a 24-h ambulatory ECG recording or had one or more runs of ventricular tachycardia (VT) of three or more consecutive ventricular complexes (1). A left ventricular ejection fraction (EF) measurement was not required or recorded in CAMIAT. The study was a double-blind, randomized comparison of amiodarone with placebo. The dosing regimen was complex and based on arrhythmia suppression, but the average daily treatment dose (300 mg by 4 months, 200 mg by 1 year) was similar to that in other contemporary trials such as EMIAT (European Myocardial Infarct Amiodarone Trial) (2). The primary endpoint was arrhythmic death or cardiac arrest and the specified analysis was an on-treatment analysis (i.e., an analysis of those actually taking amiodarone within 3 months of the event). A 2-year arrhythmic death rate of 7.5% was assumed in the control group. The sample size was calculated to be 1200 patients based on a power of 80% to detect a 50% reduction in arrhythmic death by amiodarone with a *one-sided* alpha (*p* value) of 0.05 (two-sided *p* = 0.10).

CAMIAT enrolled 1202 patients and followed them for a mean of 1.8 years. In the specified primary analysis, arrhythmic death/cardiac arrest was reduced by 49%, from 6.0% to 3.3%, one-tailed *p* = 0.016. Using a more conventional intention-to-treat, two-tailed analysis, arrhythmic death reduction was 38% (2*p* = 0.058), cardiac death reduction, 22% (2*p* = 0.22), and all-cause mortality reduction, 18% (2*p* = 0.26). A small excess of nonarrhythmic cardiac deaths was observed in the amiodarone group (19 vs. 16); noncardiac deaths were equal (13 vs. 13).

STUDY CRITIQUE

CAMIAT is the first large (>1000 patient) antiarrhythmic drug trial to achieve its primary endpoint, demonstration of a beneficial effect on arrhythmic death. The CAMIAT Investigators are to be congratulated for testing an important hypothesis using a double-blind, placebo-controlled design. Also, to their credit, given the primary objective of arrhythmic death reduction, they included an arrhythmic marker among their entry criteria: frequent VPCs and/or unsustained VT on Holter recording (this was not done in EMIAT). They hypothesized a 50% arrhythmic death reduction by amiodarone (which would be expected to translate into a 25% reduction in all-cause death). Although still overly optimistic, this was more realistic than the 35% reduction in all-cause mortality that formed the basis for EMIAT (which in turn would require a 70% reduction in sudden death, assuming arrhythmic death prevention to be the major mechanism of the a survival benefit of amiodarone). The primary result of CAMIAT, that amiodarone reduces sudden arrhythmic death or cardiac arrest, is of interest and importance. However, there are several design features of CAMIAT that may limit the reliability and generalizability of its results.

The first design problem with CAMIAT is that arrhythmic death rather than all-cause mortality was chosen as the primary endpoint. The use of sudden, rather than total, death recently has been openly criticized (3,4). If a therapy merely causes the mode of death to change, it is unlikely that it would be considered clinically worthwhile. For example, the therapy could simply convert arrhythmic to nonarrhythmic (e.g., heart failure, bradyarrhythmic) cardiac death. Another problem with not using total mortality is that noncardiac deaths, including those that may be therapy-related (e.g., pulmonary fibrosis with amiodarone), do not count toward the endpoint. Also, the exact cause and mechanism of death is notoriously difficult to determine. Specifically, the clinical determination of sudden arrhythmic death has been shown to be poorly reproducible, even when performed by panels of experts and dedicated endpoint committees. For example, Pratt et al. found that a fourfold range in sudden arrhythmic death rates could be generated from the same database using different criteria (3). Their study of 109 deaths among 834 patients with implantable cardioverter defibrillators (ICDs) was unique in providing not only clinical but also ICD telemetric and autopsy data. Classification of deaths from each of a number of perspectives using several seemingly reasonable definitions of sudden death could then be made and compared. Thus, whereas total mortality is straightforward and objective, determination of sudden death is not, and its estimate may introduce noise or even bias of a degree that is difficult to determine. Because of these problems, most clinical trialists now believe that total mortality ideally should be the primary endpoint in antiarrhythmic trials (3–5). Total mortality was successfully used in the recently reported Antiarrhythmics Versus Implantable Defibrillators (AVID) Study (6).

A second design problem is that the primary analysis of the study was not intention to treat. The on-treatment analytical approach as was used in CAMIAT is known to be fraught with problems. The advantage to the trialist of eliminating patients no longer taking active therapy (and who no longer contribute to the benefit of therapy) is the reduction of "noise" in the study and an increase in ("optimization" of) the observed treatment effect. The argument for this approach is that it more accurately assesses the full pharmacological potential of therapy. The problem is that the approach is subject to bias. The reason for patients dropping out may not be random; dropouts may be due to an adverse effect of therapy, for example. This is of particular concern with amiodarone, given its known organ-toxic potential, including potentially fatal pulmonary fibrosis (7). A delayed death from amiodarone-induced pulmonary toxicity would not contribute to the on-treatment analysis endpoint.

A third concern is the choice of a one-tailed p test. Of course, the consequence of a one-tailed test is a smaller sample size for any postulated effect size. However, with a one-tailed test, only the possibility of benefit can be statistically tested, not the possibility of harm. In CAMIAT, the investigators did not commit to "spending alpha" to assess the possibility that amiodarone might *increase* mortality (i.e., might be worse than placebo). To be sure, trials are generally undertaken with the hope that active therapy will result in a better outcome than placebo. Trialists also may claim only to be interested in testing whether a drug is of benefit. However, if an adverse result is observed, it clearly would be of interest and should be reported. If no "alpha" is preserved for the "other tail," however, the statistical handling of an adverse result is unspecified and its statistical significance is unclear. Given the poor track record of antiarrhythmic drug therapy after MI (8–10), the choice of a one-tailed p value appears to be inappropriate. Despite the promise that amiodarone might differ from other antiarrhythmics in the post-MI setting (9), investigators have a responsibility to evaluate harm as well as benefit. Because of these and other arguments, the use of a two-tailed test is generally accepted as strongly preferred if not "required" as a component of study design. Had amiodarone's toxic potential (e.g., from lung, thyroid, liver disease, etc.) led to increased morbidity/mortality, it could not have been evaluated statistically within the study design.

Fourth, the study is underpowered to test the stated hypothesis, given reasonable assumptions. It can be vigorously argued that a reduction in arrhythmic deaths of 25 to 40% is clinically worthwhile. Optimistically assuming that sudden arrhythmic deaths make up one-half of all deaths and that total mortality is the appropriate endpoint, with the other caveats discussed above, then a "definitive" study should be able to detect a reduction in all-cause mortality of 15 to 20% using an intention-to-treat approach with a two-tailed p test of significance. A study at least several times the size of CAMIAT would be required to test this hypothesis with adequate power. Unfortunately, inadequate sizing of clinical trials more often is caused by practical clinical and fiscal constraints than misunderstanding of scientific or statistical issues. Likely, resource limitations played a role in CAMIAT design planning.

Given the limitations in study design, a reasonable (conservative) interpretation is that CAMIAT only showed a trend in amiodarone's favor, even for its primary endpoint of sudden death: using an intention-to-treat approach with a two-tailed analysis, arrhythmic death reduction was 38% with a p value of 0.058, and all-cause mortality reduction, a more objective and, arguably, a clinically more relevant endpoint, was only 18%, $p = 0.26$.

A final criticism is that the study population was not characterized as to left ventricular function. Ejection fraction was not routinely measured or reported. Given the importance of EF to cardiac mortality, including sudden death, and its strong interaction with ventricular arrhythmia (11–13), this omission is unfortunate. The consequence is that the study population cannot be accurately characterized and, hence, cannot be readily compared with other studies (such as EMIAT) or with the general population of post-MI patients. Even if the results of CAMIAT are accepted to provide evidence of a beneficial clinical effect, uncertainty remains as to whom in the general post-MI population they apply. This concern is of more than theoretical interest: in SWORD, which used another class III drug, d-sotalol, therapy was adverse in arrhythmia patients post-MI or with heart failure in the LVEF stratum of 31 to 40% but neutral in those with LVEF $\leq 30\%$ (10). Dofetilide, another class III drug, also showed a neutral mortality effect in a population with poor ventricular function (14). Differences in outcome by LVEF (but in a different direction) also have been postulated for amiodarone in the other direction (i.e., greater benefit with preserved LV function) (15).

Despite the study design and statistical concerns expressed, the study data do appear to be internally consistent. They raise an issue of drug intolerance during long-term therapy but not of an important off-setting adverse risk of irreversible morbidity or mortality. In that sense, the study provides useful, if not definitive, evidence for a benefit of amiodarone.

In summary, CAMIAT falls short of establishing a prophylactic role for amiodarone in preventing cardiac mortality (by reducing sudden death) in high-risk patients after myocardial infarction. However, CAMIAT does suggest that amiodarone is a relatively *safe* antiarrhythmic when used in this population and with the dosing schedule studied. CAMIAT is thus supportive of amiodarone's use for the accepted indications of treatment of highly symptomatic or life-threatening arrhythmias.

CAMIAT leaves open the question as to whether amiodarone might be useful in reducing total mortality in addition to cause-specific sudden death mortality in post-MI patients with certain high-risk markers (including, but not limited to, frequent or complex VPCs on ambulatory ECG). This question could be definitively answered by a substantially larger, more carefully designed study. The author believes, however, that such a study is unlikely to be performed in the near future. Meanwhile, additional information may be obtained from a careful meta-analysis of all data from relevant randomized trials. Such a meta-analysis has recently been performed and published (16). Overall, that analysis is supportive of the CAMIAT results. However, in the author's view, given the many limitations of meta-analysis, it still falls short by itself of providing an adequate basis for recommending general prophylactic use of amiodarone after MI in all high-risk patients. The issue of how best to select high-risk patients for therapeutic trials also remains: should it be by Holter, EF, heart rate variability, signal averaging, baroreceptor reflex testing, electrophysiological study, a combination of these, or other tests? Additional insights into patient and drug selection thus will be required along with additional, prospective, clinical trials before the controversy of amiodarone's use in primary prevention after MI can be firmly resolved.

REFERENCES

1. Cairns JA, Connolly SJ, Roberts R, Gent M, for the Canadian Amiodarone Myocardial Infarction Arrhythmia Trial Investigators. Randomized trial of outcome after myocardial infarction in patients with frequent or repetitive ventricular premature depolarizations: CAMIAT. Lancet 1997;349:675–682.
2. Julian DG, Camm AJ, Frangin G, Janse MJ, Munoz A, Schwartz PJ, Simon P, for the European Myocardial Infarct Amiodarone Trial Investigators. Randomized trial of effect of amiodarone on mortality in patients with left ventricular dysfunction after recent myocardial infarction: EMIAT. Lancet 1997;349:667–674.
3. Pratt CM, Greenway PS, Schoenfeld MH, Hibben ML, Reiffel JA. Exploration of the precision of classifying sudden cardiac death. Implications for the interpretation of clinical trials. Circulation 1996;93:519–524.
4. Gottlieb SS. Commentary: Dead is dead—artificial definitions are no substitute. Lancet 1997;349:662–663.
5. Epstein AE, Carlson MD, Fogoros RN, Higgins SL, Vendetti FJ, Jr. Classification of death in antiarrhythmia trials. J Am Coll Cardiol 1996;27:433–442.
6. The Antiarrhythmics Versus Implantable Defibrillators (AVID) Investigators. A comparison of antiarrhythmic-drug therapy with implantable defibrillators in patients resuscitated from near-fatal ventricular arrhythmias. N Engl J Med 1997;337:1576–1583.
7. Vorperian-VR; Havighurst-TC; Miller-S; January-CT. Adverse effects of low dose amiodarone: a meta-analysis. J Am Coll Cardiol 1997;30:791–798.
8. Epstein AE, Hallstrom AP, Rogers WJ, Liebson PR, Seals AA, Anderson JL, Cohen

JD, Capone RJ, Wyse DG, for the CAST Investigators. Mortality following ventricular arrhythmia suppression by encainide, flecainide, and moricizine after myocardial infarction: The original design concept of the Cardiac Arrhythmia Suppression Trial (CAST). JAMA 1993;270:2451–2455.

9. Teo KK, Yusuf S, Furberg CD. The effects of prophylactic antiarrhythmic drug therapy in acute myocardial infarction. JAMA 1993;270:1589–1595.

10. Waldo AL, Camm AJ, deRuyter H, et al, for the SWORD Investigators. Effect of d-sotalol on mortality in patients with left ventricular dysfunction after recent and remote myocardial infarction. Lancet 1996;348:7–12.

11. Bigger JT, Jr, Fleiss JL, Kleiger R, Miller JP, Rolnitzky LM. The relationships among ventricular arrhythmias, left ventricular dysfunction, and mortality in the 2 years after myocardial infarction. Circulation 1984;69:250–258.

12. Mukharji J, Rude RE, Poole WK, Gustafson N, Thomas LJ, Strauss HW, Jaffe AS, Muller JE, Roberts R, Raabe DS, Croft CH, Passamani E, Braunwald E, Willerson JT, and the MILIS Study Group. Risk factors for sudden death after myocardial infarction: two-year follow-up. Am J Cardiol 1984;54:31–36.

13. Maggioni AP, Zuanetti G, Franzosi MG, Rovelli F, Santoro E, Staszewsky L, Tavazzi L, Tognoni G. Prevalence and prognostic significance of ventricular arrhythmias after acute myocardial infarction in the fibrinolytic era. GISSI-2 result. Circulation 1993;87:312–322.

14. Moller M. Dofetilide as an antiarrhythmic agent for patients with severe heart failure (the Diamond CHF Study). Presented at the XIXth Congress of the European Society of Cardiology, August 26, 1997, Stockholm, Sweden.

15. Pfisterer M, Kiowski W, Burckhardt D, Follath F, Burkart F. Beneficial effect of amiodarone on cardiac mortality in patients with asymptomatic complex ventricular arrhythmias after acute myocardial infarction and preserved but not impaired left ventricular function. Am J Cardiol 1992;69:1399–1402.

16. Amiodarone Trials Meta-analysis Investigators. Effect of prophylactic amiodarone on mortality after acute myocardial infarction and in congestive heart failure: meta-analysis of individual data from 6500 patients in randomised trials. Lancet 1997; 350:1412–1424.

13
The Danish Investigation of Arrhythmia and Mortality ON Dofetilide–CHF (DIAMOND–CHF) Trial

Bradley Marchant*

Pfizer Limited, Kent, England

INTRODUCTION

The Danish Investigations of Arrhythmias and Mortality ON Dofetilide (DIA-MOND) comprise two parallel studies using a single protocol and infrastructure. Patients in both studies had left ventricular dysfunction corresponding to a left ventricular ejection fraction (LVEF) less than or equal to 35%. However, the primary diagnosis was different in the two studies: DIAMOND–CHF included patients hospitalized with congestive heart failure, while DIAMOND–MI included patients with a recent myocardial infarction. This chapter will review the rationale, patient population, and study results of DIAMOND–CHF, and will complement the previously published publications of the study design and results.

Cardiac arrhythmias are common in patients with congestive heart failure and contribute both to morbidity and mortality. Atrial fibrillation is the most common rhythm abnormality in such patients, which leads to further deterioration in cardiac function and substantial morbidity. In addition, life-threatening ventricular arrhythmias are a well-documented cause of death in patients with severe left ventricular impairment. Thus the treatment of atrial and ventricular arrhythmias in patients with congestive heart failure may reduce morbidity and/or prolong life.

* The DIAMOND–CHF Investigators: Bradley Marchant, A. John Camm, Lars Køber, Christian Torp Pedersen, Paul Erik Bloch Thompson, Chris Hilton, Jan Carlsen, and Erik Sandøe.

269

Treatment with antiarrhythmic drugs has been severely limited by safety concerns. Several class I drugs (flecainide, encainide, quinidine, mexilitene) and a class III drug (d-sotalol) can convert and maintain sinus rhythm in patients with atrial fibrillation but have been shown to increase mortality (CAST, SWORD, IMPACT, Quinidine Meta-Analysis). Amioradone may be used to treat both supraventricular and ventricular arrhythmias and appeared to prolong life in one study (GESICA), but this finding was not confirmed in a number of double-blind placebo-controlled studies that showed no benefit on mortality (CHF-STAT, EMIAT, CAMIAT). However, the considerable side effects of amiodarone limit its use in nonlife-threatening arrhythmias such as atrial fibrillation. Digoxin did not increase mortality in the DIG study and is commonly used for rate control in atrial fibrillation associated with congestive heart failure. However, it neither promotes sinus rhythm nor provides rate control during exercise. Thus, there is a need for an effective and safe antiarrhythmic drug without systemic adverse effects.

Dofetilide is a highly selective agent that specifically inhibits the rapid component of the delayed rectifier potassium current (I_{kr}) in cardiac tissue without effect on other potassium currents. Unlike other nominal class III agents, dofetilide is devoid of activity on other cardiac receptors. It does not have a negative inotropic effect, even in patients with a markedly reduced left ventricular ejection fraction, and is without influence on cardiac conduction or sinus node function, even in patients with preexisting conduction abnormalities. Dofetilide demonstrated efficacy in the treatment of both supraventricular and ventricular arrhythmias. In two large clinical trials, which included over 900 patients, dofetilide maintained 62 and 70% of patients with persistent atrial fibrillation in sinus rhythm for 6 months. Given this pharmacological profile, there is a clear rationale to expect that dofetilide may have a beneficial effect on morbidity and mortality in patients with impaired left ventricular function and symptomatic congestive heart failure.

Thus the objectives of DIAMOND–CHF were twofold. First, it set out to deterimine if long-term treatment with dofetilide could benefit patients with impaired left ventricular function and CHF in terms of morbidity and mortality. Second, it attempted to determine if dofetilide could be tolerated long term and used safely in patients with severe structural heart disease who may be most at risk for proarrhythmia.

TARGET PATIENT POPULATION

Patients in DIAMOND–CHF were required to: (1) be enrolled within 7 days of hospitalization with congestive heart failure (CHF) which was classified as

NYHA class III/IV within the preceding month; (2) have wall motion index (WMI) $\leq$1.2 (equivalent to LVEF $\leq$35%) as assessed by a core laboratory.

These criteria were chosen to ensure that patients were at high risk of dying from their disease and it was anticipated that the 1-year mortality of the study population would be 25%. Thus, patients over 18 years of age of nonchild-bearing potential hospitalized with CHF were screened as above. Care was taken to ensure that screening was consecutive in order to avoid selection bias. In addition, patients who fulfilled these criteria were enrolled consecutively, provided informed consent was given.

Exclusion criteria were kept to a minimum. Only those exclusion criteria thought necessary for safety reasons were implemented (e.g., patients with creatinine clearance as low as 20 mL/min were allowed in the study.

Patients were excluded if they fulfilled the following criteria:

1. Resting heart rate <50 beats/min, sick sinus syndrome or second or third degree A-V block (without pacemaker).
2. A history of proarrhythmia with QT-prolonging drugs or with other drugs that have been shown to be associated with the genesis of TdP ventricular tachycardia.
3. Prolonged QTc interval at baseline (exceeding 460 ms$^{1/2}$ or 500 ms$^{1/2}$ in patients with bundle branch block).
4. Uncontrolled hypertension (diastolic blood pressure >115 mmHg) or profound hypotension (systolic blood pressure <80 mmHg).
5. Patients likely to die from other causes during the course of the study.
6. Serum potassium <3.6 mmol/L or >5.5 mmol/L at time of randomization.
7. Concomitant therapy with ICD, class I, or class III antiarrhythmic drugs or amiodarone treatment (within 3 months).
8. Creatinine clearance <20 mL/min or clinically significant liver dysfunction (e.g., cirrhosis).
9. Acute myocarditis or hemodynamically significant aortic stenosis; planned or recent (within 4 weeks) cardiac surgery, including cardiac transplantation.

Patients who had a myocardial infarction (MI) within 7 days were screened for the DIAMOND–MI study.

The sample size was chosen to allow a 25% reduction of relative mortality risk in dofetilide-treated patients to be demonstrated at the 5% significance level with a 90% power. Assumptions included a 1-year mortality of 25% in the placebo group and a mean duration of follow-up of 2 years. Thus, 1050 patients were needed in the CHF study based on a method for estimating survival times from two independent groups with limited recruitment and censoring. In order to take into account the potential for a lower level of placebo mortality than initially expected, and that a proportion of deaths were of nonarrhythmic etiology, a target of 1500 patients (750 on dofetilide and 750 on placebo) was set with a minimum follow-up of 1 year. All patients in the trial were followed until the last randomized patient had completed 1 year of treatment.

Protocol

Screening

Screening for the study comprised an echocardiogram, which was performed locally by trained staff, recorded on videotape, and sent to a core laboratory for central blinded evaluation. The core laboratory reviewed all screened echos within 1 working day to determine eligibility, and the results were relayed immediately to the investigating center. For evaluation of wall motion index (WMI), a 16-segment model was employed, using a scoring system: -1 = paradoxical movement; 0 = akinesia; 1 = hypokinesia; 2 = normokinesia; and 3 = hyperkinesia. Patients with a WMI ≤ 1.2 (equivalent to a left ventricular ejection fraction $\leq 35\%$) were potentially eligible.

All eligible patients with no exclusion criteria were invited to participate in the study and written informed consent was sought. Consenting patients were assigned to treatment by means of a computer-generated pseudorandom code stratified according to center and degree of LV dysfunction (wall motion index <0.8 and wall motion index ≥ 0.8).

Dosing

Patients in sinus rhythm were allocated to dofetilide 500 μg b.i.d. or placebo and patients with atrial fibrillation were allocated to dofetilide 250 μg b.i.d. or placebo. If creatinine clearance was reduced, calculated by the Cockcroft and Gault formula (17), patients received an adjusted dose as follows:

	CrCl $\geq$ 60 mL/min	40 $\leq$ CrCl < 60 mL/min	20 $\leq$ CrCl < 40 mL/min	CrCl < 20 mL/min
Sinus rhythm	500 μg b.i.d.	250 μg b.i.d.	250 μg o.d.	excluded
Atrial fibrillation or flutter	250 μg b.i.d.	250 μg b.i.d.	250 μg o.d.	excluded

Dose reductions were made if there was an increase in QTc interval exceeding 20% from baseline or exceeding 550 ms$^{1/2}$ on treatment. Patients could have dose reduction on two occasions (to 250 μg b.i.d. and 250 μg o.d.). If the QTc remained prolonged at the lowest dose, study drug was discontinued.

Dose reduction was also allowed for an adverse event or at the discretion of the investigator. Dose increases were not allowed and a drug pause of more than 21 days resulted in permanent discontinuation of study drug.

When the DIAMOND studies commenced, dose adjustment on the basis of renal function was not required. However, after recruitment of 288 patients in DIAMOND–CHF, a multivariate analysis of the global dofetilide safety database (without cases from DIAMOND) supported by a study of plasma dofetilide concentrations in patients with reduced renal function highlighted the importance of renal function in dosing patients with dofetilide. Subsequently, all patients were dosed based on their calculated creatinine clearance according to the algorithm above.

Monitoring and Follow-Up

All patients were monitored in hospital by continuous telemetry for the first 3 days of study treatment to ensure that the QT interval was monitored and arrhythmic events were detected and treated. When feasible, Holter monitoring was performed on the day prior to inclusion and on the third day of treatment.

Follow-up out-patient visits were scheduled for 1 and 3 months after inclusion and every 3 months thereafter until 12 months after recruitment of the final patient. Mortality data were available from the Danish Central Persons Register until the end of the study for all randomized patients, ensuring 100% follow-up for all mortality endpoints.

Conduct of the Study

DIAMOND–CHF was conducted in 34 hospitals throughout Denmark between November 1993 and December 1996. The area covered by participating hospitals encompassed more than half the Danish population. The study was supervised by an independent steering committee. A separate and independent Data and Safety Monitoring Board (DSMB) received regular safety updates, along with four preplanned interim analyses of mortality after 50, 100, 200, and 300 deaths. These interim analyses were not available to the steering committee, investigators, or sponsor. The DSMB were charged with recommending continuation, extension, or premature termination to the steering committee at the time of each interim analysis.

Two further committees were responsible for the classification of events; the mortality events committee classified all deaths and the arrhythmic events committee classified all cases of documented ventricular arrhythmia.

Mortality Events Committee

All deaths that occurred in the study were classified, on a blinded basis, as being of cardiac or noncardiac origin. Cardiac deaths were classified as being arrhythmic or nonarrhythmic, with arrhythmic deaths being subdivided into presumed or documented, according to the available evidence. The committee comprised four members and a chairperson. All available data were sent to two members of the committee, selected at random, who classified the death based on a preprogrammed computer algorithm. Both assessments were sent to the chairperson, who ruled on the cause of death only where the two opinions were discordant.

The committee classified deaths as cardiac unless there was specific evidence of a noncardiac cause. As in the CAST trial, cardiac deaths were classified as presumed arrhythmic unless a positive diagnosis could be made of a nonarrhythmic cause.

Arrhythmic Events Committee

All documented ventricular arrhythmias were reviewed by the three members of this committee. Cases of torsade de pointes (TdP), ventricular tachycardia (VT), and ventricular fibrillation (VF) were identified. TdP was defined as polymorphic VT of >10 beats associated with twisting of the axis and prolonged repolarization that need not be continuously present and recorded in the absence of rate correction.

Endpoints

The primary endpoint was all-cause mortality. Secondary endpoints included cardiac death; arrhythmic death (documented and presumed); cardiac death and resuscitated cardiac arrest; hospitalization with worsening CHF (requiring an increase in therapy in addition to hospitalization with worsening symptoms); myocardial infarction; and incidence of arrhythmia requiring treatment and withdrawal of study drug.

PATIENT POPULATION ENROLLED

A total of 5548 patients with CHF were screened for entry, including 246 patients who were screened on more than one occasion. Of those screened, 2531 (45%) were eligible for entry according to their left ventricular function. In total, 1518 (27% of screened, 60% of eligible) were randomized to dofetilide (762) or placebo (756). Inclusion of such a high proportion of eligible patients was a result of consecutive screening, consecutive randomization, and ensured that included patients were likely to be representative of the target population.

The population was, in general, elderly, with approximately one in four

Table 1 Demographic Characteristics of the Patient Population at Baseline

Characteristic	Dofetilide ($n = 762$)	Placebo ($n = 756$)
Median duration of heart failure (months)	12	12
Mean age [year (range)]	70 (26–94)	70 (32–92)
Male sex (%)	546 (72)	568 (75)
Current smokers (%)	254 (33)	268 (35)
History (%)		
myocardial infarction	389 (51)	390 (52)
ischemic heart disease	509 (67)	508 (67)
diabetes	152 (20)	140 (19)
hypertension	111 (15)	115 (15)
Mean renal clearance (mL/min SD)	57 (23)	57 (25)
Atrial fibrillation at randomization (%)	190 (25)	201 (27)
Median wall-motion index (range)	0.9 (0.3–1.2)	0.9 (0.3–1.2)
Treatment at randomization (%)		
beta-blocker	72 (9)	80 (11)
ACE inhibitor	552 (72)	571 (76)
calcium antagonist	153 (20)	170 (22)
NYHA class (%)		
I	16 (2)	17 (2)
II	268 (35)	297 (39)
III	423 (56)	385 (51)
IV	49 (6)	52 (7)
Not available	6 ($<$1%)	5 ($<$1%)

being female. The majority of patients were classified NYHA class III and 25% were in atrial fibrillation at the time of entry to the study. The groups were well balanced for important baseline characteristics as shown in Table 1.

The level of concomitant cardiac medication was somewhat low at baseline (Table 1), but increased during the study (89% taking ACE inhibitors, 33% taking calcium antagonists, and 23% taking beta-blockers).

RESULTS

Tolerance to Treatment

The duration of treatment was almost identical in the two treatment groups (median of 383 days on dofetilide and 371 days on placebo), suggesting that dofetilide was well tolerated. At 1 year, 421 patients continued to take dofetilide and 398 continued on placebo (75.3% and 73.4% of those alive, respectively). The high

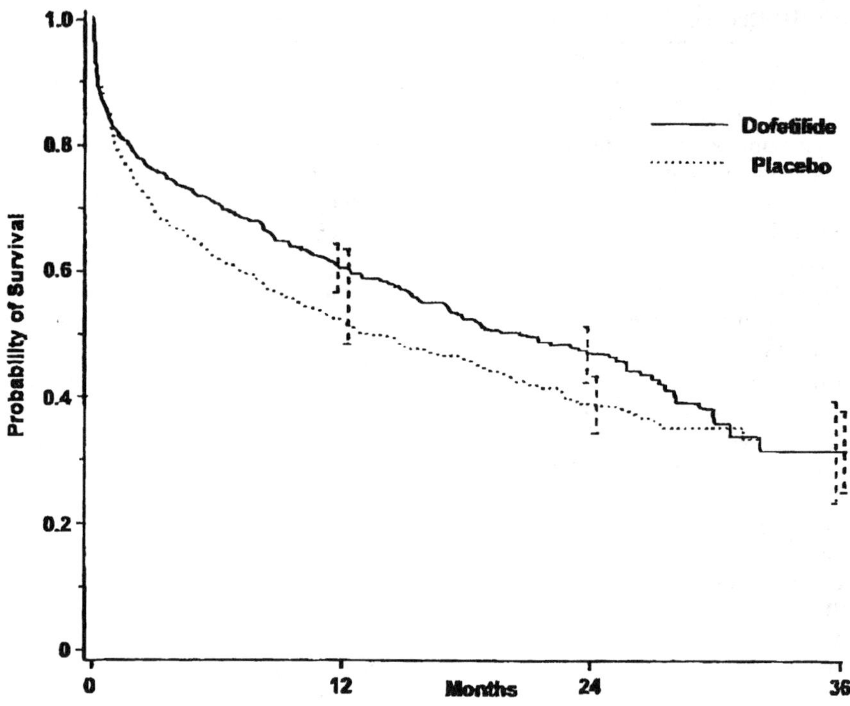

Figure 1 Kaplan-Meier plot of time to first event of worsening heart failure or death (95% CI): intent-to-treat population. Hazard ratio = 0.75. CI 0.63–0.87.

tolerance of dofetilide is confirmed when the reasons for withdrawal are examined in more detail; 14 patients were withdrawn from dofetilide for asymptomatic QT/QTc prolongation compared to three subjects from the placebo group.

Primary Endpoint: All-Cause Mortality

Over the entire duration of the study, there were slightly fewer deaths on dofetilide: 311 compared with 317 on placebo. A Kaplan–Meyer survival analysis showed 1-year survival on dofetilide of 73.4% (95% Cl: 70.2–76.5%) compared to 71.7% (95% Cl: 68.5–74.9%) on placebo. There were no differences in mortality between the treatment groups at any time during the study (Fig. 1) and applying the Cox proportional hazards regression model to the data, the hazard ratio is 0.94 on dofetilide compared to placebo, with 95% Cl ranging from 0.81 to 1.11. This neutral result is seen consistently in all predefined subgroups (Fig. 2). In addition, an analysis of the primary endpoint looking at all deaths that occurred on treatment also showed a neutral result, with slightly fewer deaths on dofetilide (82/762; 11%) compared to placebo (92/756; 12%) during active treatment. Similarly, there were no differences between dofetilide and placebo in mortality in this on-treatment analysis between the groups at any time during the study (log rank estimate of 1-year survival for both groups was 89%; 95% Cl: 86.4–91.6%).

Other Mortality Endpoints

All other mortality secondary endpoints showed the same neutral result. Of the 628 deaths, the mortality events committee classified 122 (19%) as noncardiac, 199 (32%) as cardiac–nonarrhythmic, and 307 (49%) as cardiac–arrhythmic. Of the cardiac–arrhythmic deaths, and ECG diagnosis was made in 18% and the remainder were presumed arrhythmic. The times to cardiac and arrhythmic death are shown in Figure 3. The endpoints that did not relate to mortality were similarly neutral, with the single exception of hospitalization with worsening CHF.

Hospitalization with Worsening CHF

To achieve this endpoint, patients were required to have symptoms of heart failure severe enough to require hospitalization for at least 24 h and a concomitant intensification of heart failure therapy (i.e., introduction of ACE inhibitors, digoxin, or diuretics not previously received, or an increase in diuretic therapy). Patients on dofetilide showed a reduction both in the number of patients hospitalized [231 (30.3%) versus 290 (38.4%)] and the total number of hospitalizations (352 events on dofetilide compared to 422 events on placebo). Analysis of the time to first event of hospitalization showed a significant benefit favoring dofetilide ($p <$ 0.001). The probability of remaining event-free for 12 months in the dofetilide treatment group was 70.5% (95% CI: 66.9–74.2%) compared to 59.9% (95% CI: 56.0–63.8%) in patients given placebo with a hazard ratio of 0.75 on dofetilide. In clinical terms, this translates to a delay in hospitalization of approximately 6 months.

Since 25% of patients were in atrial fibrillation at the time of randomization, the beneficial effect of dofetilide on the progression of CHF may be partially explained by the hemodynamic improvement associated with normal sinus rhythm. The effect of dofetilide on rhythm was therefore explored further.

At the time of randomization, 190 patients on dofetilide were in atrial fibrillation/flutter compared to 201 on placebo. During the study, 84 patients on

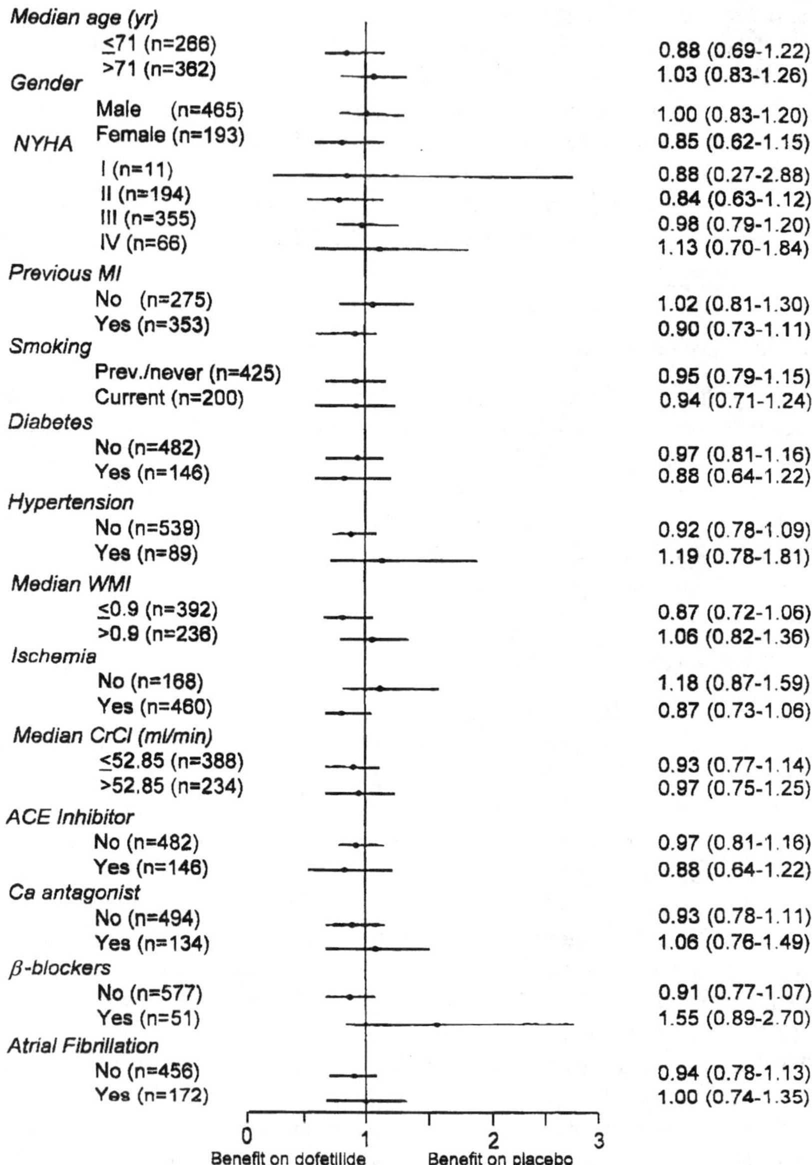

Figure 2 Cox's proportional hazards for total mortality in predefined subgroups.

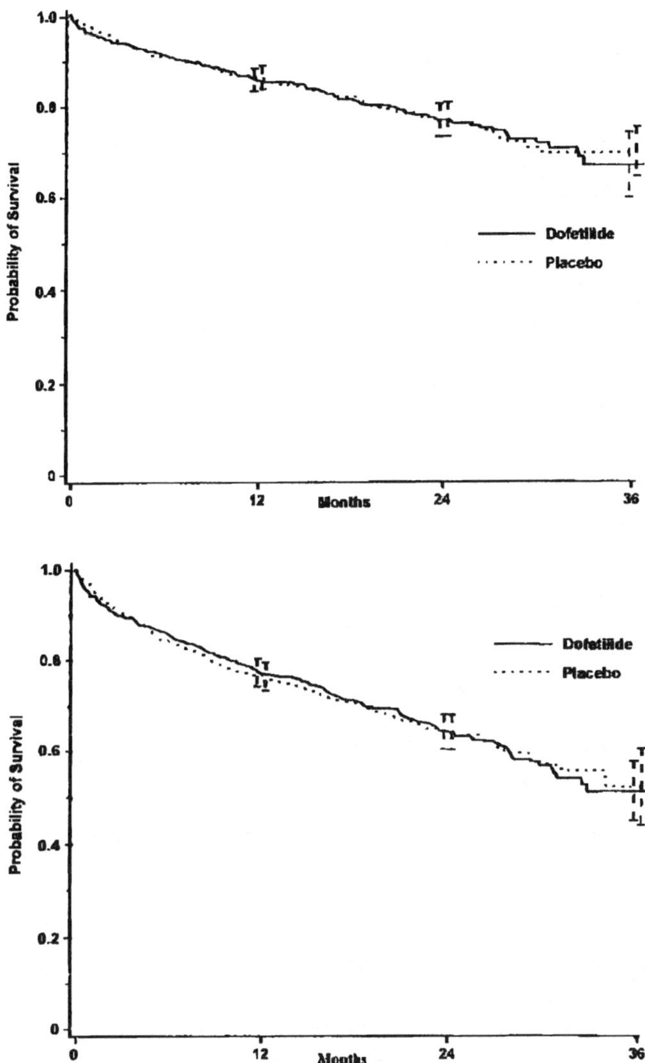

Figure 3   (top) Kaplan-Meier plot of arrhythmic mortality (95% CI): intent-to-treat population. (bottom) Kaplan-Meier plot of cardiac mortality (95% CI): intent-to-treat population.

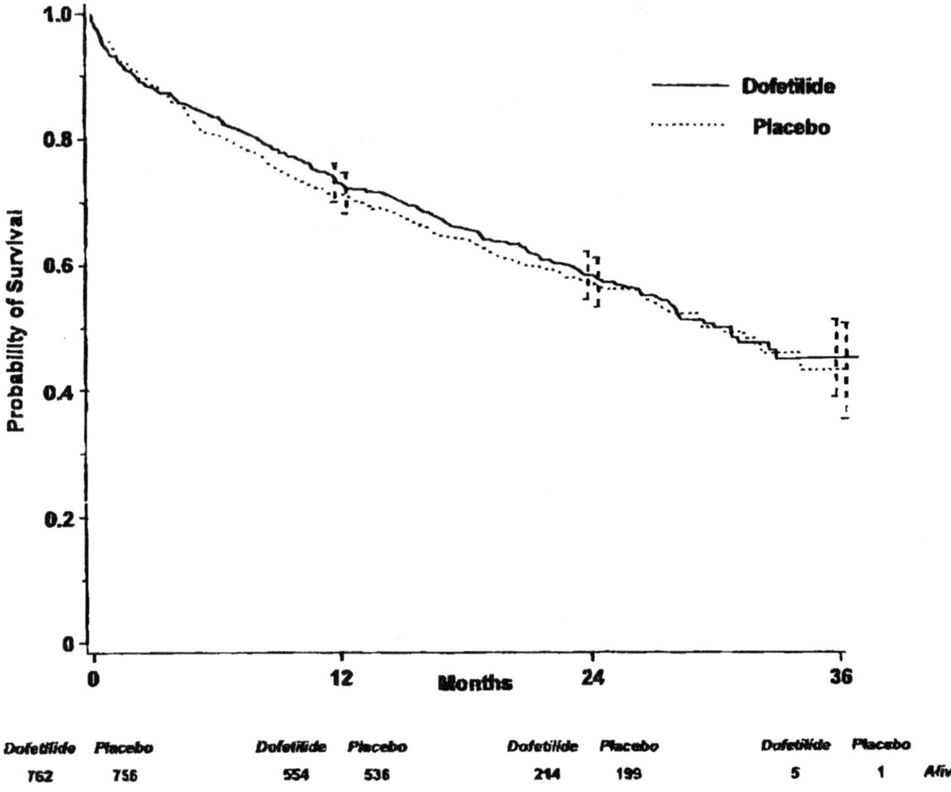

Figure 4   Kaplan-Meier plot of total mortality (95% CI): intent-to-treat population.

dofetilide (44%) and 28 (14%) on placebo converted to sinus rhythm without DC cardioversion ($p < 0.001$).

There was also a significant difference favoring dofetilide in the maintenance of sinus rhythm regardless of how sinus rhythm was induced. Including subjects who had a successful DC cardioversion, 119 patients on dofetilide and 69 patients on placebo who had AF/AFl at baseline achieved sinus rhythm. Of these, the probability of remaining in sinus rhythm for 1 year was 77.7% on dofetilide compared with 42.8% on placebo ($p < 0.002$).

Dofetilide was also effective in preventing atrial fibrillation in patients with AF at baseline. Of 556 patients in sinus rhythm on dofetilide, 11 developed AF during the study compared with 35 of 534 patients on placebo ($p < 0.001$).

Table 2 Ventricular Arrhythmias

	Dofetilide $n = 762$	Placebo $n = 756$
TdP[a]	25 (14–2)	0 (0–0)
Mono VT[a]	11 (4–2)	13 (1–5)
Poly VT[a]	3 (2–0)	4 (2–0)
VF[a]	14 (1–11)	12 (3–7)
Other RCA[a]	18 (17–1)	8 (8–0)
Total RCA	38	14
Total Death	16	12

[a] Numbers with resuscitated cardiac arrest–death for each rhythm are shown in parenthesis.

RCA = resuscitated cardiac arrest; Mono VT = sustained monomorphic ventricular tachycardia; Poly VT = sustained polymorphic ventricular tachycardia; VF = ventricular fibrillation.

Adverse Effects and Proarrhythmia

As with all class III antiarrhythmic drugs, dofetilide may cause proarrhythmia, which usually manifests as torsade de pointes ventricular tachycardia (TdP). In order to detect and promptly treat any possible proarrhythmia, patients were monitored intensively with continuous telemetry for the first 3 days of therapy. All ventricular arrhythmias recorded during the study were classified by the arrhythmic events committee and are presented in Table 2. TdP occurred in 25 patients on dofetilide and none on placebo. However, the incidence of sustained ventricular arrhythmias other than TdP are similar in the two treatment groups. Importantly, the occurrence of TdP or other possible proarrhythmias did not result in an increased mortality.

Of the 25 cases of TdP, ten did not require DC cardioversion and 19 occurred within the first 3 days of therapy.

As described above, dosing according to renal function was introduced *after* the enrollment of 288 patients. This dosing strategy had an impact on the incidence of TdP. Incidence was 4.8% (7/146) for patients on dofetilide included *before* dosing by renal function was introduced; this subsequently dropped to 2.9% (18/616) for those dosed according to calculated creatinine clearance (a decline of 40%).

As a result of the specific mode of action of dofetilide there was no difference in the incidence of systemic adverse effects between dofetilide and placebo.

CONCLUSION

The DIAMOND study included 1518 patients with moderate-to-severe CHF and left ventricular dysfunction. If demonstrated that dofetilide is well tolerated in this population and can be used safely when initiated with appropriate monitoring.

As well as demonstrating safety, two important benefits of dofetilide are seen in atrial fibrillation and progression of heart failure. A beneficial effect of dofetilide on conversion of atrial fibrillation and maintenance of sinus rhythm was clearly observed in these patients with marked left ventricular dysfunction (LVEF $\leq 35\%$). In addition, patients on dofetilide had a reduced need for hospitalization with worsening CHF, providing a substantial benefit on morbidity in this severely compromised population.

Craig M. Pratt
Baylor College of Medicine, Houston, Texas

The Danish Investigation of Arrhythmia and Mortality ON Dofetilide (DIA-MOND) trial was conducted to study the effect of dofetilide, an I_{kr} blocker on a population selected for the presence of congestive heart failure (CHF) (1). The patient population was composed of a group of patients primarily with NYHA class II, III CHF, approximately two-thirds of which had underlying ischemic heart disease. The primary endpoint of this trial was total mortality. The DIA-MOND–CHF study showed that an I_{kr} blocker, dofetilide, compared to placebo, did not alter mortality in this heart failure population.

Importantly, the study design mandated inpatient initiation in all patients, with telemetry monitoring for 72 h. In addition, scrutiny of renal function was important to adjust dosage, both at the time of drug initiation and if any changes occurred in renal function during the trial. Although 500 µg dofetilide bid was the target dose in some patients, dosage was frequently 250 µg bid in patients whose creatinine clearance was 40–60 cc/h, and was set at 250 µg once a day in patients whose creatinine clearance was 20–40 cc/h. After dosage adjustment based on creatinine clearance was implemented, there was a 40% reduction in the observed incidence of torsades de pointes ventricular tachycardia (VT).

CLINICAL BENEFITS OF DOFETILIDE

The most important clinical results of the DIAMOND trial relate to the long-term, placebo-controlled observations of patients with atrial fibrillation. Approximately one-quarter of the DIAMOND population had atrial fibrillation at randomization. Compared to placebo, dofetilide-assigned patients had a significantly higher conversion to sinus rhythm (141 vs. 106; $p < 0.001$); also, the number of patients who developed new-onset atrial fibrillation was also reduced in dofetilide-assigned as opposed to placebo-assigned patients (12 vs. 40; $p < 0.001$; dofetilide vs. placebo). An intriguing result was that a significantly greater proportion of placebo-assigned patients developed worsening CHF during the trial than did dofetilide-assigned patients (38% vs. 30%; $p < 0.001$).

FOCUS ON ADVERSE EVENTS

In the DIAMOND–CHF trials, the most important toxicity of dofetilide was, as one would expect, the development of torsade de pointes ventricular tachycardia. By requiring inpatient initiation of drug with telemetry monitoring as well as modifying dosing by the results of creatinine clearance, this proarrhythmia did not adversely affect the primary outcome of the trial. Approximately three-quarters of the torsade de pointes VT cases occurred in the first 3 days. Modifying the dofetilide dose based upon renal function decreased the torsades rate from 4.8 to 2.9%. Of the 25 cases of observed torsade de pointes VT, 15 required resuscitation and three patients died. This was in comparison to two cardiac arrests on placebo. These results are not unexpected with an I_{kr} blocker and point to the importance of initiating dofetilide by: (1) inpatient telemetry monitoring; (2) the use of the creatinine clearance algorithm for dosing; and (3) careful attention to serum potassium, magnesium, and concomitant therapies. Otherwise, dofetilide is well tolerated, and its side-effect profile during long-term dosing was comparable to placebo.

GENERALIZABILITY OF THE DIAMOND–CHF PATIENT POPULATION

A minor limitation is that this trial was performed in one country, Denmark, with an almost exclusively Caucasian population. However, the gender distribution was quite similar to the gender distribution in CHF as reported throughout the world (75% male). In my view, this study can be extrapolated to typical heart failure populations, and certainly to the atrial fibrillation population. This was a high-risk population of heart failure patients with a high mortality and a mean left ventricular ejection fraction <30%. The study offers the perspective of long-term follow-up in a large placebo-controlled population to estimate risk and benefit. The study itself was run with great attention to detail as evidenced by the fact that there was 100% follow-up of all patients in the trial. Thus, the results are interpretable and quite believable.

COMPARISON WITH OTHER MORTALITY TRIALS

Up until the report of the DIAMOND–CHF trial, only mortality trials utilizing amiodarone had reported results compatible with antiarrhythmic drug safety. These included the Congestive Heart Failure–Survival Trial of Antiarrhythmic Therapy (CHF-STAT) (2) as well as the European Myocardial Infarct Amiodarone Trial (EMIAT) (3) and Canadian Amiodarone Myocardial Infarction Arrhythmia Trial (CAMIAT) (4) trials. These trials were reported after the results of smaller trials had shown a trend to a mortality benefit on amiodarone, including

Basel Antiarrhythmic Study of Infarct Survival (BASIS) (5), the Polish Amiodarone Trial (6), as well as the Grupo de Estudio de la Sobrevida en la Insuficiencia Cardiaca en Argentina (GESICA) (7) trial. It should be emphasized that in all of these trials, amiodarone was administered with a loading regimen, gradually tapered over many months, and all included outpatient drug initiation. In contrast to dofetilide, long-term tolerability of amiodarone is limited by significant noncardiac side effects such as pulmonary and thyroid toxicity, such that approximately twice as many patients in the amiodarone-treated group discontinued therapy compared to placebo [e.g., 40% dropout rate in EMIAT (3)]. This is in distinct contrast to a nearly equal number of placebo-treated and dofetilide-treated patients remaining on study drug in the DIAMOND–CHF study.

A very intriguing question is why the results of the Survival With ORal D-sotalol (SWORD) (8,9) trial and the DIAMOND–CHF trial are so discrepant. Despite the fact that both dofetilide and d-sotalol are I_{kr} blockers, the SWORD trial reported a d-sotalol-associated increase in mortality (relative risk = 1.6), whereas the DIAMOND–CHF trial was consistent with dofetilide safety (relative risk = 0.95) (8,9). The SWORD population closely resembled the DIAMOND–CHF population. In the SWORD population, the major group experiencing increased mortality were patients enrolled many years after myocardial infarction who had NYHA class II, III CHF. One potential explanation for the difference in outcome of the trials was the inpatient initiation of dofetilide with telemetry monitoring, which eliminated a substantial number of patients who might have had adverse mortality consequences from dofetilide. In both protocols, dosage adjustment due to renal impairment was mandatory. Interesting results that may have improved the prognosis in the DIAMOND–CHF trial was the reduction in atrial fibrillation and the reduction in hospitalizations for CHF. Perhaps a combination of these factors accounts for the differences in outcome in the two trials or other unappreciated differences in these two I_{kr} blockers.

LESSONS FROM THE DIAMOND–CHF TRIAL

1. Dofetilide can be used safely in patients with significant clinical CHF when initiated as an inpatient with telemetry monitoring for 3 days. Careful attention to baseline creatinine clearance, changes in creatinine clearance as well as electrolytes, during dosing, minimizes the occurrence of torsade de pointes ventricular tachycardia.
2. In DIAMOND, dofetilide therapy reduced the incidence of new-onset atrial fibrillation; it also significantly increased the rate of conversion to sinus rhythm in those patients who had atrial fibrillation at baseline.
3. Dofetilide administration resulted in a reduction in hospitalizations for clinical CHF and reduction in the development of clinical CHF as compared to placebo.
4. These results in atrial fibrillation are fairly powerful observations be-

cause of the severity of CHF, the long-term follow-up and safety data relative to total mortality. These results will be combined with the results of placebo-controlled trials of patients selected for the presence of atrial fibrillation. The combined information will provide a powerful data set to interpret the role of dofetilide in the treatment of atrial fibrillation.

5. Dofetilide appears to be a safe, effective alternative in patients with atrial fibrillation to maintain sinus rhythm.

REFERENCES

1. DIAMOND Study Group. Dofetilide in patients with left ventricular dysfunction and either heart failure or acute myocardial infarction: rationale, design, and patient characteristics of the DIAMOND studies. Clin Cardiol 1997;20:704–710.
2. Singh SN, Fletch RD, Fisher SG, Singh BN, Lewis HD, Deedwania PC, Massie BM, Colling C, Lazzeri, for the Survival Trial of Antiarrhythmic Therapy in Congestive Heart Failure. Amiodarone in patients with congestive heart failure and asymptomatic ventricular arrhythmia. N Engl J Med 1995;333:77–88.
3. Julian DG, Camm AJ, Fragin G, Janse MJ, Munoz A, Schwartz PJ, Simon P, for the European Myocardial Infarct Amiodarone Trial Investigators. Randomised trial of effect of amiodarone on mortality in patients with left-ventricular dysfunction after recent myocardial infarction: EMIAT. Lancet 1997;349:667–674.
4. Cairns JA, Connolly SJ, Robert R, Gent M, for the Canadian Amiodarone Myocardial Infarction Arrhythmia Trial Investigators. Randomized trial of outcome after myocardial infarction in patients with frequent or repetitive ventricular premature depolarisations: CAMIAT. Lancet 1997;349:675–682.
5. Burkart F, Pfisterer M, Kiowski W, Follath F, Burckhardt D. Effect of antiarrhythmic therapy on mortality in survivors of myocardial infarction with asymptomatic complex ventricular arrhythmias: Basel Antiarrhythmic Study of Infarct Survival (BASIS). J Am Coll Cardiol 1990;16:1711–1718.
6. Budaj A, Kokowicz P, Smielak-Korombel W, Kuch J, Krzeminska-Pakuoa M, Maciejewicz J, Nartowicz E, Zaleska T, Dyduszynski A, Ceremuznski L. Lack of effect of amiodarone on survival after extensive infarction. Polish Amiodarone Trial. Coron Artery Dis 1996;7:315–319.
7. Doval HC, Nul DR, Grancelli HO, Perrone SV, Bortman GR, Curiel R for Grupo de Estudio de la Sobrevida en la Insuficiencia Cardiaca en Argentina (GESICA). Randomized trial of low-dose amiodarone in severe congestive heart failure. Lancet 1994; 344:493–98.
8. Waldo AL, Camm AJ, deRuyter H, Friedman PL, MacNeil DJ, Pauls JF, Pitt B, Pratt CM, Schwartz PJ, Veltri EP, for the SWORD Investigators. Effect of d-sotalol on mortality in patients with left ventricular dysfunction after myocardial infarction. Lancet 1996;348:7–12.
9. Pratt CM, Camm AJ, Cooper W, Friedman PL MacNeil DJ, Moulton KM, Pitt B, Schwartz PJ, Veltri EP, Waldo AL, for the SWORD Investigators. Mortality in the survival with oral d-sotalol (SWORD) trial: Why did patients die? Am J Cardiol 1998; 81:869–876.

14

The Cardiac Arrest Study Hamburg (CASH) Trial

Steven N. Singh
*Georgetown University Medical Center
and Veterans Affairs Medical Center, Washington, D.C.*

Raymond L. Woosley
Georgetown University Medical Center, Washington, D.C.

In 1987, the Cardiac Arrest Study Hamburg (CASH) was initiated. Survivors of cardiac arrest were prospectively randomized to four treatment groups: amiodarone, propafenone, metoprolol, or ICD. The primary endpoint was total mortality.

METHODS

Survivors of cardiac arrest were recruited from several centers. All patients underwent complete physical examination, laboratory analyses, chest x-ray, 12-lead ECG, echocardiogram, exercise testing, 24-h ambulatory ECG, and coronary angiography. All patients also underwent programmed electrical stimulation before and after randomization. After informed consent, patients received either amiodarone (1000 mg daily for 7 days, 400–600 mg daily thereafter), metoprolol (12.5 to 25 mg/daily, up to 200 mg if tolerated), profanenone (450 mg/daily, up to 900 mg), or the ICD. The ICD was set at a cut-off rate between 170 to 200 bpm. Shock delivery was chosen as primary therapy, but, if available, ATP pacing was individualized.

RESULTS

In March 1992, after 11 months of follow-up, it was noted that a significantly higher incidence of total mortality and cardiac arrest recurrence was seen in the propafenone arm compared to the ICD arm (1).

The main results of the 349 enrolled patients were presented at the 47th Scientific Sessions of the American College of Cardiology, Atlanta, Georgia, in March, 1998. The 2-year mortality in the ICD arm was 12.1% versus 19.6% in the combined amiodarone and metoprolol arms ($p = 0.047$). There was no significant difference in survival between the two drug groups. The authors concluded that in survivors of cardiac arrest the ICD is superior to drug therapy.

REFERENCES

1. Siebels J, Cappato R, Ruppell, Schneider M, Kuck K and the CASH investigators. Am J Cardiol 1993;72:109F–113F.

CASH: Critique

Steven N. Singh

*Georgetown University Medical Center
and Veterans Affairs Medical Center, Washington, D.C.*

Raymond L. Woosley

Georgetown University Medical Center, Washington, D.C.

The Cardiac Arrest Study Hamburg (CASH) trial was an intent to test the effects of ICD, amiodarone, propafenone or metoprolol on total mortality in survivors of cardiac arrest. After a mean follow-up period of 11 months, an interim analysis in 1992 showed that propafenone compared to ICD was harmful, and this arm was terminated. The trial continued comparing the three remaining arms. The final results were presented at the 47th Scientific Sessions of The American College of Cardiology, Atlanta, Georgia, in March 1998. Three hundred and forty-nine patients were enrolled: 99–ICD, 92–amiodarone, and 99–metoprolol. The mean EF for the entire group was about 46%. The 2-year mortality was 12% in the ICD arm versus 19% on the combined amiodarone and metoprolol arms (i.e., a 37% reduction in mortality; $p = 0.047$). There was no significant difference in mortality between amiodarone and metoprolol.

The population studied included survivors of cardiac arrest from ventricular tachycardia or ventricular fibrillation. This definition of cardiac arrest is less specific than desired and could have the potential of creating imbalances across groups. Because the primary endpoint was total mortality, the propafenone arm may have been prematurely discontinued since there was no difference in the total number of deaths (8-ICD; 9-propafenone). Moreover, some deaths occurred when the patients were not taking propafenone. The decision to discontinue the propafenone arm was probably based on higher incidence of freedom from sudden death survival and recurrence of cardiac arrest. In patients assigned to the ICD group, the mean ejection fraction (~46%) was surprisingly higher than expected. Of note, in the AVID study there was no improvement in mortality in the group with EF $>35\%$ treated with the ICD.

Even though the primary endpoint was total mortality, a major weakness is that the three drugs were assigned in an open-label fashion, creating the potential for bias due to differences in patient management. Moreover, the study lacks power to detect differences in survival. There was no mention in the published reports whether differences were sought among all arms in the trial or just by comparison of the ICD arm versus the drug arms. To combine the results of the amiodarone and metoprolol arms against ICD may not be appropriate. Moreover, to conclude that there is no difference between amiodarone and metoprolol based on the small samples could be erroneous. Finally, to use a one-tailed test and a p value of <0.05 is of questionable validity. Using the more appropriate two-tailed test, this trial would have had neutral results.

15

The Canadian Implantable Defibrillator Study (CIDS)

Steven N. Singh
*Georgetown University Medical Center
and Veterans Affairs Medical Center, Washington, D.C.*

Raymond L. Woosley
Georgetown University Medical Center, Washington, D.C.

The Canadian Implantable Defibrillator Study (CIDS) tested the hypothesis that the ICD will reduce the risk of arrhythmic death when compared to amiodarone in patients who have (1) documented VF; (2) survived cardiac arrest; (3) symptomatic (chest pain or dizziness) sustained monomorphic VT (rate >150 bpm, depressed EF <35%); (4) sustained VT with syncope; or (5) syncope with spontaneous or EP-induced sustained VT. Once entrance criteria were met, patients were randomized to the ICD or amiodarone (1200 mg daily for 7 days, 400 mg daily for 10 weeks, 300 mg daily thereafter). In the event of intolerable side effects, the minimum dose was 200 mg daily. All patients were seen at 2 months, 6 months, and every 6 months thereafter (1).

RESULTS

The results were presented at the 47th Scientific Sessions of the American College of Cardiology, Atlanta, Georgia, March 1998. Three hundred and twenty patients received the ICD and 331 received amiodarone. After 4 years, there was a trend toward reduction in all-cause mortality with use of the ICD compared to amiodarone (27% ICD vs. 33% amiodarone; $p = 0.07$). The authors concluded that the ICD was modestly better than amiodarone in the high-risk population.

REFERENCES

1. Connolly SJ, Gent M, Roberts RS, Dorian PD, Green MS, Klein GI, Mitchell B, Sheldon RS, Ross D on behalf of the CIDS Investigators. Am J Cardiol 1993;72: 103F–108F.

CIDS: Critique

David J. Wilber
University of Chicago, Chicago, Illinois

The Canadian Implantable Defibrillator Study (CIDS) is one of a series of multicenter randomized trials comparing the efficacy of implantable defibrillators (ICD) to antiarrhythmic drug therapy in patients with a history of sustained ventricular arrhythmias (1). The CIDS study population was limited to patients thought to be at high risk for arrhythmic death: cardiac arrest survivors, patients with syncopal ventricular tachycardia, and patients with symptomatic (but not syncopal) ventricular tachycardia associated with a left ventricular ejection fraction (LVEF) $\leq$ 35%. The study also permitted enrollment of patients with unmonitored syncope who subsequently had inducible sustained monomorphic ventricular tachycardia during electrophysiological testing, or spontaneous self-terminating runs of ventricular tachycardia ($\geq$10 s) during monitoring. Enrolled patients were randomized to receive either an ICD or amiodarone therapy ($\geq$1200 mg daily loading dose for 1 week, $\geq$300 mg daily chronic maintenance). A total of 659 patients were randomized between October 1990 and December 1996. A minimum 1-year follow-up was completed in December, 1997. Preliminary results of the completed trial were presented in early 1998 (2). At 3 years of follow-up, survival in ICD-treated patients was 75%, and survival in amiodarone-treated patients was 70%. The 19.6% reduction in all-cause mortality associated with ICD therapy did not reach statistical significance ($p = 0.072$). The goal of this commentary is to provide an initial perspective on the results of CIDS, and to assess the significance of these preliminary results in the context of other recently completed trials evaluating the efficacy of ICDs relative to antiarrhythmic drug therapy in patients with hemodynamically compromising sustained ventricular arrhythmias.

The trend toward improved survival with ICD therapy in CIDS is consistent with the results of two other randomized trials in similar patient populations,

293

each of which demonstrated a significant reduction in all-cause mortality in ICD-treated patients. In the Antiarrhythmics Versus Implantable Defibrillator (AVID) trial, 1016 patients with cardiac arrest or hemodynamically compromising sustained ventricular tachycardia were randomized to ICD therapy or amiodarone (3,4). Guided sotalol therapy was initially planned as an alternative therapeutic option in patients assigned to drug therapy. However, only 2.6% of all patients randomized to drug therapy were actually discharged on sotalol. The trial was terminated prematurely in 1997 because of significantly improved survival associated with ICD therapy. At 3 years of follow-up, survival was 75% in ICD-treated patients, and 64% in amiodarone-treated patients, a 31% reduction in mortality ($p < 0.02$) (4).

The final results of the Cardiac Arrest Study Hamburg (CASH) were also reported recently. In this study, 400 cardiac arrest survivors were randomized to one of four treatment arms: ICD, amiodarone, metoprolol, or propafenone (5). Enrollment began in 1987. An interim analysis of the study was reported in 1993, after treatment in the propafenone limb was prematurely terminated due to excess mortality (29% in propafenone-treated patients at 11 months, compared to 11% in the remaining treatment groups) (6,7). The final results of follow-up in the remaining 349 patients assigned to ICD therapy, amiodarone, or metoprolol were reported in early 1998 (7). At 2 years of follow-up, survival was 88% in ICD-treated patients, and 80% in patients treated with either amiodarone or metoprolol, a 37% reduction in all-cause mortality ($p = 0.047$).

Collectively, these three studies provide a clear and consistent picture of improved survival with ICD therapy in patients with a previous history of sustained ventricular arrhythmias. What remains less clear, and is likely to be the subject of continued discussion and debate, is the overall magnitude of the survival benefit associated with device therapy, and potential differences between subgroups of patients in the degree of survival benefit. Several aspects of CIDS specifically (which showed the least survial benefit of the three trials), and of the three as a whole, are important to review in this regard.

COMPARISON OF CIDS AND THE AVID TRIAL

The survival benefit associated with ICD therapy was less in CIDS than in the study it most closely resembled, AVID. The two trials differed in statistical design and assumptions. The design of the AVID trial was relatively robust (3). It was planned as a two-sided trial (no a priori assumption of which treatment was superior). The large, planned sample size of 1200 patients allowed preservation of a high degree of power (>80%) to detect a 30% treatment effect over a broad range of mortality and crossover rates. The trial was stopped prematurely prior to completion of planned enrollment and follow-up by the Data and Safety Monitoring Board when sequential monitoring of differences between treatment groups in the primary study endpoint, total mortality, crossed the statistical boundary for early termination (4). In CIDS, the original planned enrollment was 400 patients, and the primary endpoint was arrhythmic death (1). Enrollment was subsequently increased to improve the power of the study to detect treatment differences in total mortality. Enrollment of 650 patients was calculated to provide a power of 90% to detect a 30% reduction in mortality with ICD therapy (single-sided trial, $\alpha = 0.05$, assumed mortality rate in amiodarone-treated patients of 30%, minimal crossover) (2). The study completed planned enrollment and follow-up, and the 20% reduction in mortality associated with ICD therapy at final follow-up was not statistically significant. However, even with the expanded enrollment, CIDS remained underpowered ($<70\%$) to detect a real treatment effect of 20% (8). The extent of crossovers may have reduced this power even further.

Overall, the baseline characteristics of the patients in each study were similar, with two notable exceptions (Table 1). CIDS enrolled patients with unexplained syncope if subsequent data from electrophysiological testing or ambulatory monitoring suggested that a hemodynamically unstable ventricular arrhythmia was a likely cause. The rationale for including such patients was the assumption that this subgroup had a high risk of future arrhythmic death similar to that of patients with documented hemodynamically compromising ventricular arrhythmias (10). However, both preliminary subgroup analysis of CIDS (2), as well as data from the AVID Registry (9), indicate that the mortality risk in such patients, while not inconsequential, is lower than in patients with documented

Table 1 Comparison of CIDS to Other Secondary Prevention Trials

	CIDS	AVID	CASH
PATIENTS (*n*)	659	1016	349
AGE (mean years)	64	65	58
LVEF (mean)	0.33	0.31	0.46
CAD	84%	81%	73%
CLASS 3–4 CHF	21%	10%	NA
INDEX ARRHYTHMIA			
VF or Cardiac Arrest	48%	45%	100%
VT with syncope	13%	21%	0%
VT, low LVEF, symptoms	25%	34%	0%
Syncope, inducible VT	14%	0%	0%
CROSSOVER TO ICD IN DRUG GROUP	25%	24%	6%
AMIODARONE WITHDRAWAL	17%	15%	9%

Data are expressed as percentages of *n*, except where indicated.
CAD = coronary artery disease; CHF = congestive heart failure; LVEF = left ventricular ejection fraction; NA = not available; VF = ventricular fibrillation; VT = ventricular tachycardia.

hemodynamically compromising ventricular arrhythmias. The inclusion of patients with unexplained syncope potentially may have contributed to the smaller survival benefit of ICDs observed in CIDS. CIDS also contained a greater proportion of patients with New York Heart Association Class III or IV heart failure. This latter group of patients faces an increased risk of death due to the competing causes of heart failure and bradyarrhythmias (11,12). Retrospective nonrandomized studies indicate that the potential survival benefit of ICDs in these patients may be more limited (13,14). Inclusion of a substantial number of these patients (21% in CIDS) may have influenced the overall apparent survival benefit of ICD therapy.

CIDS and the AVID trial were also similar with respect to most aspects of therapy. The loading dose of amiodarone was similar between the two studies, as was the chronic maintenance dose (mean 240–280 mg daily at 2 to 3 years). The rate of amiodarone withdrawal was small in both studies, considerably less than the 30% discontinuation rate noted in recent primary prevention trials (15,16), and was not likely to have contributed to differences in outcome. In the AVID trial, approximatley two-thirds of patients received angiotensin converting enzyme inhibitors, and 42% of ICD- and 17% of amiodarone-treated patients received beta-blockers at discharge. Comparable data for CIDS are not yet available. Coronary revascularization was undertaken in approximately 30% of CIDS patients (2). In the AVID trial, approximately 30% of patients underwent revascularization prior to the index arrhythmia (17), and 11% underwent revascularization after the index arrhythmia (4). Both studies spanned the transition between epicardial and transvenous systems: 11% of CIDS patients and 5% of AVID trial patients received epicardial lead systems. The potential impact of early and late adverse events associated with the greater use of epicardial systems in CIDS awaits more complete reporting of trial data.

Both CIDS and the AVID trial demonstrated a relatively high percentage of crossover from amiodarone therapy to device therapy over the course of the trial (approximately 10% at 1 year, and 25% at 3 years) (2,4). This is somewhat greater than anticipated in both studies. Given the observed benefit of ICD therapy despite crossovers, the true magnitude of survival benefit associated with device therapy was almost certainly underestimated in both trials. It is unreasonable to suggest that the use of amiodarone in ICD patients (approximately 30% at 3 years in both trials) somehow offsets the impact of amiodarone crossover to ICD therapy. While the drug may be effective in diminishing the frequency of spontaneous ventricular arrhythmias, there is little evidence of mortality benefit either in these trials or in two recently completed placebo-controlled trials of patients after myocardial infarction (15,16), who comprise the majority of CIDS and AVID patients. It is of interest that the largest estimated reduction in mortality associated with ICDs, 37%, was reported in CASH, which also had the lowest crossover rate (6%) (7).

Data regarding the number, characteristics, and outcome of eligible, but nonrandomized, patients would allow assessment of potential enrollment bias and the representative nature of the observed mortality rates in CIDS. A registry of such patients was planned as part of the original study design (1), but no information is currently available. Preliminary data from the AVID registry indicate that randomized patients in that trial had baseline characteristics similar to eligible, but nonrandomized, patients (9,17).

CIDS, AVID, AND CASH: QUESTIONS ANSWERED AND QUESTIONS REMAINING

A positive feature of randomized trials incorporating a broad spectrum of prognostically diverse patient subgroups is generalizability. Data from CIDS, in addition to that provided by CASH and AVID, support the use of ICD therapy in patients with hemodynamically compromising sustained ventricular arrhythmias over a broad range of ventricular function and cardiac disease. The true magnitude of overall survival benefit remains unclear. The inevitable tradeoff with broad-based enrollment strategies is a reduced ability and statistical power to identify differences in treatment benefit between clinical subgroups. This latter consideration becomes important when evaluating the cost-benefit ratio of relatively expensive therapy with a modest impact on survival in the overall population. For example, it is unclear how survival benefit and cost effectiveness may differ between patients with idiopathic ventricular fibrillation relative to patients with Class III heart failure and idiopathic dilated cardiomyopathy. Meta-analysis of the three trials together may generate sufficient patient numbers in individual groups to permit more detailed comparisons of outcome.

The results of CIDS, like AVID and CASH, cannot be generalized to certain subgroups of patients that were specifically excluded from the trials, but in whom ICD therapy is often clinically applied. The largest of these groups consists of patients presenting with hemodynamically stable ventricular tachycardia, particularly those with relatively preserved ventricular function. Nonrandomized observational studies (18,19), including the AVID registry (9), suggest that while mortality is not inconsequential in these patients, mortality risk and the incidence of arrhythmia-related death appears lower than in trial-eligible patients; the potential survival benefit of ICD therapy in this setting may be less. The initial design of both CIDS and the AVID trial also excluded patients with relatively well-preserved ventricular function and significant myocardial ischemia, in whom revascularization was undertaken as the primary therapy for cardiac arrhythmia. Retrospective studies provide conflicting data regarding the adequacy of revascularization alone to reduce subsequent mortality and recurrent ventricular arrhythmias in this subgroup (20–22). Finally, limited data suggest that selected patients with the long QT syndrome may benefit from ICD therapy (23). These patients were excluded from all three trials. While ICD therapy may be appropriate and provide survival benefit in some patients from each of these subgroups, the results of CIDS and the two other secondary prevention trials provide no information to guide clinical decisions.

CONCLUSIONS

CIDS represents an important step forward in providing evidence-based guidelines for the management of patients with hemodynamically compromising sustained ventricular arrhythmias. The preliminary results of this study are best understood in the context of other recently completed randomized clinical trials of secondary prevention. Collectively, the results of these studies support the use of ICD therapy in cardiac arrest survivors and patients with other hemodynamically compromising sustained ventricular arrhythmias over a broad range of ventricular function and cardiac disease. A final perspective on CIDS awaits more extensive publication of data from both randomized patients and those in the accompanying registry.

REFERENCES

1. Connolly SJ, Gent M, Roberts RS, Dorian P, Green MS, Klein GJ, Mitchell LB, Sheldon RS, Roy D. Canadian Implantable Defibrillator Study (CIDS): Study Design and Organization. Am J Cardiol 1993;72:103F–108F.
2. Connolly SJ. The Canadian Implantable Defibrillator Study. Presented at the American College of Cardiology Scientific Sessions, Atlanta, Georgia, March 1998.
3. The AVID Investigators. Antiarrhythmics versus implantable defibrillators (AVID)—Rationale, design and methods. Am J Cardiol 1995;75:470–475.
4. The AVID Investigators. A comparison of antiarrhythmic-drug therapy with implantable defibrillators in patients resuscitated from near-fatal ventricular arrhythmias. New Engl J Med 1997;337:1576–1583.
5. Siebels J, Kuck KH. Implantable cardioverter defibrillator compared with antiarrhythmic drug treatment in cardiac arrest survivors (the Cardiac Arrest Study Hamburg). Am Heart J 1994;1139–1144.
6. Siebels J, Cappato R, Ruppel R, Schneider MA Kuck KH. Preliminary Results of the Cardiac Arrest Study Hamburg (CASII). Am J Cardiol 1993;72:109F–113F.
7. Kuck KH. The Cardiac Arrest Study Hamburg (CASH). Presented at the American College of Cardiology Scientific Sessions, Atlanta, Georgia March 1998.
8. Friedman LM, Furberg CD, DeMets DL. Fundamental of Clinical Trials. St Louis: Mosby, 1996.
9. Anderson JL, the AVID Investigators. Long-term survival in the antiarrhythmics vs. implantable defibrillators (AVID) registry. J Am Coll Cardiol 1998;31:160A (abstr).
10. Link MS, Costeas XF, Griffith JL, Colburn CD, Estes MA, Wang PJ. High incidence

of appropriate implantable defibrillator therapy in patients with syncope of unknown etiology and inducible ventricular arrhythmias. J Am Coll Cardiol 1997;29:370–375.

11. Uretsky BF, Sheahan RG. Primary prevention of sudden cardiac death in heart failure: will the solution be shocking? J Am Coll Cardiol 1997;30:15898–1597.

12. The Defibrillator Study Group. Actuarial risk of sudden death while awaiting cardiac transplantation in patients with atherosclerotic heart disease. Am J Cardiol 1991;68:545–546.

13. Sweeney MO, Ruskin JN, Garan H, McGovern BA, Guy ML, Torchiana DF, Vlahakes GJ, Newell JB, Semigran MJ, Dec GW. Influence of the implantable cardioverter/defibrillator on sudden death and total mortality in patients evaluated for cardiac transplantation. Circulation 1995;92:3273–3281.

14. Trappe HJ, Wenzlaff P, Pfitzner P, Fieguth HG. Long-term follow-up of patients with implantable cardioverter-defibrillators and mild, moderate, or severe impairment of left ventricular function. Heart 1997;78:243–249.

15. Julian DG, Camm AJ, Frangin G. Randomized trial of effect amiodarone on mortality in patients with left ventricular dysfunction after recent myocardial infarction: EMIAT. Lancet 1997;349:667–674.

16. Cairns JA, Connolly SJ, Roberts R, Gent M. Randomised trial of outcome after myocardial infarction in patients with frequent or repetitive ventricular premature depolarizations. CAMIAT. Lancet 1997;349:675–682.

17. Kim SG, Hallstrom A, Love JC Rosenberg Y, Powell J, Roth J, Brodsky M, Moore R, Wilkoff B. Comparison of clinical characteristics and frequency of implantable defibrillator use between randomized patients in the antiarrhythmic vs implantable defibrillators (AVID) trial and nonrandomized registry patients. Am J Cardiol 1997;80:454–457.

18. Sarter B, Finkle JK, Gerszten RE, Buxton AE. What is the risk of sudden cardiac death in patients presenting with hemodynamically stable sustained ventricular tachycardia after myocardial infarction? J Am Coll Cardiol 1996;28:122–129.

19. Bhatt D, Kopp D, Kall J, Kinder C, Wilber D. Influence of clinical presentation on survival in patients with sustained ventricular arrhythmias. PACE 1995;18:883 (abstr).

20. Kelly P, Ruskin JN, Vlahakes GJ, Buckley MJ, Freeman CS, Garan H. Surgical coronary revascularization in survivors of prehospital cardiac arrest: its effect on inducible ventricular arrhythmias and long-term survival. J Am Coll Cardiol 1990;15:267–273.

21. Natale A, Sra J, Axtell K, Maglio C, Dhala A, blanck Z, Deshpande S, Jazayeri M, Akhtar M. Ventricular fibrillation and polymorphic ventricular tachycardia with critical coronary artery stenosis: does bypass surgery suffice? J Cardiovasc Electrophysiol 1994;5:988–994.

22. Daoud EG, Niebauer M, Kou WH, Man KC, Horwood L, Morady F, Strickberger SA. Incidence of implantable defibrillator discharges after coronary revascularization in survivors of ischemic sudden death. Am Heart J 1995;130:277–280.

23. Groh WJ, Silka MJ, Oliver RP, Halperin BD, McAnulty JH, Kron J. Use of implantable cardioverter-defibrillators in the congenital long QT syndrome. Am J Cardiol 1996;78:703–706.

16

The Multicenter UnSustained Tachycardia Trial (MUSTT): A Randomized, Controlled Trial of the Primary Prevention of Sudden Death in Patients with Coronary Artery Disease

Alfred E. Buxton

Brown University School of Medicine and Rhode Island Hospital,
Providence, Rhode Island

Kerry L. Lee

Duke Clinical Research Institute, Durham, North Carolina

INTRODUCTION

In spite of the continuing downward trend in overall cardiovascular disease mortality, posthospital mortality remains high for some survivors of acute myocardial infarction. Patients with significant left ventricular dysfunction are at particular risk, with a 6-month mortality of at least 10% (1). Furthermore, the long-term risk of death in all survivors of infarction remains high, with the 5-year mortality estimated at 33% (2). Approximately one-third of the late deaths in survivors of infarction occur suddenly and unexpectedly, and the risk of sudden death persists for years after the acute infarction (3,4). The appropriate management of survivors of out-of-hospital cardiac arrest has been clarified by the results of recent trials, reported elsewhere in this volume. However, only a small minority (2–30%) of cardiac arrest victims survive to benefit from such treatments (4–7). Thus, primary prevention is desirable. In our current resource-limited environment, effective primary prevention of sudden death is dependent on identifying patient populations at highest risk and then applying the best treatments to these patients. Attainment of these goals is dependent on understanding the mechanisms responsible for sudden death in each population. Since these mechanisms

301

vary, depending on the type of underlying cardiac disease, trials of primary prevention should study relatively homogeneous populations.

The Multicenter Unsustained Tachycardia Trial (MUSTT) was conceived in 1989, as an evaluation of one method to reduce the risk of sudden death in high-risk patients with coronary artery disease. This ongoing trial was designed to test two major hypotheses:

1. By treating patients with antiarrhythmic therapy guided by electrophysiological studies, we can reduce the risk of sudden death, cardiac arrest, spontaneous sustained ventricular tachycardia (VT), and overall mortality in patients with chronic coronary artery disease and diminished left ventricular function having asymptomatic nonsustained VT.
2. The signal-averaged ECG will identify those at highest risk for sudden cardiac death, enabling it to be used to predict which patients should receive antiarrhythmic therapy.

This trial differs in two major respects from prior studies in this area. First, it is not a test of a specific antiarrhythmic drug or device. Rather, it is evaluating the utility of a *method* of guiding antiarrhythmic therapy (programmed stimulation in the electrophysiology laboratory) to reduce mortality in the study population. Programmed stimulation is used in two ways in this trial: to define a high-risk population, and to choose a specific antiarrhythmic treatment. Second, antiarrhythmic therapy in this study does not aim to suppress nonsustained VT. Nonsustained VT serves only as one factor to identify a high-risk population.

Enrollment in the trial was completed in October, 1996, and follow-up was finished in October, 1998. Several preliminary analyses have been reported, describing the relationship of electrocardiographic and clinical factors to the inducibility of sustained ventricular tachycardia by programmed stimulation. This chapter will outline the major features of the study and summarize the results of the preliminary analyses.

BACKGROUND

The rationale for this trial was based on a series of studies conducted in two patient populations. First, several centers applied electrophysiological studies to survivors of recent myocardial infarction to test the hypothesis that the presence of inducible ventricular tachycardia would identify patients at high risk specifically for sudden death (i.e., in excess of overall cardiovascular mortality). Two studies from Australia involving 403 and 200 patients, respectively, indicated that between 9 and 20% of patients early after myocardial infarction have inducible ventricular tachycardia, with protocols employing 1 to 5 ventricular extrastimuli (8,9). In Canada, a small study (150 patients), using one and two ventricular extrastimuli induced sustained VT in 11% of patients (10). With follow-up periods of 10 to 12 months, studies using stimulation protocols limited to ≤2 ventricular extrastimuli have reported very low sensitivity and predictive values for sudden death (<10%) (11,12). Later studies using stimulation protocols with ≥3 ventricular extrastimuli and follow-up of at least 1 year observed arrhythmic event rates of 25 to 36% in patients with inducible sustained ventricular tachycardia (13,14). The negative predictive value has been over 90% in all reports.

The second group of patients upon which this study was based were patients with spontaneous nonsustained ventricular tachycardia in the setting of chronic coronary artery disease. At the inception of the MUSTT, five studies, of ≥35 patients each, had examined the results of programmed stimulation in such patients (15–19). Studies using stimulation protocols involving only one or two ventricular extrastimuli demonstrated inducible ventricular tachycardia in 20–30% of patients (15,16). In contrast, protocols including 1–3 ventricular extrastimuli, produced rates of inducible sustained ventricular tachycardia of 40–45% (17–19). The latter three studies (in which patients with inducible VT received antiarrhythmic therapy) reported overall event rates (sudden death, resuscitated cardiac arrest, or sustained ventricular tachycardia) in 12.5 to 23% of patients (including patients with and without inducible VT), after a mean follow-up ranging from 14 to 30 months. None of these reports incorporated a control group of patients who had inducible sustained VT, but received no antiarrhythmic therapy. This factor is critical, because to date we do not know the risk of sudden death in asymptomatic nonsustained VT patients who have inducible VT. These studies did show that the rates of arrhythmic events in patients with inducible VT who received antiarrhythmic therapy guided by serial electrophysiological studies ranged from 11 to 31%. In contrast, in the patients who received empirical antiarrhythmic therapy, arrhythmic event rates were 50 to 88%. The arrhythmic events occurred almost exclusively in patients with inducible sustained ventricular tachycardia and left ventricular ejection fractions ≤0.40. The negative predictive value of electrophysiological studies ranged from 88 to 96%. The results of these studies formed the basis for the study protocol summarized below. The high arrhythmic event rates are notable in light of the fact that these reports examined patients an average of 3 years after acute infarction.

STUDY OVERVIEW

After an electrophysiological study performed in the absence of antiarrhythmic drugs to identify ''high- and low-risk patients,'' those patients with inducible sustained VT were randomized to either no antiarrhythmic therapy or therapy guided by serial electrophysiological studies. Patients with no sustained VT in-

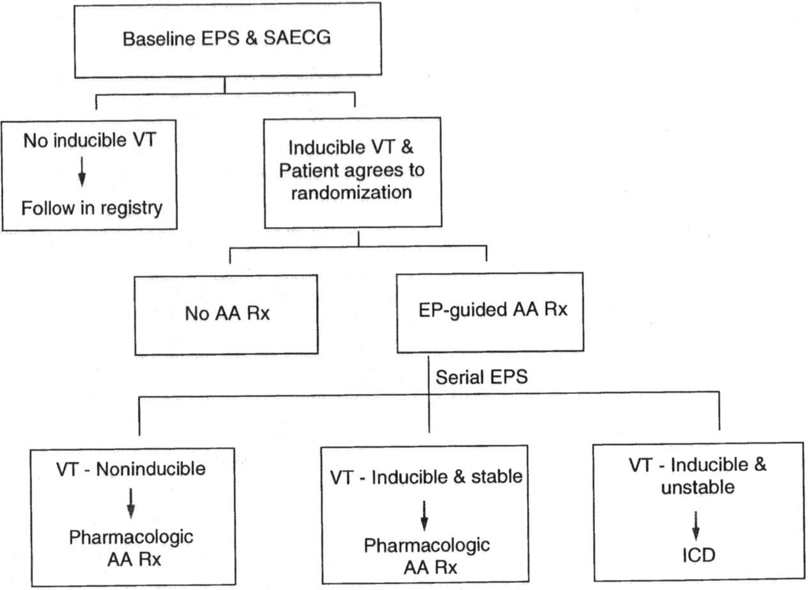

Figure 1 Schema of the MUSTT Protocol. Abbreviations: EPS-electrophysiological study; SAECG-signal-averaged electrocardiogram; VT-ventricular tachycardia; AA Rx-antiarrhythmic therapy; ICD-implantable cardioverter/defibrillator.

duced at the baseline electrophysiological study were followed without antiarrhythmic therapy in a registry (Fig. 1). It was recommended that all patients be treated with beta-adrenergic blocking agents and angiotensin converting enzyme inhibitors whenever tolerated in doses corresponding with those found effective in randomized, controlled trials demonstrating beneficial effects of these agents on survival after myocardial infarction. This applied to all patients in the trial, regardless of the presence or absence of inducible sustained ventricular tachycardia, or assignment to specific antiarrhythmic therapy (for patients with inducible sustained ventricular tachycardia).

ENTRY CRITERIA

1. Patients all had chronic coronary artery disease. Enrollment (performance of baseline EPS) occurred at least 4 days after the most recent

myocardial infarction, and at least 72 h after the last evidence of hemo-dynamic instability or myocardial ischemia. The presence of coronary artery disease was documented by catheterization or documented myo-cardial infarction.

2. All patients had a left ventricular ejection fraction ≤ 0.40 quantified by contrast ventriculogram, gated blood pool scan, or echocardiogram within 1 year of the study.

3. All patients had nonsustained VT causing no or minimal symptoms within 6 months of enrollment, and at least 4 days after the most recent myocardial infarction, or revascularization procedure, in the absence of antiarrhythmic drug therapy. Nonsustained VT was documented by Holter monitor, telemetry, or standard electrocardiogram.

4. Within 6 months prior to enrollment, patients had to complete a symptom-limited exercise test, combined with thallium scans or radionuclide ventriculography if the exercise ECG was uninterpretable. If the exercise test demonstrated evidence of ischemia, catheterization was performed, if clinically appropriate. Patients in whom revascularization was anticipated were not to be enrolled until 4 days after the procedure. The persistence of spontaneous nonsustained VT had to be documented at least 4 days after revascularization. If the patient was unable to exercise, a dipyridamole–thallium scan (or other pharmacological ''stress'' test) was performed. If a cardiac catheterization had been performed within 12 months, and the results of the stress test would not alter the patient's clinical management, the stress test could be omitted.

EXCLUSION CRITERIA

1. Patients with a history of syncope, or sustained VT or fibrillation >48 h after the onset of acute myocardial infarction.

2. Patients with nonsustained VT occurring only in the setting of drug-induced long QT syndrome, acute myocardial ischemia, acute metabolic disorders, or drug toxicity.

3. Patients could not have symptoms due to nonsustained VT that required treatment.

4. History of noncompliance.

5. A systemic disease likely to be fatal in less than 2 years.

6. Unstable angina. Such patients could be enrolled if, after angina became stable, nonsustained VT persisted.

7. Anticipation of the need for cardiac surgery for valvular or coronary artery disease in the near future.

8. Patients who had received amiodarone within the 6 months prior to enrollment.
9. Severe, uncontrolled congestive heart failure. Patients with a history of heart failure that was compensated on a stable medical regimen could be enrolled.
10. Patients with recurrent atrial fibrillation requiring antiarrhythmic drugs for treatment.

BASELINE STUDY PROTOCOL

After obtaining written informed consent, all antiarrhythmic drugs were discontinued. At least five half-lives after antiarrhythmic drugs were stopped, a signal-averaged electrocardiogram and an electrophysiological study were performed within 48 h of each other.

Electrode catheters were placed at the right ventricular apex and outflow tract. Ventricular stimulation was performed at twice diastolic threshold using a pulse width of 1 or 2 ms, an 8-beat drive train, cycle lengths of 600 (or the longest possible in patients whose sinus cycle length was close to or less than 600) and 400 ms, at both right ventricular sites with one to three extrastimuli, plus rapid pacing (bursts) of synchronized bursts of 15 cycles at cycle lengths of 350 to 250 ms. A 2-s pause was inserted after each pacing sequence. The sequence of pacing sites, cycle lengths, and extrastimuli was specified precisely, as was the method to be used in progressively decrementing extrastimuli. At least three standard surface ECG leads were recorded simultaneously during the electrophysiology study.

Potential endpoints for the protocol of programmed stimulation included: (1) the reproducible (≥ 2 times) induction of sustained uniform VT; (2) refractoriness of all three extrastimuli (2 RV sites, ≥ 2 paced cycle lengths); (3) if >15 complexes of polymorphic VT or flutter were reproducibly (at least twice) initiated with three extrastimuli, stimulation was to be stopped at that point. If cardioversion was required to terminate an induced arrhythmia, reproduction was not required. However, every effort was made to demonstrate reproducible induction of sustained ventricular tachycardia. Ventricular flutter and fibrillation were counted as polymorphic VT.

Following the baseline study, each patient with induced uniform sustained VT, or sustained polymorphic VT or VF induced by one or two extrastimuli, was randomized, using a random number generator, to one of two groups: (1) electrophysiological study to guide antiarrhythmic therapy or (2) no antiarrhythmic therapy. ''Randomizable'' patients (those with inducible sustained VT) who refused to be randomized after the baseline study were also followed, and their treatment (or lack of treatment) noted.

ASSIGNMENT OF ANTIARRHYTHMIC THERAPY BY ELECTROPHYSIOLOGICAL STUDY

Patients randomized to electrophysiologically guided therapy underwent serial drug testing. Antiarrhythmic drugs were chosen randomly for each patient (1) since there was no evidence that any one drug is more effective than any other in this group of patients; and (2) to ensure the results of this trial were not inappropriately influenced by one or two agents. The first round of antiarrhythmic drugs included a ''group IA'' drug (procainamide, quinidine, disopyramide), propafenone, and sotalol (Fig. 2). The second round of potential drug choices included all the above, plus the combination of: quinidine or disopyramide plus mexiletine. At least two failed drug trials had to be performed before amiodarone was begun. Because of its unique pharmacokinetics, amiodarone was not one of the first two

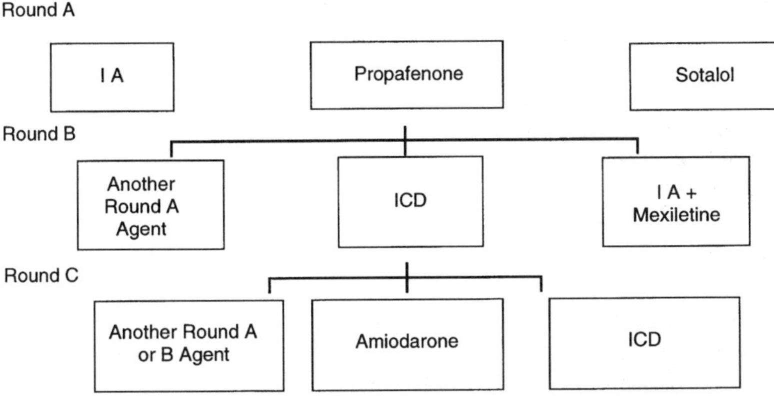

Figure 2   Schema of therapy for patients randomized to EP-guided therapy. All antiarrhythmic agents were assigned randomly, in each treatment round. If patients were randomized to a Group IA antiarrhythmic agent, the investigator chose among quinidine, procainamide, or disopyramide. After failing at least on trial of pharmacological therapy (''round A''), the investigator could choose to implant an ICD. A patient had to fail trials of at least two pharmacological agents before undergoing a trial of amiodarone. If an investigator and patient wished, further trials of pharmacological therapy could be undertaken beyond ''round C.'' Abbreviations as in Figure 1.

drugs chosen. It was not mandatory to use amiodarone. Drugs were administered with the aim of achieving a serum level or dose approximating those doses or serum levels usually found effective in the past. If a group 1A drug was specified by the randomization scheme, the investigator chose the specific 1A agent that he or she thought would be most appropriate for that patient. After four to five half-lives (i.e., 2 days of oral therapy in most cases, except amiodarone, which was tested after at least 1 week of loading), programmed stimulation was repeated. If sustained VT was induced during a drug trial, the patient was observed for 5 min during VT (if clinically appropriate) to assess hemodynamic stability (i.e., no angina, severe dyspnea, or loss of consciousness). If none of these symptoms were present, and the systolic blood pressure was >80 mmHg during VT, the patient was said to be hemodynamically stable.

The programmed stimulation protocol for drug testing was the same as that utilized in the baseline study. A drug was said to prevent induction of uniform sustained VT enough to permit chronic therapy and discharge on that regimen if <15 complexes were induced by the stimulation protocol. If no drug regimen could be found that rendered the tachycardia noninducible, the investigator could choose to discharge the patient on a drug regimen that resulted in hemodynamic stability during induced VT, as defined above.

No empiric antiarrhythmic drug therapy was utilized in this trial, including amiodarone. In order to be discharged on an antiarrhythmic drug, one of the criteria for success, as defined above by electrophysiological testing, had to be met.

After one unsuccessful drug trial, implantation of an FDA-approved implantable cardioverter/defibrillator device could be recommended to the patient. Patients receiving a device were not given antiarrhythmic agents, except as necessary to control nonsustained VT that triggered the device inappropriately, or to control supraventricular rhythms, such as atrial fibrillation that caused spurious device discharges.

Implantation of FDA-approved cardioverter/defibrillator devices was performed in the standard fashion in operating rooms using a uniform testing procedure. Intraoperative testing of ventricular fibrillation energy requirements was performed in all patients. Defibrillation test pulses were delivered after 10 s of ventricular fibrillation, and at least 1 min was allowed to elapse between defibrillation tests. Successful defibrillation was demonstrated using <20 J (or at least a 10-J margin between the DFT and the maximum output of the ICD) on at least three consecutive trials. If the defibrillation threshold was >20 J, four consecutive trials had to demonstrate successful defibrillation, using energy values less than the output of the device. Confirmation of normal and appropriate functioning of the device with adequate defibrillation was repeated prior to hospital discharge if the defibrillation energy requirement determined in the operating room was >20 J.

If a patient refused device implantation, he or she remained in the protocol and was discharged on no antiarrhythmic drugs.

FOLLOW-UP

All patients (including those without inducible sustained VT) were seen at one of the participating centers' outpatient facilities 1 month after discharge, and every 3 months thereafter. Patients living too far to return for routine outpatient visits were followed by telephone contact at the same intervals with the patient and their primary physician. At each visit, a 12-lead ECG and serum drug levels were checked in order to assess patient compliance.

STUDY ENDPOINTS

The primary endpoint in this study is sudden death, or cardiac arrest from which the patient is resuscitated. Secondary endpoints include total mortality, cardiac-related deaths, and spontaneous sustained VT. Other analyses will include: non-sudden cardiac deaths and noncardiac deaths. The occurrence of events such as syncope or nonsustained VT associated with symptoms considered to warrant therapy are being tracked.

QUALITY CONTROL

A number of checks were performed during this trial in order to ensure the accuracy of reported data. Three experienced nurses appointed by the Data Coordinating Center visited each study center to compare data entered on the study forms with patients' hospital charts and office records for all randomized patients, and a large sample of the nonrandomized (registry) patients. During the first year of the study, the principal investigator visited a majority of study centers to review the calibration of the stimulating equipment to confirm stimulator pulse widths, review the recording equipment, and the data collection methods with the clinical coordinator at each study center. The ECG recording of the qualifying nonsustained VT for each patient was reviewed by members of the study executive committee to verify the diagnosis. The executive committee reviewed all recordings of induced sustained VT to ensure that induction methods conformed with the protocol, and to confirm reported VT morphologies for the baseline electrophysiological study and drug follow-up studies.

ANALYSIS OF EVENTS

Investigators at each study center provided a narrative description (including electrocardiographic recordings, relevant hospital records, and laboratory data) of the clinical circumstances surrounding any study patients who died or experienced cardiac arrest. The Data Coordinating Center then edited the narrative in a manner such that the members of the events committee were blinded with regard to whether the patient had inducible VT and to the state of randomization of each patient. This edited description of each event, including supporting source documents, was reviewed by two of the events committee members, who then classified the event's mechanism. If both committee members agreed on the classification, the event was recorded by the Data Coordinating Center as such. If both committee members disagreed on the classification of the event, that case report was presented to the entire committee, which then ruled on the classification by consensus.

STUDY DURATION AND SIZE

Our original study plan called for recruitment of patients to take place over a period of 3 years, with minimum follow-up to be 2 years. Therefore, we planned for the study to last a total of 5 years. However, patient recruitment actually required 5 years, and, allowing for a minimum follow-up of 2 years, follow-up of patients was completed in October, 1998.

The study size was based on estimates derived from survival in prior reports (quoted above) of similar (but not the same) patient populations enrolled in this trial. Given the study duration requirements outlined above, we anticipated a 2-year arrhythmic event rate of 15% in the untreated group of patients with inducible VT, and a reduction in arrhythmic events of at least 33% in the group with antiarrhythmic therapy guided by electrophysiological study. Using these outcome rates, assuming an alpha error of 0.05, and a power of >0.80 of demonstrating this outcome, we planned to randomize 900 patients with inducible sustained VT. We encountered difficulty in meeting the targeted sample size, and patient enrollment was terminated in October 1996, after 704 patients with inducible sustained VT had been randomized.

OUTCOME ANALYSIS

The major purpose of this trial will be to analyze, on an intention to treat basis, the rates of the primary and secondary endpoints outlined above, in the group with inducible sustained VT receiving no antiarrhythmic therapy versus these rates in the group receiving electrophysiologically guided antiarrhythmic therapy. The other primary points of analysis will be to compare the rates of the primary and secondary endpoints in the patients without inducible sustained VT with the event rates in the two subgroups of patients with inducible sustained VT. In addition, we will compare the occurrence rates of sustained VT and "appropriate" implanted defibrillator/cardioverter discharges in patients with electrophysiologically guided therapy with the rates of sustained VT in patients with inducible sustained VT randomized to no therapy, and patients without inducible sustained VT. The pattern of events in each group will be depicted by Kaplan–Meier curves. The statistical comparisons will be performed using the Cox proportional hazards model.

RESULTS

At the time of this writing, outcome data are not available. However, data regarding characteristics of patients recruited into the study are available. A total of 2202 patients were enrolled into the trial. This included 704 patients with inducible sustained VT who were randomized, and an additional 62 "randomizable" patients, who refused randomization, but who are being followed in the registry. Thus 766, or 35% of patients meeting the entry criteria, had inducible sustained VT. Therefore, the registry includes 1442 patients meeting the entry criteria but not having randomizable VT.

As would be expected from a group of patients with coronary artery disease, the majority are male (Table 1). Given that entry into the trial required the left

Table 1 Clinical Characteristics of 2208 Patients Enrolled in MUSTT

Variable	% (categorical variables) or median (25th, 75th percentiles)
Gender (female)	14
Race (white)	86
Age (years)	65 (58,72)
Prior thrombolytic therapy	21
Prior coronary bypass grafting	60
Prior angioplasty	23
History of myocardial infarction	89
Ejection fraction	30 (22,35)
Time from most recent myocardial infarction to enrollment (years)	2.5 (0.2,8.4)

ventricular ejection fraction to be ≤0.40, it is not surprising that the majority had a previously documented myocardial infarction, and the average time from the most recent acute myocardial infarction to enrollment was over 2 years. Approximately one-fifth of the study population had received thrombolytic therapy, and about one-fifth had previously undergone coronary angioplasty. Over half of the study population had prior coronary artery bypass surgery.

Analysis of the 351 patients randomized to electrophysiologically guided antiarrhythmic therapy reveals that approximately 43% responded to antiarrhythmic drugs (ventricular tachycardia either became noninducible, or remained inducible, but was rendered hemodynamically stable, according to the protocol criteria). While this figure may appear high, previous reports of electrophysiological studies in patients with nonsustained ventricular tachycardia have cited a higher rate of response to antiarrhythmic drugs than observed in patients with spontaneous sustained ventricular tachycardia (16–19). In addition, this figure is inflated somewhat by patients in whom tachycardia remained inducible, but was associated with hemodynamic stability. Forty-six percent of the patients failed to respond to drugs and were discharged after implanting a cardioverter/defibrillator. Eight percent of patients were discharged without antiarrhythmic therapy. The latter do not represent protocol violations. When the study was designed and initiated (and for the first 3 years of the study), the only defibrillators available required thoracotomy for implantation. We predicted that some patients (or their physicians) who failed to respond to drugs would refuse implantation of defibrillators, since they were asymptomatic. As the purpose of the study was to ascertain the ability of electrophysiologically guided therapy to reduce mortality, we felt that if we could not demonstrate a clear-cut benefit of antiarrhythmic therapy in this population, it would be prudent to avoid therapy. In this case, the electrophysiological study was guiding treatment—to avoid drugs in which objective evidence of benefit could not be demonstrated.

Although outcome data are not available at this time, we have performed analyses of the relationship of a number of factors to inducible sustained ventricular tachycardia (20–24). These analyses have demonstrated that electrocardiographic characteristics of spontaneous nonsustained ventricular tachycardia, such as rate, morphology, frequency, and duration of episodes do not correlate with inducibility of sustained ventricular tachycardia or characteristics of induced tachycardias (20,22). However, this analysis did reveal that the characteristics of spontaneous nonsustained ventricular tachycardia are virtually identical (with regard to rate, frequency and rate of episodes) to those of patients enrolled in the Cardiac Arrhythmia Suppression Trial (CAST) (25).

Another analysis has demonstrated that a large number of clinical variables, including markers of left ventricular dysfunction and ischemia, extent of coronary artery disease, and congestive heart failure have no clinical utility in this population in predicting which patients will have inducible sustained ventricular tachycardia (21). Furthermore, although we have found that signal-averaged ECG parameters, although more abnormal in patients with inducible sustained ventricular tachycardia, as expected, are poor predictors of inducible sustained ventricular tachycardia in this population (24). Finally, we have now demonstrated that clinical variables cannot predict patients with inducible ventricular tachycardia in this population who will respond to antiarrhythmic drugs, although electrophysiological characteristics of ventricular tachycardia induced in the baseline state do correlate with drug responsiveness (23).

SUMMARY

The Multicenter UnSustained Tachycardia Trial is the first randomized, controlled study to test the utility of therapy guided by electrophysiological testing for primary prevention of sudden death in high-risk patients with coronary artery disease. This study will provide an estimate of the prognostic implications of inducible ventricular tachycardia in patients without symptomatic arrhythmias. The outcome data resulting from this study will place into perspective the results of trials such as the Multicenter Automatic Defibrillator Implantation Trial (MADIT) and other primary prevention studies. Together, the results of these studies should provide a rational approach for prevention of sudden death in survivors of acute myocardial infarction.

ACKNOWLEDGMENTS

This work was supported by Grants No. UO1 HL45700 and UO1 HL45726 from the National Heart, Lung, and Blood Institute, National Institutes of Health, and by grants from C.R. Bard, Inc., Berlex Laboratories, Inc., Boehringer-Ingelheim Pharmaceuticals, Inc., Cardiac Pacemakers, Inc./Guidant, Knoll Pharmaceutical Co., Medtronic, Inc., Searle Pharmaceutical, Ventritex, and Wyeth-Ayerst Laboratories.

REFERENCES

1. Tavazzi L, Volpi A, the GISSI Investigators. Remarks about postinfarction prognosis in light of the experience with the Gruppo Italiano per lo Studio della Sopravvivenza nell' Infarto Miocardico (GISSI) Trials. Circulation 1997;95:1341–1345.
2. De Vreede-Swagemakers JJM, Gorgels APM, Verstraaten GMP, Vermeer F, Dassen WRM, Wellens HJJ. Did prognosis after acute myocardial infarction change during the past 30 years? A meta-analysis. J Am Coll Cardiol 1991;18:698–706.

3. Rouleau JL, Talajic M, Sussex B, Potvin L, Warnica W, Davies RF, Gardner M, Stewart D, Plante S, Dupuis R, Lauzon C, Ferguson J, Mikes E, Balnozan V, Savard P. Myocardial infarction patients in the 1990s—their risk factors, stratification and survival in Canada: The Canadian Assessment of Myocardial Infarction (CAMI) Study. J Am Coll Cardiol 1996;27:1119–1127.

4. De Vreede-Swagemakers JJM, Gorgels APM, Dubois-Arbouw WI, Van Ree JW, Daemen MJAP, Houben LGE, Wellens HJJ. Out-of-hospital cardiac arrest in the 1990s. A population-based study in the Maastricht area on incidence, characteristics and survival. J Am Coll Cardiol 1997;30:1500–1505.

5. Liberthson RR, Nagel EL, Hirschman JC, Nussenfeld SR. Prehospital ventricular defibrillation: Prognosis and follow-up course. N Engl J Med 1974;291:3317–321.

6. Weaver WD, Hill D, Fahrenbruch CE, Copaass MK, Martin JS, Cobb LA, Hallstrom AP. Use of the automatic external defibrillator in the management of out-of-hospital cardiac arrest. N Engl J Med 1988;319:11:661–716.

7. Becker LB, Han BH, Meyer PM, Wright FA, Rhodes KV, Smith DW, Barrett J. CPR Chicago Project. Racial differences in the incidence of cardiac arrest and subsequent survival. N Engl J Med 1993;329:600–606.

8. Denniss AR, Richards DA, Cody DV, Russell PA, Young AA, Cooper MJ, Ross DL, Uther JB. Prognostic significance of ventricular tachycardia and fibrillation induced at programmed stimulation and delayed potentials detected on the signal-averaged electrocardiograms of survivors of acute myocardial infarction. Circulation 1986;74:731–745.

9. Richards D, Taylor A, Fahey P, Irwig L, Koo CC, Ross D, Cooper M, Kiat H, Skinner M, Uther J. Identification of patients at risk of sudden death after myocardial infarction: The continued Australian experience. In: Brugada P, Wellens HJJ. Cardiac Arrhythmias: Where to Go From Here? Mount Kisco, NY: Futura Publishing Company, Inc., 1987.

10. Roy D, Marchand E, Theroux P, Waters DD, Pelletier GB, Bourassa MG. Programmed ventricular stimulation in survivors of an acute myocardial infarction. Circulation 1985;72:487–494.

11. Bhandari AK, Rose JS, Kotlewski A, Rahimtoola SH, Wu D. Frequency and significance of induced sustained ventricular tachycardia or fibrillation two weeks after acute myocardial infarction. Am J Cardiol 1985;56:737–742.

12. Roy D, Marchand E, Theroux P, Waters DD, Pelletier GB, Carter R, Bourassa MG. Long-term reproducibility and significance of provocable ventricular arrhythmias after myocardial infarction. J Am Coll Cardiol 1986;8:32–39.

13. Iesaka Y, Nogami A, Aonuma K, Nitta J, Chun Y, Fujwara H, Hiraoka M. Prognostic significance of sustained monomorphic ventricular tachycardia induced by programmed ventricular stimulation using up to triple extrastimuli in survivors of acute myocardial infarction. Am J Cardiol 1990;65:1057–1063.

14. Bourke JP, Richards ADB, Ross DL, Wallace EM, McGuire MA, Uther JB. Routine programmed electrical stimulation in survivors of acute myocardial infarction for prediction of spontaneous ventricular tachyarrhythmias during follow-up: Results, Optimal stimulation protocol and cost-effective screening. J Am Coll Cardiol 1991; 18:780–788.

15. Gomes JAC, Hariman RI, Kang PS, EI-Sherif N, Chowdhry I, Lyons J. Programmed electrical stimulation in patients with high-grade ectopy: Electrophysiologic findings and prognosis for survival. Circulation 1984;70:43–51.

16. Manolis AS, Estes NAM. Value of programmed stimulation in the evaluation and management of patients with nonsustained ventricular tachycardia associated with coronary artery disease. Am J Cardiol 1990;65:201–205.

17. Buxton AE, Marchlinski FE, Flores BT, Miller JM, Doherty JU, Josephson ME. Nonsustained ventricular tachycardia in patients with coronary artery disease: Role of electrophysiologic study. Circulation 1987;75:1178–1185.

18. Klein RC, Machell C. Use of electrophysiologic testing in patients with nonsustained ventricular tachycardia: Prognostic and therapeutic implications. J Am Coll Cardiol 1989;14:155–161.

19. Wilber DJ, Olshansky B, Moran JF, Scanlon PJ. Electrophysiological testing and nonsustained ventricular tachycardia: Use and limitations in patients with coronary artery disease and impaired ventricular function. Circulation 1990;82:350–358.

20. Buxton AE, Lee KL, DiCarlo L, Echt DS, Fisher JD, Greer GS, Josephson ME, Packer D, Prystowsky EN, Talajic M, for the Multicenter Unsustained Tachycardia Trial Investigators. Nonsustained ventricular tachycardia in patients with coronary artery disease: relationship to inducible sustained ventricular tachycardia. Ann Intern Med 1996;125:35–39.

21. Buxton AE, Greer GS, Gold MS, DiCarlo L, O'Toole MF, Fisher JD, Prystowsky EN, Hook BG, Bernstein RC, Hafley G for the Multicenter UnSustained Tachycardia Trial Investigators. Can clinical characteristics predict inducible sustained ventricular tachycardia in potentially high risk patients with coronary artery disease? Circulation 1995;92:98.

22. Prystowsky EN, Buxton AE, Lee K, Coromilas J, Tang AS, Hafley G. Nonsustained ventricular tachycardia characteristics: Do they correlate with cardiac function and sustained ventricular tachycardia? Circulation 1997;96;l:33.

23. Gold MR, Hafley GE, DiCarlo LA, Lehmann MH, Page RL, Lee KL, Buxton AE. Clinical predictors of antiarrhythmic drug response in the MUSTT Trial. J Am Coll Cardiol 1998;31:159A.

24. Cain ME, Gomes JA, Hafley GE, Lee KL, Gold MR, MUSTT Investigators. Performance of the signal-averaged ECG in identifying patients inducible into sustained ventricular tachycardia. Circulation 1996;94:8;I-451–452.

25. Denes P, Gillis AM, Pawitan Y, Kammerling JM, Wilhelmsen L, Salerno DM, and the CAST Investigators. Prevalence, characteristics and significance of ventricular premature complexes and ventricular tachycardia detected by 24-hour continuous electrocardiographic recording in the Cardiac Arrhythmia Suppression Trial. Am J Cardiol 1991;68:887–896.

MUSTT: Critique

John P. DiMarco

University of Virginia Health Sciences Center, Charlottesville, Virginia

The Multicenter Unsustained Tachycardia Trial (MUSTT) (1) is an ambitious clinical study that hopes to answer several questions concerning the value of electrophysiological (EP) studies with programmed ventricular stimulation in a high-risk population. The study's two primary hypotheses are that: (1) induction of sustained ventricular tachycardia (VT) or ventricular fibrillation (VF) will have prognostic significance; and (2) antiarrhythmic therapy guided by repeat EP studies will improve survival in patients with inducible arrhythmias. A second hypothesis concerning the value of a signal-averaged electrocardiogram is also listed but will not be discussed here. The population chosen for study was patients with known coronary artery disease, a depressed left ventricular ejection fraction (EF $\leq$ 0.40), and documented spontaneous nonsustained VT. At this point in time, no endpoint data from MUSTT have been reported. Therefore, this chapter will discuss what the author believes are the major strengths and weaknesses in the MUSTT design.

Prior small studies (2–5) have suggested that programmed ventricular stimulation had a high negative predictive value for sustained VT or sudden death in patients after myocardial infarction, but the positive predictive value of EP studies remains controversial. Most studies that dealt with patients with chronic coronary disease and nonsustained VT treated all patients with inducible VT and therefore the positive predictive value of EP studies in such patients cannot be accurately estimated. MUSTT includes untreated groups with and without inducible VT, so an accurate estimate of the value of both negative and positive programmed stimulation will now be available. This question is of critical importance since two recent trials for primary prevention of arrhythmic death have yielded discordant results. The Multicenter Automatic Defibrillator Implantation Trial (MADIT) (6) did show a highly significant benefit with implantable cardioverter-defibrillator (ICD) implantation among patients with induced VT, but the comparison group received antiarrhythmic therapy in a nonstandardized fashion. In contrast, the much larger Coronary Artery Bypass Graft (CABG) Patch Trial (7) failed to show benefit with ICD therapy compared to no antiarrhythmic therapy, but this study did not include any EP study criteria for trial entry. MUSTT should resolve finally the prognostic value of induced VT or VF in this population.

Limited preliminary data from MUSTT are already available. The study has shown that VT inducibility at EP study cannot be predicted by ECG characteristics or clinical variables (8–10). The former observation suggests either that ECG characteristics (length, duration, and morphology) are highly variable and any single episode is of little value or that the nonsustained VT represents only an initiating event not self-terminating reentry through the VT circuit itself. The MUSTT study group was already selected based on two key variables that influence VT induction, coronary disease and ejection fraction ≤ 0.40, so it is not surprising that other clincial variables are of little additional value.

The treatment portion of MUSTT is likely to yield fewer clear answers. The stated goal of the study was to examine the value of EP-guided antiarrhythmic therapy. The MUSTT drug selection cascade, however, does not reflect common practice among electrophysiologists. In view of results from the Endocardial Stimulation Versus Electrocardiographic Monitoring (ESVEM) trial (11), and the Cardiac Arrest in Seattle: Conventional versus Amiodarone Drug Evaluation (CASCADE) trial (12), the class III agents, sotalol and amiodarone, with or without EP study guidance, are the drugs preferred for treating sustained ventricular arrhythmias. In a population with low ejection fractions, amiodarone is overwhelmingly the number one choice (13). In MUSTT, more than 50% of the patients treated long term with drugs received class I agents and amiodarone was not supposed to be used until after two failed trials. This drug selection strategy was commonly used when the MUSTT protocol was being developed, but seems to be less relevant to current clinical practice. It is likely that many MUSTT investigators ''bailed out'' to ICD therapy as soon as possible rather than laboriously continuing to do serial drug studies. In view of data supporting ICD use over drug therapy from MADIT (6) and the Antiarrhythmic Versus Implantable Defibrillators (AVID) trial (13), which were reported after MUSTT enrollment concluded, this practice might have favorably influenced survival in the treated group even though only a limited effort to select a drug with EP studies—a primary question for the trial—was made.

During the course of MUSTT, it became clear that enrollment would lag behind schedule. The Cardiac Arrest Suppression Trial (CAST) (14) results decreased the routine use of Holter monitoring in ambulatory asymptomatic populations. Therefore, the qualifying episode of nonsustained VT in MUSTT patients was often detected from telemetry monitoring during hospitalizations for heart failure, myocardial infarction, unstable angina, or a revascularization procedure. Although the arrhythmia had to be documented 3 or 4 days after the last acute event, the natural history of a group of patients who have recently required hospitalization for ischemia or heart failure is likely to be different from that of stable outpatients with the same arrhythmia. If these less stable patients have a higher risk of recurrent ischemia or progressive heart failure, the ability of MUSTT to detect any change in arrhythmic deaths or cardiac arrest may be compromised. This is presumably what happened in the CABG-Patch trial, where 78% of deaths occurred in an institutional setting (hospital, chronic care facility, or hospice) (15). As expected, ICD therapy failed to improve survival in such a population. If MUSTT also observes that a large proportion of randomized patients have end-stage disease, its ability to detect an effect of therapy directed primarily at arrhythmic mortality will be compromised.

Several other minor limitations of the MUSTT study design should be recognized. Total mortality is the unequivocal endpoint now used in most trials of antiarrhythmic therapy. IN MUSTT, the primary endpoint is a compendium of arrhythmic events. This required adjudication of deaths by an events committee (this author was a member), and many of the decisions about the role of arrhythmias were uncertain, usually because of progressive heart failure or systemic disease as confounding factors. Although MUSTT has a well-defined stimulation protocol, it was impossible to ensure that every investigator at every site for every study followed it exactly. For a trial in which an EP study response is a major acute endpoint, this may be a significant problem. Finally, we do not yet know what the long-term adherence to prescribed therapy in MUSTT will be. Due to side effects of drugs, investigators' bias in favor of ICDs, and patients' reluctance to take prophylactic therapy, it is highly likely that a large fraction of patient-years of exposure will actually be off prescribed therapy. This will highlight the limitations of the antiarrhythmic drugs we have available, but will do little to help us evaluate the role of EP studies for selecting drug therapy.

In conclusion, MUSTT is likely to provide highly valuable information concerning the prognostic value of EP studies in patients with coronary artery disease. It is much less likely to provide sufficient data to determine whether or not EP-guided drug therapy is of benefit for those patients with inducible arrhythmias.

REFERENCES

1. Buxton AE, Fisher JD, Josephson ME, Lee KL, Pryor DB, Prystowsky EN, Simson MB, DiCarlo L, Echt DS, Packer D, Greer GS, Talajic M, and the MUSTT Investigators. Prevention of sudden death in patients with coronary artery disease: the

Multicenter Unsustained Tachycardia Trial (MUSTT). Prog Cardiovasc Dis 1993; 36:215–226.

2. Denniss AR, Richards DA, Cody DV, Russell PA, Young AA, Cooper MJ, Ross DL, Uther JB. Prognostic significance of ventricular tachycardia and fibrillation induced at programmed stimulation and delayed potentials detected on the signal-averaged electrocardiograms of survivors of acute myocardial infarction. Circulation 1986;74:731–745.

3. Buxton AE, Simson MB, Falcone RA, Marchlinski FE, Doherty JU, Josephson ME. Results of signal-averaged electrocardiography and electrophysiologic study in patients with nonsustained ventricular tachycardia after healing of acute myocardial infarction. Am J Cardiol 1987;60:80–85.

4. Gomes JA, Hariman RI, Kang PS, El-Sherif N, Chowdhry I, Lyons J. Programmed electrical stimulation in patients with high-grade ventricular ectopy: electrophysiologic findings and prognosis for survival. Circulation 1984;70:43–51.

5. Wilber DJ, Olshansky B, Moran JF, Scanlon PJ. Electrophysiological testing and nonsustained ventricular tachycardia. Use and limitations in patients with coronary artery disease and impaired ventricular function. Circulation 1990;82:350–358.

6. Moss AJ, Hall WJ, Cannom DS, Daubert JP, Higgins SL, Klein H, Levine JH, Saksena S, Waldo AL, Wilber D, Brown MW, Heo M. Improved survival with an implanted defibrillator in patients with coronary disease at high risk for ventricular arrhythmia. Multicenter Automatic Defibrillator Implantation Trial Investigators. N Engl J Med 1996;335:1933–1940.

7. Bigger JT Jr. Prophylactic use of implanted cardiac defibrillators in patients at high risk for ventricular arrhythmias after coronary-artery bypass graft surgery. Coronary Artery Bypass Graft (CABG) Patch Trial Investigators. N Engl J Med 1997;337: 1569–1575.

8. Buxton AE, Lee KL, DiCarlo L, Echt DS, Fisher JD, Greer GS, Josephson ME, Packer D, Prystowsky EN, Talajic M, for the Multicenter Unsustained Tachycardia Trial Investigators. Nonsustained ventricular tachycardia in patients with coronary artery disease: relation to inducible sustained ventricular tachycardia. Ann Intern Med 1996;125:35–39.

9. Buxton AE, Greer GS, Gold MR, DiCarlo L, O'Toole MF, Fisher JD, Prystowsky EN, Hook BG, Bernstein RC, Hafley G, for the Multicenter Unsustained Tachycardia Trial Investigators. Can clinical characteristics predict inducible sustained ventricular tachycardia in potentially high risk patients with coronary artery disease? Circulation 1995;92(suppl I):I-98 (abstr).

10. Prystowsky EN, Buxton AE, Lee KL, Coromilas J, Tang AS, Hafley G. Nonsustained ventricular tachycardia characteristics: do they correlate with cardiac function and sustained ventricular tachycardia? Circulation 1997;96(suppl I):I-334 (abstr).

11. Mason JW. A comparison of electrophysiologic testing with Holter monitoring to predict antiarrhythmic-drug efficacy for ventricular tachyarrhythmias. Electrophysiologic Study Versus Electrocardiographic Monitoring Investigators. N Engl J Med 1993;329:445–451.

12. Anonymous. Cardiac Arrest in Seattle: Conventional Versus Amiodarone Drug Evaluation (the CASCADE study). Am J Cardiol 1991;67:578–584.

13. Anonymous. A comparison of antiarrhythmic-drug therapy with implantable defibrillators in patients resuscitated from near-fatal ventricular arrhythmias. The Antiarrhythmics Versus Implantable Defibrillators (AVID) Investigators. N Engl J Med 1997;337:1576–1583.

14. Echt DS, Liebson PR, Mitchell LB, Peters RW, Obias-Manno D, Barker AH, Arensberg D, Baker A, Friedman L, Greene HL, Huther ML, Richardson DW, and the CAST Investigators. Mortality and morbidity in patients receiving encainide, flecainide, or placebo. The Cardiac Arrhythmia Suppression Trial. N Engl J Med 1991;324:781–788.

15. Bigger JT Jr, Whang W, Rottman JN, Kleiger RE, Gottlieb CD, Namerow PB, Steinman RC, Estes NA, for The CABG Patch Trial Investigators and Coordinators. Mechanisms of death in The CABG Patch trial: A randomized trial of implantable cardiac defibrillator prophylaxis in patients at high risk of death after coronary artery bypass graft surgery. Circulation 1999;99:1416–1421.

17

The Sudden Cardiac Death–Heart Failure Trial (SCD-HeFT)

Gust H. Bardy*

University of Washington, Seattle, Washington

INTRODUCTION

Congestive heart failure (CHF) is a common and lethal disease. A new diagnosis of congestive heart failure is made in 400,000 Americans each year. Those with moderate left ventricular dysfunction have a substantial risk of premature death, approximately 25% over 2.5 years. Fifty percent of these deaths are thought to be sudden, due to arrhythmias, and may be preventable. As a consequence, CHF patients represent the largest single identifiable population of patients that can be targeted for primary prevention of sudden cardiac death (SCD).

STUDY DESIGN AND GOALS

In this paper, we present the rationale for the conduct of a primary SCD prevention trial in patients with CHF. The central hypothesis of this study is that amiodarone or an implantable cardioverter-defibrillator (ICD) will improve survival compared to placebo in patients with NYHA class II and class III CHF and reduced left ventricular ejection fraction ($\leq$35%).

The principal goal of this three-arm, randomized, primary prevention trial is to identify therapy that will significantly reduce death rates in patients with CHF resulting from ischemic cardiomyopathy or nonischemic dilated cardiomy-

---

* The SCD-HeFT Investigators: Gust H. Bardy, Kerry L. Lee, Daniel B. Mark, Jeanne E. Poole, Daniel P. Fishbein, Steven N. Singh, Charles L. Troutman, Victoria L. Christian, Jill Anderson, George W. Johnson, Nancy Clapp-Channing, Michael Domanski, and Derek Exner.

323

opathy. We will attempt to achieve this goal by reducing arrhythmic deaths in patients with CHF and a reduced ejection fraction ($\leq 35\%$) and no record of sustained ventricular tachycardia (VT) or ventricular fibrillation (VF).

The study will be a prospective, clinical trial with 2500 patients randomly allocated in equal proportions to three different treatment arms over 2.5 years. The first arm of the study will be a control arm that consists of conventional heart failure therapy and placebo. Placebo therapy is a critical aspect of this trial that is needed to prevent bias in favor of active therapy. Conventional CHF therapy will require the use of appropriate dose angiotensin converting enzyme (ACE) inhibitors. The second arm of the study will combine conventional therapy with the use of amiodarone. Placebo and amiodarone will be delivered in a double-blind fashion. The third arm of the study will employ conventional therapy together with a single lead, pectoral ICD inserted on an outpatient basis. Treatment arms will be compared using an intention-to-treat analysis.

By using readily available clinical measures of CHF and eliminating the need for specialized screening tests to identify subjects, the study is designed to facilitate ease of enrollment and to be broadly applicable as a primary prevention strategy implemented on an outpatient basis.

The primary, specific aim is to compare all-cause mortality in the three arms of the study. Four secondary specific aims follow:

1. To compare arrhythmic and nonarrhythmic cardiac mortality in the three arms of the study.
2. To compare morbidity in the three arms of the study, defined as all-cause mortality, and rehospitalization for CHF.
3. To compare health-related quality of life in the three arms of the study.
4. To compare cost of care for each treatment group and calculate incremental cost-effectiveness ratios for the two intervention arms.

We also will determine the incidence of VT/VF and profound bradyarrhythmias (rates less than or equal to 34 bpm) in CHF patients in the ICD arm via the ICD memory log.

STATEMENT OF THE PROBLEM

Congestive heart failure has a profound effect on public health and use of health care resources. Approximately 1 to 2 million people in the United States have CHF, with 400,000 new cases occurring annually (1–4). Heart failure is the most common cardiovascular discharge diagnosis in elderly patients. Its incidence more than doubles each decade after age 45. In 1989, it accounted for approximately 5 million person-days of hospitalization (5). In light of this, with the aging of the U.S. population, its prevalence is anticipated to increase markedly.

Although the use of angiotensin converting enzyme inhibitors has improved survival, patients with moderately symptomatic heart failure still have at least a 25% probability of dying over 2.5 years. One-half of these deaths occur suddenly and without warning and are probaly caused by ventricular arrhythmias or, less commonly, bradyarrhythmias. Therefore, developing an effective primary prevention strategy for SCD in CHF patients should result in a significant reduction in death rates in this large patient population.

RELEVANT STUDIES ON THE RELATIONSHIP OF SUDDEN CARDIAC DEATH AND LEFT VENTRICULAR DYSFUNCTION

SCD, like CHF, is a major public health problem in the United States, affecting 200,000 to 400,000 Americans each year (6–10). The relationship between SCD and CHF is inextricable. Epidemiological studies of SCD (11–13) have shown that the most important preexisting condition in cardiac arrest victims is left ventricular dysfunction due to coronary artery disease or primary cardiac muscle disease. Left ventricular dysfunction is known to be the strongest predictor of SCD (14–18). Thus, patients with CHF represent a prime target population in which to undertake a primary SCD prevention trial.

RELEVANT STUDIES ON TOTAL MORTALITY AND MECHANISM OF DEATH IN CHF

The natural history of heart failure has been thought to be characterized by an inexorable deterioration in ventricular function, with death occurring from progressive pump failure, ventricular tachyarrhythmias, or bradyarrhythmias. Several moderate-sized, randomized multicenter trials (19–20a) have confirmed that ACE inhibitors reduce mortality in patients with moderate and severe congestive heart failure. The definitive mechanisms by which ACE inhibitors reduce mortality are not known, but ACE inhibitors presumably do so by reducing death from pump failure (CONSENSUS; SOLVD) and may reduce the risk of sudden cardiac death (V-HeFT II). However, despite the beneficial effect of ACE inhibitors, patients with moderate CHF treated with ACE inhibitors continue to have a significantly increased risk of dying (SOLVD 1991; V-HeFT II 1991) (21). Survival data from the ACE inhibitor treatment arms of three recent trials, SOLVD, V-HeFT II and the VA study of amiodarone vs. placebo, CHF-STAT (21) best reflect the prognosis of patients with congestive heart failure of moderate severity (i.e., those most pertinent to SCD-HeFT). The 2.5-year mortality rate in the ACE inhibitor treatment groups was approximately 27% in SOLVD, 25% in V-HeFT II, and 36% in CHF-STAT.

In SOLVD, V-HeFT II, and CHF-STAT, historical information was used to characterize the mechanism of death. In SOLVD, 23% of deaths were characterized as ''arrhythmic without worsening CHF.'' In V-HeFT II, 31% of deaths were characterized as ''sudden with no warning symptoms,'' and 43% of deaths were ''sudden with or without warning symptoms.'' In CHF-STAT, 52% of the deaths in the control population were characterized as sudden. These data suggest that up to half of the deaths in patients with CHF may be preventable with effective prophylaxis against tachyarrhythmias and, possibly, bradyarrhythmias.

The mortality data from the V-HeFT trials provides information about the natural history of patients with congestive heart failure (22). First, sudden deaths tended to occur earlier than pump-failure deaths. Second, total mortality, and both pump-failure death and sudden death were related to the severity of left ventricular dysfunction measured by ejection fraction, plasma norepinephrine levels, or the severity of functional impairment measured by peak exercise oxygen consumption. Third, sudden death occurred at similar rates in patients with ischemic cardiomyopathy versus nonischemic dilated cardiomyopathy. Fourth, the presence of ventricular arrhythmias on Holter monitoring was associated with a higher overall mortality but not an increased proportion of sudden versus pump failure deaths. V-HeFT data did not identify a clinical marker specific for sudden death. Rather, sudden death and pump failure death were both predicted by the severity of left ventricular dysfunction and functional impairment. These findings have direct pertinence to the SCD-HeFT trial design. The data suggest that we cannot predict which patients with heart failure will succumb to cardiac arrhythmias. As a consequence, we believe that SCD-HeFT can remain unencumbered by screening and risk stratification tools of unproven value. This approach fosters the development of a broadly applicable prevention strategy based on easily identifiable clinical measures of left ventricular dysfunction. In turn, the cost and complexity of the study will be minimized and enrollment will be facilitated.

THE ROLE OF BETA-BLOCKER THERAPY

Beta-blocker therapy for the prevention of SCD in CHF is under intense investigation. Several trials are currently evaluating the value of pure beta-blockers (e.g., bucindolol) and those with vasodilatory effects (e.g., carvedilol) on mortality. Although there is increasing evidence to suggest that beta-blockers may improve survival in CHF, that evidence is insufficient to mandate beta-blocker therapy as part of SCD-HeFT. That said, it is important for the eventual interpretation of SCD-HeFT results to have no disparities in beta-blocker use in the three arms of the study. Consequently, to avoid such disparities in beta-blocker use in the three arms of SCD-HeFT, we have recommended that enrolling sites have a consistent approach to whether or not beta-blockers are used in their heart failure patients. This recommendation will be tempered of course by the results of adequately powered prospective, randomized mortality trials that will provide more definitive data on the use of beta-blocker therapy in CHF. Pending these beta-blocker trial results, the issue for now with respect to SCD-HeFT is safety of using beta-blocker therapy with amiodarone. Recent meta-analyses of the amiodarone trials have suggested that the concomitant administration of beta-blocker therapy with amiodarone may actually decrease mortality compared to either therapy used alone (23,24). Thus, although there are no definitive data to strongly recommend the use of combined beta-blocker/amiodarone therapy, we also believe that there are no compelling data to prohibit the use of beta-blocker therapy in SCD-HeFT patients receiving amiodarone.

If a SCD-HeFT investigator elects to use beta-blocker therapy in their heart failure patients on a routine basis, we recommend waiting 2 weeks after the last anticipated increase in beta-blocker dosage or waiting 2 weeks after their patient's maximally tolerated dose prior to SCD-HeFT randomization.

We have recommended the following approach to the use of carvedilol or metoprolol in SCD-HeFT patients.

Carvedilol: 3.125 mg bid for first 2 weeks; 6.25 mg bid for weeks 2–4; 12.5 mg bid for weeks 4–6; and 25 mg bid for weeks 6–8.

Metoprolol (Toprol XL): 12.5 mg qd for first 2 weeks; 25 mg qd for weeks 2–4; 37.5 mg qd for weeks 4–6; and 50 mg qd for weeks 6–8.

THE ROLE OF AMIODARONE IN SCD PREVENTION

In patients resuscitated from VF, empiric amiodarone has been shown to be more effective in the prevention of recurrent cardiac arrest and death than conventional antiarrhythmic drug therapy guided by electrophysiological studies or Holter monitoring (25). These data, together with its favorable history in preventing death in other studies like BASIS (26), the Polish post-MI study (27), and in meta-analyses (28), has made amiodarone the most promising antiarrhythmic agent for sudden death prevention in CHF patients. These studies notwithstanding, amiodarone's ability to prevent death from any cause, either as a primary prevention agent or as a secondary prevention agent, continues to be vigorously debated in light of more recent studies.

The two most relevant studies on the use of amiodarone in patients with CHF are CHF-STAT (29), with 674 patients, and GESICA (30), with 516 patients. CHF-STAT was a placebo-controlled, double-blind study of the effect of moderate-dose amiodarone (300–400 mg q.d.) on total mortality in patients with class II–IV CHF treated with ACE inhibitors or vasodilators having left ventricular ejection fractions ≤40% and >10 VPDs/h. This study found no difference in mortality in the amiodarone treatment arm compared to the placebo arm. Mortality from all causes at 3 years was 42% for both arms. Sudden death rates estimated from historical information were also similar in both groups—52% of the deaths in the placebo group and 49% of the deaths in the amiodarone group.

CHF-STAT is the only placebo-controlled study in heart failure patients to suggest that amiodarone does not have a favorable effect on survival. As such, its findings are contrary to the traditional experience with amiodarone for secondary prevention of death in survivors of cardiac arrest (25,31). It is possible, though, that the poor outcome with amiodarone in CHF-STAT is a consequence of the inclusion of class IV patients in the study. Class IV patients appear to have more cardiac arrests associated with bradyarrhythmias than with ventricular tachyarrhythmias (32). Because amiodarone induces sinus bradycardia and slows atrioventricular conduction, it is logical to postulate that amiodarone may have promoted bradyarrhythmic deaths in CHF-STAT, especially in class IV patients. At the same time, amiodarone may have decreased deaths from ventricular tachyarrhythmias. We speculate that the two effects may have canceled. In addition, CHF-STAT was a study of American Veterans, mostly male, and therefore did not represent the general population. It may be that women would fare better on amiodarone than men. Consequently, one cannot yet dismiss amiodarone as a viable therapeutic alternative in a broad population of CHF patients, especially those with less severe cardiac dysfunction who are less likely to suffer bradyarrhythmic deaths. Finally, and perhaps most importantly, drug noncompliance was high in this study, with only 59% on amiodarone. Noncompliance was purportedly because of side effects. It is difficult to conclude, however, that these side effects were genuinely related to amiodarone given the near identical rates of side effects in the placebo arms. Therefore, to conclude that amiodarone has failed as a prophylactic agent in view of the high rate of noncompliance is premature.

In considering the role of amiodarone in primary SCD prevention, one must also examine the results of the GESICA study, the findings of which contradict those of CHF-STAT and argue in favor of prophylactic amiodarone (30). This smaller, unblinded randomized study examined the benefit of prophylactic, moderate-dose amiodarone (300 mg q.d.) compared to conventional therapy in the prevention of death from any cause in patients with class II, III, and IV CHF, having enlarged hearts and/or left ventricular ejection fractions ≤ 35%. Cumulative mortality rates at 2 years were 33% in the amiodarone arm and 41% in the control arm ($p = 0.024$). The percentage of deaths that were sudden was estimated from historical data to be identical, 37% in both arms. The limitations of this study are that it was not blinded and that the patient population was unusual: 32% were alcoholics and 9% had Chagasic cardiomyopathy. The strength of this study was the high compliance rate with the test therapy: 96% were on amiodarone. Thus, although the findings of GESICA cannot be used at the present time to advocate the use of amiodarone as a prophylactic agent in North American patients with mild-to-moderate CHF, the study suggests that amiodarone may be beneficial if compliance is high.

The value of amiodarone in prevention of death is further confused by the findings in two large post-MI primary prevention trials: EMIAT and CAMIAT (33,34). In the case of EMIAT and CAMIAT, total mortality rates in both trials were no different in the amiodarone and the placebo arms using an intention-to-treat analysis. That said, it is difficult to dismiss the role of amiodarone as a prophylactic agent because the studies were powered under the presumption that the patients would actually take the drug. In EMIAT, only 61.5% were on the drug at the end of the trial. Similarly, with CAMIAT, only 63.5% were on amiodarone at trial end. These findings are comparable to the off-treatment rates in CHF-STAT, thus leaving open the issue of amiodarone use as a prophylactic agent.

Although there remains no clear consensus regarding the prophylactic use of amiodarone for prevention of death in CHF patients, the apparent efficacy of this drug in preventing death in patients following resuscitated SCD (25), its ease of use, and its modest cost argue strongly that it be considered for further evaluation. The SCD-HeFT investigators therefore feel that it merits reexamination in a larger heart failure trial endeavoring to maintain a high compliance rate for drug therapy.

Sotalol was considered as an alternative to amiodarone, but the findings of increased mortality in patients treated with the d-isomer over placebo in the SWORD study (35) has raised concerns about its efficacy. The negative inotropic effect of the racemic form of sotalol will also limit its use in patients with CHF. Finally, sotalol is difficult to use without in-hospital monitoring because of its tendency to prolong the QT interval with its relatively high incidence of pro-arrhythmia. Consequently, it is a much less suitable agent for SCD-HeFT than amiodarone.

THE ROLE OF ICD THERAPY IN SCD PREVENTION

The AVID trial of ICD therapy versus conventional drug therapy (mostly amiodarone) evaluated survival in patients who had already been resuscitated from VT or VF and, unlike SCD-HeFT, represents a secondary prevention trial. AVID unequivocally favored ICD therapy (36). Moreover, in oral presentations (publications not available), the Canadian ICD Study (CIDS), and the German ICD study (CASH) for secondary prevention have suggested ICD therapy prolongs survival over drug therapy (37,38). These findings, coupled to the host of uncontrolled studies showing ICD therapy likely beneficial for the secondary prevention of SCD (39–41), the investigative field now turns to ICD use for primary prevention.

Currently, no prospective, controlled, randomized study has been done to evaluate ICD therapy for primary prevention of SCD in patients with CHF. Although not a heart failure trial per se, there has, however, been one large, randomized ICD primary prevention trial for patients with reduced ejection fraction undergoing coronary artery bypass graft (CABG) surgery. This study, CABG-Patch (42) is described in detail elsewhere in this text. In this study, ICDs were randomized against control (CABG alone) immediately following CABG. There were no mortality differences in the two arms. It is believed that the failure of ICD therapy to improve survival in this population relates to the fact that the primary mortality risk in this population was ischemia, which was relieved with CABG. Moreover, the benefit of ICD therapy may have been obscured by a high ICD-related mortality rate and the fact that most of the ICDs used in that trial did not have backup antibradycardia pacing, a potential cause of SCD in such patients.

The MADIT study, also described elsewhere in this text, raised the possibility that, for select populations, ICDs can indeed be used to reduce mortality. In this study, patients with nonsustained VT (NSVT) with inducible sustained VT/VF before and after infusion of intravenous procainamide treated with ICD therapy appeared to have better survival than patients treated with drugs. The study focused on a small population of patients and was hampered by the fact that there were significant disparities in beta-blocker use in the two arms as well as substantial amiodarone noncompliance and use of drugs suspected of proarrhythmia in the drug arm. These objections notwithstanding, MADIT has increased attention on the potential value of prophylactic ICD use.

SCD-HeFT offers the first opportunity to evaluate ICD therapy referenced to a true placebo control. Unlike secondary SCD prevention trials, a placebo control group is possible in SCD-HeFT because there are presently no ethical constraints to withholding antiarrhythmic drug or device therapy in this patient population. Placebo therapy also avoids the inherent bias in favor of an active therapy incurred in an open control study. Placebo therapy best duplicates clinical practice where both the patient and the physician believe active therapy is being given. Not only is this not possible in open control trials but the patient fails to benefit from the positive attitude of receiving therapy, and therefore the well-known beneficial placebo effect.

CONTROL OF ICD TECHNOLOGY

Another unique feature of SCD-HeFT is the manner in which ICD technology and device programming is strictly controlled. This is an important design consideration not done in other ICD trials. SCD-HeFT employs the new paradigm for ICD therapy: easy to use, single-lead, pectoral systems (43,44) that can be inserted on an outpatient basis. The SCD-HeFT investigators view the type of ICD used and the selection of detection and therapeutic algorithms to be comparable to the type and dosage of antiarrhythmic drugs. Just as all antiarrhythmic drugs are not alike, so is the case with ICDs and their programming. Previous ICD studies have treated the lead system, pulsing methods, detection, and therapy algorithms under the rubric of a single therapeutic maneuver. Such an approach belies the multiple ways devices can be considered as therapeutic instruments. Representation of ICDs as a single therapeutic entity is an oversimplification, similar to calling all antiarrhythmic drugs the same. It would be inconceivable to design a study that allows indiscriminate use of and dosing of amiodarone, sotalol, disopyramide, propafenone, procainamide, quinidine, mexiletine, flecainide, diltiazem, and beta-blockers in a prophylactic drug study. The SCD-HeFT investigators believe it is important not to make the parallel mistake with ICDs. Thus, SCD-HeFT is the first ICD clinical trial to control for the important clinical variables of ICD shock method and detection and therapy algorithms.

ECONOMICS AND QUALITY OF LIFE

While the prevention of SCD is a major national public health goal, in the current era of restrained spending on health care, new therapies must not only produce evidence of efficacy but also must show that their extra or incremental health benefits are produced in proportion to their incremental costs (i.e., they must be cost effective) in order to be acceptable for large-scale implementation (45). In this project, since the ICD therapy arm is associated with substantially greater costs than the other two arms, it must provide significant incremental quality-adjusted survival benefits if it is to be viewed as a viable prevention strategy for death in patients with CHF. It is also important to establish that any extra survival produced by the two investigational arms in this trial is not counterbalanced by significant morbidity resulting in diminished health-related quality of life. Thus, without careful prospective analysis of the economic and quality of life aspects of the investigational therapies being evaluated in SCD-HeFT, the mortality results of the trial would be insufficient to address the clinical and health policy questions about whether these therapies are ''worthwhile.''

We feel that inclusion of both economic and quality of life data are a core requirement of the SCD-HeFT research effort. If postualted efficacy is demonstrated for the primary clinical endpoint (all-cause mortality), then these data will clearly be pivotal in determining how the results of this study are viewed and whether the superior therapeutic strategy (or strategies) recieve widespread implementation.

STATISTICAL ISSUES AND DATA ANALYSIS

Sample Size

The sample size for this trial will be 2500 patients enrolled over a 2.5-year period, with a subsequent minimum follow-up period of 2.5 years after the last patient enters the study (Fig. 1). Detailed sample size and power calculations have been performed to guide the design and planning of the trial. A major guiding factor in arriving at the proposed study size is our estimate that the *total* death rate over 2.5 years in class II and class III CHF patients with ejection fractions $\leq 35\%$ will be approximately 25%. This expected event rate is based on the data from SOLVD, V-HeFT II, and CHF-STAT that were presented. The mean EF in those studies was 25–29%. With the SCD-HeFT entry criterion of a left ventricular ejection fraction $\leq 35\%$, our study population may even prove to be at slightly higher risk. Notwithstanding this possibility, the sample size calculations were performed with the more conservative estimate of 25% mortality in 2.5 years. With 2500 patients randomized in equal proportions across the three arms, the study will have > 90% power for detecting a 25% reduction in mortality if the event rate at 2.5 years in the control arm is 25% or higher. Furthermore, if these mortality assumptions should prove to be optimistic, 2500 patients will still provide excellent power. For example, if the effect of either amiodarone or the ICD intervention is to reduce mortality by as little as 21% (instead of 25%), the power for detecting this smaller benefit is still 80%. Moreover, if the control arm mortality rate at 2.5 years should only be 20% (rather than the expected 25%), the power is still greater than 80% for detecting a treatment benefit amounting to a 25% reduction in mortality. Thus the chosen sample size preserves excellent

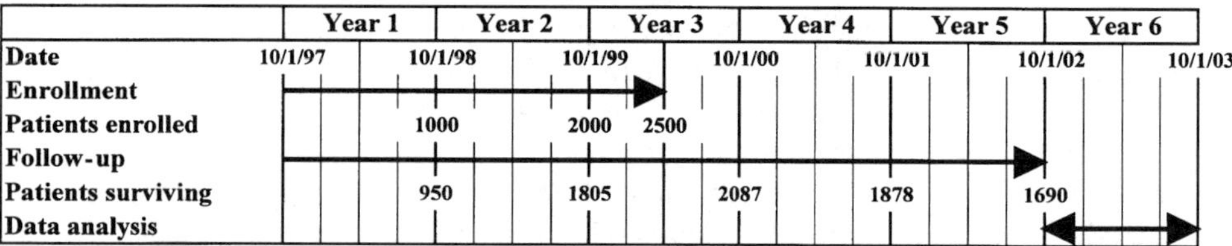

Figure 1 SCD-HeFT study timetable.

power even under relatively conservative assumptions regarding the control arm event rate and the magnitude of the benefit from the intervention arms.

In the process of choosing the population to study, there was no attempt made to stratify patients according to Holter, EPS, SAECG, heart rate variability, $VO_{2\,max}$, etc., given their debatable or only modest positive predictive value for SCD in the SCD-HeFT population. Moreover, the use of these various ''risk stratification tools'' removes the study from the near intuitive level that currently is operative. Stratification will be done, however, on the basis of structural heart disease (ischemic vs. nonischemic) and on the basis of functional class (NYHA II vs. NYHA III).

Statistical Data Analysis

Treatment comparisons between the randomized groups in this trial will be performed according to the principle of ''intention-to-treat''; that is, subjects will be analyzed (and endpoints attributed) according to the treatment arm to which patients are randomized, regardless of subsequent crossover. Statistical comparisons will be performed using two-sided significance tests. Additional perspective regarding the interpretation of the data will be provided through extensive use of confidence intervals and graphical displays.

Treatment comparisons for the primary efficacy endpoint of all-cause mortality will consist of pairwise comparisons of each intervention arm versus the control arm, with each comparison performed with alpha equals 0.025. These comparisons will be performed using the log-rank test (46). This procedure can accommodate varying lengths of follow-up, it uses information for each patient on the time from study entry until the occurrence of the endpoint, and it accommodates ''censored'' survival times that arise because many patients will be alive when the analyses are performed, and the length of time they will survive without an event is known only to be greater than the length of their current follow-up. The analysis strategy will be to first perform treatment comparisons that are adjusted only for the stratification factors of ischemic versus nonischemic cardiomyopathy and NYHA class II vs. NYHA class III. These standard group comparisons, separately contrasting each intervention arm versus the control arm, will constitute the primary analysis to assess treatment differences. Supplementary analysis involving a small number of predefined baseline characteristics (e.g., age, sex, race, presence of atrial fibrillation, and ejection fraction) will also be performed using the Cox proportional hazards model (47,48) to allow adjustment for other relevant covariates. Kaplan-Meier (49) survival curves will be calculated to graphically display the mortality patterns of each treatment arm. If the data provide evidence of an overall difference in outcome between treatment groups, analyses will examine whether the therapeutic effect is similar for all patients, or whether it varies according to specific patient characteristics. These analyses will be carefully executed by testing for interactions between the treatments and specific baseline characteristics.

The log-rank test and Cox proportional hazards model will also be used in the analysis of the secondary clinical endpoints of cardiac death, arrhythmic death, and morbidity. Other specialized analytical techniques for the nonfatal morbidity outcomes will also be used. Appropriate interim analyses of the key clinical endpoints, using specific group-sequential methodology (e.g., O'Brien-Fleming boundaries generated using the flexible Lan-DeMets (51) methodology, will be employed for those interim analyses presented to the Data and Safety Monitoring Board (DSMB). The DSMB, responsible for patient safety in this trial, will be independent of all SCD-HeFT investigators and will be under the direct aegis of the National Institutes of Health (NIH). The DSMB will be responsible for review of patient morbidity and mortality data approximately every 6 months as the data are classified by the SCD-HeFT events committee and provided to the DSMB by the data coordinating center.

PHILOSOPHY OF SCD-HeFT TRIAL DESIGN

Some have argued that SCD in CHF patients is a humane end for those with a limited lifespan due to an inexorable disease process. This attitude does not, however, accurately reflect the quality of life affordable to ambulatory patients with CHF using state-of-the-art heart failure management. A nihilistic approach may be understandable in class IV patients who are not candidates for transplantation, especially in a time of fiscal constraint. However, such an approach is not reasonable in the majority of less severely ill CHF patients in whom a benefit from therapies directed toward SCD prevention might be achieved.

SCD victims do not represent, in any substantial numbers, the group of patients with end-stage, class IV CHF or those of advanced age where the SCD prevention strategies outlined in this proposal would probably be unwise as a broad national public health measure. It is important to recognize that most people who suffer SCD have been active and productive members of the community in the 55 to 65 year age range (52,53). The value of SCD-HeFT to the nation's health, therefore, lies with our target population of ambulatory patients with CHF, where a focused intervention of modest-to-moderate cost will be more acceptable.

We have intentionally excluded patients with class IV heart failure from SCD-HeFT because of their limited prospects for long-term survival [PROMISE (54), CONSENSUS 1987]. Although event rates are higher in this population, therapies directed toward sudden death prevention are less likely to meaningfully prolong life in these patients.

As an integral part of this study design, it is our opinion that any broad-

Table 1 Inclusion Criteria

1. Patients must be 18 years of age or older.
2. Heart failure must be present for at least 3 months.
3. Patinets must have symptomatic CHF (NYHA class II and III) due to ischemic or nonischemic dilated cardiomyopathy on the day of enrollment.
4. The left ventricular ejection fraction must be ≤35% as measured by nuclear imaging, echocardiography, or catheterization within 3 months of enrollment.
5. CHF must be present for at least 3 months prior to randomization and treated with an ACE inhibitor and a beta-blocker if tolerated. Use of an appropriate dose of an ACE inhibitor must be administered for at least 1 month (e.g., enalapril 10 mg bid.).
6. All patients should have had a coronary angiogram to document the nature of their disease unless clinically unreasonable to do so. The definition of ischemic cardiomyopathy will be systolic LV dysfunction in the presence of ≥75% luminal coronary artery narrowing in one or more major coronary arteries or ≥50% in the left main coronary artery *or* insignificant coronary artery disease with definitive evidence of myocardial infarction (e.g., ruptured plaque, acute thrombosis on a modest plaque.) Patients with ischemic cardiomyopathy who have not had coronary angiography within 3 years of enrollment should have clinical findings consistent with stable coronary artery disease prior to inclusion into the study.
7. All patients with chronic atrial fibrillation must be anticoagulated with warfarin with documeneted INRs of at least 2.0 for ≥21 days prior to randomization.
8. Referring physicians to the participating study sites must be willing to allow joint patient management over the course of the study.
9. All patients must have performed a 6-min walk at the time of randomization unless they are unable to walk due to amputation, stroke, or other disability.
10. All patinets must have had a 24-h Holter tape recording within 1 week prior to randomization and forwarded to the Data Coordinating Center. The Holter tape will not be read for clinical use.
11. All patients must have a 12-lead ECG obtained at the time of randomization.

scale attempt to prevent SCD has to be within the conceptual and practical reach of general medical practitioners, not just electrophysiologists and heart failure experts. It is our opinion that the general medical community of family practitioners, internists, and general cardiologists have the most opportunity to easily identify those individuals at risk. SCD-HeFT, then, has true public health importance in that a simple and broadly applicable identification strategy can be implemented on a comprehensive scale in the same manner as ACE inhibitors in CHF and beta-blockers after myocardial infarction. Thus, this study is designed to be reduced to practice by generalists rather than highly specialized electrophysiologists and heart failure experts, although someone skilled in pacemaker insertion

Table 2   Permanent Exclusion Criteria

1. Patients with left ventricular ejection fractions >35%.
2. Asymptomatic patients with left ventricular dysfunction.
3. Patients unable to conduct activities of daily living (i.e., those with NYHA class IV CHF).
4. Patients with a history of cardiac arrest or a spontaneous episode of sustained ventricular tachycardia ($\geq$30 s at rates $\geq$100 bpm) not associated with an acute Q-wave MI. (Sustained VT or an aborted cardiac arrest within 48 h of a myocardial infarction is *not* an exclusion criterion.)
5. Patients younger than 18 years of age.
6. Patients likely to die from any noncardiac cause within 12 months.
7. Females who are pregnant or have child-bearing potential and are not using reliable methods of contraception. (A pregnancy test should be done in the week prior to enrollment on all females with child-bearing potential.)
8. Patients with restrictive, infiltrative, or hypertrophic cardiomyopathy, constrictive pericarditis, acute myocarditis, congenital heart disease, surgically correctable valvular disease, and/or inoperable obstructive valvular disease.
9. Patients with mechanical prosthetic cardiac valves because of the risk in altering anticoagulation status for ICD surgery.
10. Patients with a history of a major psychiatric disorder, active alcohol/drug abuse, or noncompliance.
11. Patients in whom amiodarone is contraindicated for any reason.
12. Patients currently taking amiodarone.
13. Patients requiring antiarrhythmic drugs other than calcium blockers, beta-blockers, or digoxin.
14. Patients concomitantly participating in any investigational clinical trial.
15. Patients with atrial fibrillation requiring catheter ablation of the atrioventricular conduction system or amiodarone for rate control.
16. Patients with unexplained syncope within the last 5 years.
17. Patients unable to accommodate ICD placement in the left infraclavicular region.
18. Patients expected to undergo cardiac transplantation within 12 months.
19. Patients with pacemakers.
20. Patients with liver function tests $\geq$2.5 times normal or a serum creatinine >2.5 mg/dL.
21. Patients unable to provide informed consent.

would have to insert the ICD should this therapy prove useful. We do not view this as a major problem, though, as almost every community of modest size has this capability. Consequently, if one of the two treatment arms of this study proves useful, then the primary physician need only determine heart failure class and ejection fraction to make a decision about SCD prophylaxis and have it implemented with relative ease.

The inclusion criteria for this trial are shown in Table 1. The permanent

Table 3 Temporary Exclusion Criteria[a]

1. Patients having had amyocardial infarciton or cerebrovascular accident within 30 days.
2. Patients with unstable angina within 30 days.
3. Patients having had any cardic surgery or catheter revascularization (angioplasty/ stent or atherectomy) within 30 days.
4. Patients with atrial fibrillation/flutter and an uncontrolled ventricular rate defined as an average resting ventricular rate <120 bpm.
5. Patients with congestive heart failure for less than 3 months and who have not been on an adequate dose of ACE inhibitor (e.g., enalapril 10 mg bid) for a least 1 month.
6. New-onset atrial fibrillation on ECG obtained on date of randomization.

[a] If any patient satisfies a temporary exclusion criterion, that patient will be ineligible for immediate enrollment but may be reappproached when stable for entry into the study.

and temporary exclusion criteria for SCD-HeFT are shown in Tables 2 and 3, respectively. Its administrative structure is shown in Figure 2.

SIGNIFICANCE OF SCD-HeFT

The significance of SCD-HeFT is fourfold.

This study tests two widely applicable SCD prevention strategies in otherwise functional individuals with CHF who have reasonable intermediate-term survival prospects and reasonable expectations for living productive lives. Enrollment of class IV patients is specifically excluded in our study because these patients do not have these reasonable expectations of survival and productivity from therapies directed to SCD prevention.

SCD-HeFT is unique in its ability among present ICD trials to define state-of-the-art ICD therapy in reference to a true control. In AVID, CASH, and CIDS, use of a control arm would be ethically untenable.

This study has the potential to define clinical mechanisms of death and teach us more about the natural history of CHF by virtue of the ICD electrogram and R-R interval memory log. Specifically, the relative incidence of bradyarrhythmic and tachyarrhythmic events will be determined in the 833 patients randomized to ICD therapy. This information will improve our understanding of SCD in patients with CHF and help us interpret the relative value of the two treatment arms in reference to control therapy. These data will also help in the design of future studies on CHF.

This study is designed to provide accurate economic and quality of life information for the three arms of the study. These data will have broad public health implications.

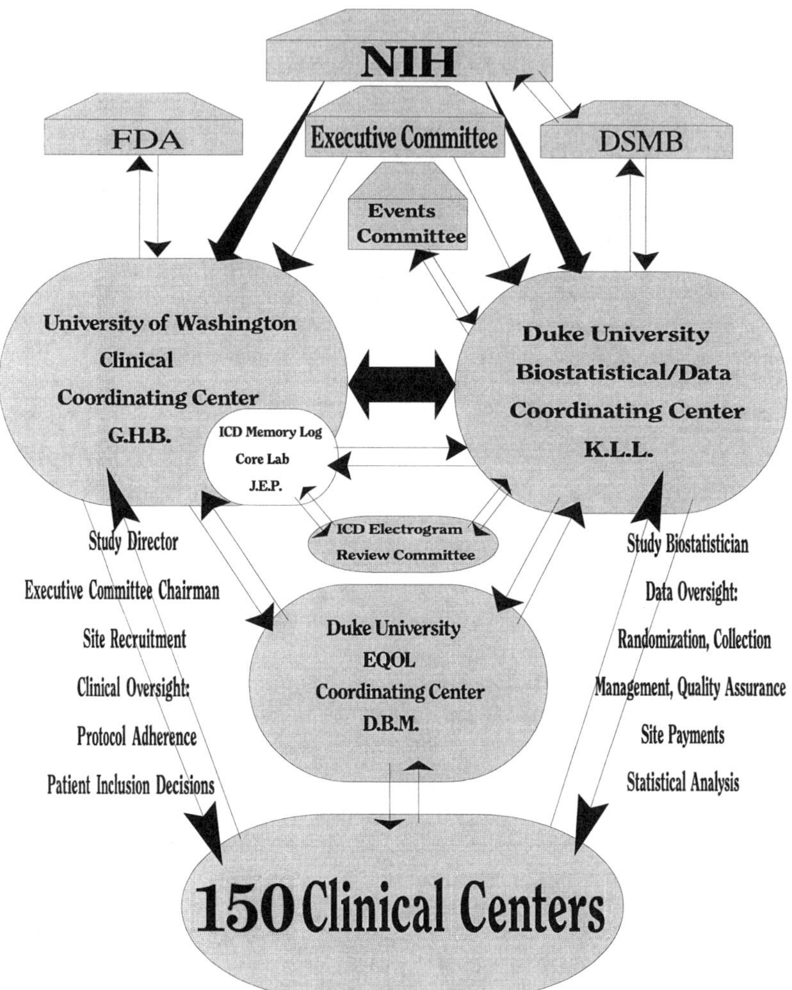

Figure 2 SCD-HeFT organization.

ACKNOWLEDGMENTS

This work supported by a grant from the National Heart, Lung and Blood Institute, UO1 HL55788-01, with subsidiary funding by Medtronic and Wyeth-Ayerst.

REFERENCES

1. McFate-Smith W. Epidemiology of congestive heart failure. Am J Cardiol 1985;55: 3A–8A.
2. Francis GS. Development of arrhythmias in the patient with congestive heart failure: Pathophysiology, prevalence, and prognosis. Am J Cardiol 1986;57:3B–7B.
3. Parmley WW, Chatterjee K, Francis GS, Firth BG, Kloner RA. Congestive heart failure-new frontiers. West J Med 1991;154:427–441.
4. Schocken DD, Arrieta MI, Leaverton PE, Ross EA. Prevalence and mortality rate of congestive heart failure in the United States. J Am Coll Cardiol 1992;20:301–306.
5. Graves EJ. 1989 Summary: National Discharge Survey. Adv Data Vital Health Stal 1989;199:1–11.
6. Gillum RF. Sudden coronary death in the United States: 1980–1985. Circulation 1989;79:756–765.
7. Gordon T, Kannel WB. Premature mortality from coronary heart disease. The Framingham study. JAMA 1971;215:1617–1625.
8. Gordon T, Thom T. The recent decrease in coronary heart disease mortality. Preventive Med 1975;4:115–125.
9. Kuller LH, Lilienfeld A, Fisher R. Epidemiological study of sudden and unexpected deaths due to arteriosclerotic heart disease. Circulation 1996;34:1056–1068.
10. Kuller LH, Traven ND, Rutan GH, et al. Marked decline of coronary heart disease mortality in 35–44 year old white men in Allegheny County, Pennsylvania. Circulation 1989;80:261–266.
11. Ritchie JL, Hallstrom AP, Trobaugh GB, Caldwell JH, Cobb LA. Out-of-hospital sudden coronary death: rest and exercise radionuclide left ventricular function in survivors. Am J Cardiol 1985;55:645–651.
12. Myerburg RJ, Conde CA, Sung RJ, Mayorga-Cortes A, Maallon SM, Scheps DS, Appel RA, Castellanos A. Clinical, electrophysiologic and hemodynamic profile of patients resuscitated from prehospital cadiac arrest. Am J Medicine 1980;68:568–576.
13. Greene HL. Sudden arrhythmic cardiac death-mechanisms, resuscitation and classification: The Seattle Perspective. Am J Cardiol 1990;65:4B–12B.
14. Bigger JT, Fleiss JL, Kleiger R, et al. The Multicenter Post Infarction Program: The relationship between ventricular arrhythmias, left ventricular dysfunction and mortality in the years after myocardial infarction. Circulation 1984;69:250–258.
15. Cupples A, Gagnon DR, Kannel WB. Long-and short-term risk of sudden coronary death. Circulation 1992;85:(suppl I):I-11–18.
16. Hammermeister KE, DeRouen TA, Dodge HT. Variables predictive of survival in patients with coronary disease. Circulation 1979;59:421–430.
17. Mukharji J, Rude RE, Poole WK, et al. The MILIS Study Group. Risk factors for sudden death after acute myocardial infarction: Two year follow-up. Am J Cardiol 1984;54:31–36.
18. Schlant, RC, Forman S, Stamler J, et al. The natural history of coronary heart disease:

Prognostic factors after recovery from myocardial infarction in 2789 men. Circulation 1982;66:401–414.

19. CONSENSUS Trial Study Group. Effects of enalapril on mortality in severe congestive heart failure. Results of the Cooperative North Scandinavian Enalapril Survival Study (CONSENSUS). N Engl J Med 1987;316:1429–1435.

20. Cohn JN, Johnson G, Ziesche S, Cobb F, Francis G, Tristani F, Smith R, Dunkman WB, Loeb H, Wong M, Bhat G, Goldman S, Fletcher RD, Doherty J, Hughes CV, Carson P, Cintron G, Shabetal R, Haakenson C. A comparison of enalapril with hydralazine-isosorbide dinitrate in the treatment of chronic congestive heart failure. N Engl J Med 1991;325:303–310.

20a. SOLVD Investigators. Effects of enalapril on survival in patients with reduced left ventricular ejection fraction and congestive heart failure. N Engl J Med 1991;325:293–302.

21. SOLVD Investigators. Effect of enalapril on mortality and the development of heart failure in asymptomatic patients with reduced left ventricular ejection fractions. N Engl J Med 1992;327:685–691.

22. Goldman S, Johnson G, Cohn JN, Cintron G, Smith R, Francis G. Mechanisms of death in heart failure: The vasodilator-heart failure trials. The V-HeFT VA Cooperative Studies Group. Circulation 1993;87:VI24–V131.

23. Amiodarone Trials Meta-Analysis Investigators. Effect of prophylactic amiodarone on mortality after acute myocardial infarction and in congestive heart failure: meta-analysis of individual data from 6500 patients in randomised trials. Lancet 1997;350:1417–1424.

24. Sim I, McDonald KM, Lavori PW, Norbutas CM, Hlatky MA. Quantitative overview of randomized trials of amiodarone to prevent sudden cardiac death. Circulation 1997;96:2823–2829.

25. Greene HL, et al. The CASCADE Investigators. Randomized antiarrhythmic drug therapy in survivors of cardiac arrest (The CASCADE Study). Am J Cardiol 1993;72:280–287.

26. Pfisterer M, Kiowski W, Burckhardt D, Follath F, Burkart F. Beneficial effect of amiodarone on cardiac mortality in patients with asymptomatic complex ventricular arrhythmias after acute myocardial infarction and preserved but not impaired left ventricular function. Am J Cardiol 1992;69:1399–1402.

27. Ceremuzynski L, Kleczar E, Krzeminska-Pakula M, Kuch J, Nartowicz E, Smielak-Korombel J, Dyduszynski A, Maciejewicz J, Zaleska T, Lazarczyk-Kedzia E, et al. Effect of amiodarone on mortality after myocardial infarction: a double-blind, placebo-controlled, pilot study. J Am Coll Cardiol 1992;20:1056–1062.

28. Teo KK, Yusuf S, Furberg CD. Effects of prophylactic antiarrhythmic drug therapy in acute myocardial infarction. An overview of results from randomized controlled trials. JAMA 1993;270:1589–1595.

29. Singh SN, Fletcher RD, Fisher SG, Singh BN, Lewis HD, Deedwania PC, Massie BM, Colling C, Lazzeri D for the Survival Trial of Antiarrhythmic Therapy in Congestive Heart Failure. Amiodarone in patients with congestive heart failure and asymptomatic ventricular arrhythmia. N Engl J Med 1995;333:77–82.

30. Doval HC, Nul DR, Grancelli HO, Perrone SV, Bortman GR, Curiel R for Grupo de Estudio de la Sobrevida en la Insuficiencia Cardiaca en Argentina (GESICA).

Gary S. Francis
The Cleveland Clinic Foundation, Cleveland, Ohio

As the population of patients with heart failure continues to grow with the aging population, the identification of patients at risk for sudden death becomes even more compelling. Although there is much enthusiasm for the greater use of implantable cardioverter-defibrillators (ICDs) (1,2,), the real question is not whether they can prolong life, but rather, which patients will benefit the most (3). For example, ICDs are life saving in very high-risk groups, such as patients with a combination of unsustained ventricular tachycardia, previous myocardial infarction, and left ventricular dysfunction (the Multicenter Automatic Defibrillator Trial—MADIT) (4). They are also superior to antiarrhythmic drugs among survivors of ventricular fibrillation or sustained ventricular tachycardia with severe symptoms (the Antiarrhythmic Versus Implantable Defibrillator trial—AVID) (5). On the contrary, there is no evidence to support improved survival among patients with coronary heart disease, a low left ventricular ejection fraction, and an abnormal signal-averaged electrocardiogram in whom an ICD is prophylactically implanted at the time of elective coronary bypass surgery (the Coronary Artery Bypass Graft Patch Trial—CABG Patch Trial) (6).

The benefits from an ICD may be limited in patients with heart failure, since the majority of the deaths ($\cong$ two-thirds) are nonsudden (7). Moreover, the strategy of using ICDs is expensive, with the estimated cost per life-year saved being \$133,000 for patients who are New York Heart Association (NYHA) functional class II and \$62,000 for those in class III (7). The question of selecting the patients most likely to benefit then becomes critical, and only a large broad-based study such as Sudden Cardiac Death in Heart Failure (SCD-HeFT) will have the potential to provide the answer.

Like most clinical trials, SCD-HeFT went through a lengthy and careful planning process. Following peer review and final approval at the NIH, the trial was launched in 1997. The central hypothesis is that amiodarone or an ICD will improve survival compared to placebo in patients with NYHA class II and class III heart failure with an ejection fraction of 35% or less. Patients with either ischemic or nonischemic dilated cardiomyopathy are eligible to enter the trial. The principal aim is to reduce overall death rate by reducing arrhythmic deaths. The study has three arms, including a control arm that consists of conventional therapy for heart failure, including digitalis, diuretics, and angiotensin converting enzyme (ACE) inhibitors. This is referred to as the "placebo arm." Hydralazine and nitrates can be used if ACE inhibitors are not well tolerated. There is also an "amiodarone arm" and an "ICD" arm of the trial. Patients in all three arms receive "conventional therapy," which may or may not include beta-adrenergic blockers. The sample size (2500) assumes a mortality reduction of 20% in the ICD arm, with an estimated 25% annual mortality rate. This assumed annual mortality rate may be too high, given the recent improvements in medical therapy. An annual mortality rate of 12 to 15% may be more realistic for class II and III patients. Therefore, it is possible that the SCD-HeFT sample size is underestimated.

Very importantly, in SCD-HeFT the use of beta-adrenergic blockers has been left to the discretion of the managing physician. At the time SCD-HeFT was being planned, beta-adrenergic blockers were considered primarily nonconventional therapy. However, there is now a large data base to suggest that beta-blockers may improve survival and hospitalization rate in patients with heart failure (8). Specifically, the large carvedilol data base (8–12) was instrumental in prompting the Food and Drug Administration (FDA) to provide approval for carvedilol for the prevention of progression of heart failure for patients with NYHA class II and III symptoms. A recent meta-analysis has confirmed that beta-adrenergic blocking drugs may improve patient survival for patients with heart failure (13). There are several national and international beta-blocker trials currently ongoing or in the late planning stages that will further test the hypothesis that beta-blockers can interrupt the natural history of patients with heart failure, thus providing clinicians with a definitive answer to the beta-blocker and heart failure question. There is also a growing awareness among cardiologists that beta-adrenergic blockers may retard progression of heart failure and thereby reduce mortality and the need for hospitalization (14).

A potential key problem with SCD-HeFT is that patients entering the trial might become imbalanced with regard to the use of beta-adrenergic blocking drugs. Rather than being randomized, the assignment of beta-blockers will be left to chance. If any arm of the study has an excess or deficiency of patients being treated with beta-adrenergic blocking drugs, it could directly influence the outcome of the study. If, on the other hand, all three arms of the study are by chance equally balanced with regard to the use of beta-adrenergic blocking drugs, or only a small minority of patients are being treated with these drugs, it is less likely that beta-blockers will have a significant impact on study outcome. What will happen remains to be seen.

The problem of novel therapy being approved during the planning or conduct of large clinical trials has plagued clinical investigators since the earliest trials were performed. Even though carvedilol has been approved by the FDA for treatment of heart failure, its emergence into practice has been rightfully cautious. Several additional large-scale survival trials with beta-adrenergic blocking drugs, including those with carvedilol, are being planned. This would suggest that their use for the treatment of heart failure has not yet been universally embraced. It might have been prudent, in retrospect, for SCD-HeFT investigators to have mandated the use of beta-blocking drugs, but this was not possible at the time of planning since carvedilol was not yet approved by the FDA. On the other hand, if the SCD-HeFT investigators had insisted that beta-blockers be excluded, recruitment of patients into the trial might be far more difficult. Many cardiologists are now convinced of the safety and efficacy of beta-blockers in NYHA class II and III patients. Although perhaps too late for a new randomization scheme, the stratification for beta-adrenergic-blocker use might ensure a better balance. For now, SCD-HeFT investigators must simply hope that the use of beta-adrenergic blockers will be evenly spread among all three treatment arms.

Since the design and implementation of SCD-HeFT, new information has also become available regarding the combined use of amiodarone and beta-blockers. The SCD-HeFT investigators were rightfully concerned about the combined use of beta-adrenergic blocking drugs and amiodarone, since symptomatic bradycardia is a well-known complication of either treatment. Data from the European Myocardial Infarct Amiodarone Trial (EMIAT) suggest that there may be an important interaction between amiodarone and beta-adrenergic blockers (15). In this study there were fewer cardiac deaths among amiodarone-treated patients who were receiving concomitant beta-blockers than among those who were not. This is possibly because beta-adrenergic blockers were not prescribed for patients at high risk of cardiac death, but there is no way to be sure. The fact remains that those patients who received beta-blockers had a substantial reduction in cardiac and arrhythmic mortality if they were also treated with amiodarone. Despite the fact that EMIAT findings do not support the use of systematic prophylactic use of amiodarone in all patients with depressed left ventricular function following myocardial infarction, the potentially positive interaction between beta-adrenergic blockers and amiodarone was unanticipated by the investigators, and was also not apparent to the planners of SCD-HeFT.

In support of the notion of a positive interaction between amiodarone and beta-adrenergic blockers, the Canadian Amiodarone Myocardial Arrhythmia Trial (CAMIAT) also found the two drugs had favorable additive effects (16). In CAMIAT, 60% of the patients receiving amiodarone and 50% of the patients in the placebo group were also taking beta-adrenergic blockers at the time of enrollment into the study. Of interest, the reduction in death rate clustered among the amiodarone-treated patients, and was even greater in those patients who were taking beta-adrenergic blockers (16). These findings support the hypothesis that the benefit of amiodarone is likely to be additive to that of beta-adrenergic blockers. Still, there will be a natural reluctancy to combine beta-blockers and amiodarone by some SCD-HeFT investigators, fearing unwanted heart block and bradyarrhythmias. Though SCD-HeFT is a blinded study, the addition of a study pill (amiodarone?) to a patient knowingly receiving a beta-blocker may ''unblind'' some investigators by provoking severe bradycardia. It is uncertain how this might affect the trial.

Many amiodarone trials have been associated with adverse side effects which have forced discontinuation of the drug (17). The high rate of discontinuation of amiodarone would suggest that although the primary analysis should still be intention to treat, a secondary ''on-treatment'' efficacy analysis might also be considered. This is because the effects of amiodarone continue long after discontinuation of the drug. Such an ''on-treatment'' analysis could be done by censoring patients from further analysis for 3 months after permanent early discontinuation of study medications. If a very large proportion of patients discontinues study medication, such a secondary analysis would prove more difficult.

An imbalance of baseline beta-adrenergic blocker therapy was observed in patients entering MADIT (4). In this trial, beta-adrenergic blockers were used more frequently in the defibrillator group, which conceivably might have accounted for an improved survival pattern in this group. However, the investigators state that less than 30% of patients in the defibrillator group received beta-blockers during the course of the study, suggesting that its role was not substantial. In MADIT, only 62 patients in the ''conventional therapy'' limb were being treated with what might be considered effective therapeutic agents, in terms of their impact on mortality. In contrast, of the 86 ICD patients remaining in the study at the last point of contact, 38% were taking antiarrhythmic agents that might have favorably affected mortality. Additionally, patients in the ICD limb of MADIT seemed to increase their use of potentially effective antiarrhythmic drugs and other cardioactive drugs such as digoxin, ACE inhibitors, and diuretics. This may have improved myocardial function and possibly had an impact on mortality. The vagaries of the MADIT experience point out the importance of achieving therapeutic balance in all treatment arms throughout the study.

The Antiarrhythmic Versus Implantable Defibrillator (AVID) trial was terminated prematurely because of the positive result on mortality during first year (5,18–20). The difference between device therapy and medical therapy (essentially empiric amiodarone) does not seem to be as striking as was found in MADIT. It will be important that the AVID trial results be analyzed carefully to include an estimate of the contribution that drug therapy, in addition to the ICD, might have made toward the improved mortality benefit. For example, 42%

of the patients in the ICD limb of AVID were initially taking beta-blockers, whereas only 16.5% of patients in the drug group were using beta-blockers. This finding can potentially confound the interpretation of the study.

In summary, SCD-HeFT is a well-designed and important randomized controlled trial with a central hypothesis that amiodarone or an implantable cardioverter-defibrillator will improve survival compared to placebo in patients with class II and III heart failure. The estimated mortality rate may be too high, making the sample size somewhat too small, but this remains to be seen. Somewhat unfortunately, ''conventional therapy'' has to some extent been left to the discretion of the managing physician. Given the emerging use of beta-adrenergic blocking drugs for the treatment of heart failure, it is conceivable that many of the patients entering SCD-HeFT will be placed on a beta-blocker. An imbalance in the use of beta-blockers in any of the three arms during the study will make interpretation of the primary endpoint more difficult. Moreover, given the results of EMIAT and CAMIAT, a positive interaction between beta-blockers and amiodarone should be anticipated. If a large number of patients assigned to amiodarone are also taking beta-adrenergic blockers, the interpretation may be further confounded. The high dropout rate of patients being treated with amiodarone will also likely plague the study to some extent. Adding ''blinded'' amiodarone therapy to a patient already relatively bradycardiac from beta-adrenergic blockers may also pose some difficulty for investigators. Last, efforts to determine the likely mechanism of death, despite the careful adjudication by an expert events committee, continues to be a problem (21). All-cause mortality is relatively easy to determine. However, the ability to make a clear distinction between an arrhythmic death and a nonarrhythmic death has been an emerging concern in heart failure trials. It appears as though about one-third of such patients who die while participating in a heart failure trial cannot be easily classified as either sudden cardiac death or nonsudden cardiac death (22). Nevertheless, SCD-HeFT addresses a very important issue in contemporary cardiology. If chance allows for excellent balance between the three arms in the usage of beta-adrenergic blocker drugs and other cardioactive drugs at entry and throughout the trial, very useful information should emerge for the practicing physician. If early and serious imbalance of therapy is observed, further stratification may become necessary.

REFERENCES

1. Sweeney MO, Ruskin JN, Garan H, Mc Govern BA, Guy ML, Torchiana DF, Vlahakes GJ, Newell JB, Semigran MJ, Dec GW. Influence of the implantable cardioverter/defibrillator on sudden death and total mortality in patients evaluated for cardiac transplantation. Circulation 1995;92:3273–3281.

2. Zipes, DP. Are implantable cardioverter-defibrillators better than conventional anti-arrhythmic drugs for survivors of cardiac arrest? Circulation 1995;91:2115–2117.

3. Josephson M, Nisam S. Prospective trials of implantable cardioverter defibrillators versus drugs: Are they addressing the right question? Am J Cardiol 1996;77:859–863.

4. Moss AJ, Hall WJ, Cannom DS, Daubert JP, Higgins SL, Klein H, Levine JH, Saksena S, Waldo AL, Wilber D, Brown MW, Heo M. Improved survival with an implanted defibrillator in patients with coronary disease at high risk for ventricular arrhythmia. N Engl J Med 1996;335:1933–1940.

5. AVID Investigators. A comparison of antiarrhythmic-drug therapy with implantable defibrillators in patients resuscitated from near-fatal ventricular arrhythmias. N Engl J Med 1997;337:1576–1583.

6. Bigger JT, Jr and the CABG Patch investigators. Prophylactic use of implanted cardiac defibrillators in patients at high risk for ventricular arrhythmias after coronary-artery bypass graft surgery. N Engl J Med 1997;337:1569–1575.

7. Uretsky BF, Sheahan RG. Primary prevention of sudden cardiac death in heart failure: will the solution be shocking? J Am Coll Cardiol 1997;30:1589–1597.

8. Packer M, Bristow MR, Cohn JN, Colucci WS, Fowler MB, Gilbert EM, Shusterman NH. The effect of carvedilol on morbidity and mortality in patients with chronic heart failure. N Engl J Med 1996;334:1349–1355.

9. Australia/New Zealand Heart Failure Research Collaborative Group. Randomized, placebo-controlled trial of carvedilol in patients with congestive heart failure due to ischaemic heart disease. Lancet 1997;349:375–380.

10. Krum H, Sackner-Bernstein J, Goldsmith RL, Kukin ML, Schwartz B, Penn J, Medina N, Yushak M, Horn E, Katz SD, Levin HR, Neuberg GW, DeLong G, Packer M. Double-blind, placebo-controlled study of the long-term efficacy of carvedilol in patients with severe chronic heart failure. Circulation 1995;92:1499–1506.

11. Packer M, Colucci WS, Sackner-Bernstein JD, Liang C, Goldscher DA, Freeman I, Kukin ML, Kinhal V, Udelson JE, Klapholz M, Gottlieb SS, Pearle D, Cody RJ, Gregory JJ, Kantrowitz NE, LeJemtel TH, Young ST, Lukas MA, Shusterman NH. Double-blind, placebo-controlled study of the effects of carvedilol in patients with moderate to severe heart failure. Circulation 1996;94:2793–2799.

12. Bristow MR, Gilbert EM, Abraham WT, Adams KF, Fowler MB, Hershberger RE, Kubo SH, Narahara KA, Ingersol H, Krueger S, Young S, Shusterman N. Carvedilol produces dose-related improvements in left ventricular function and survival in subjects with chronic heart failure. Circulation 1996;94:2807–2816.

13. Heidenreich PA, Lee TT, Massie BM. Effect of beta-blockade on mortality in patients with heart failure: a meta-analysis of randomized clinical trials. J Am Coll Cardiol 1997;30:27–34.

14. Eichhorn EJ, Bristow MR. Medical therapy can improve the biological properties of the chronically failing heart. A new era in the treatment of heart failure. Circulation 1996;94:2285–2286.

15. Julian DG, Camm AJ, Frangin G, Janse MJ, Munoz A, Schwartz, Simon P. Randomised trial of effect of amiodarone on mortality in patients with left-ventricular dysfunction after recent myocardial infarction: EMIAT. Lancet 1997;349:667–674.

16. Cairns JA, Connolly SJ, Roberts R, Gent M. Randomised trial of outcome after

myocardial infarction in patients with frequent or repetitive ventricular premature depolarizations. CAMIAT. Lancet 1997;349:675–682.

17. Vorperian VR, Havighurst TC, Miller S, January CT. Adverse effects of low dose amiodarone: a meta-analysis. J Am Coll Cardiol 1997;30:791–798.

18. Anonymous. NHLBI stops arrhythmia study—implantable cardiac defibrillators reduce deaths. NIH News Release, April 14, 1997.

19. McCarthy M. Implantable cardiac defibrillators cut deaths. Lancet 1997;349:1225.

20. Anonymous. NHLBI stops arrhythmia study: implantable cardiac defibrillators reduce deaths. Circulation 1997;95:2465.

21. Gottlieb SS. Dead is dead–artificial definitions are no substitute. Lancet 1997;349:662–663.

22. Ziesche S, Rector TS, Cohn JN. Interobserver discordance in the classification of mechanism of death in studies of heart failure. J Cardiac Failure 1995;1:127–32.

18
Future Clinical Trials

Eleanor B. Schron and Lawrence M. Friedman

National Heart, Lung and Blood Institute,
National Institutes of Health, Bethesda, Maryland

H. Leon Greene

University of Washington, Seattle, Washington

INTRODUCTION

Clinical trials conducted over the past decade have made important contributions to guide the management of ventricular arrhythmias in patients with coronary heart disease (CHD) and/or congestive heart failure (CHF). Implantable cardioverter defibrillators (ICDs) have been proven to decrease mortality in patients resuscitated from cardiac arrest or sustained ventricular tachycardia and patients who have had a myocardial infarction who are at high risk of sudden death, identified by nonsuppressibility on electrophysiological testing (1,2). Amiodarone also has reduced sudden cardiac death in some patients with myocardial infarction or heart failure (3–6), although there is still question about its generalizability to all heart failure patients (7). Other antiarrhythmic agents, with the exception of beta-blockers, have either had little or no clinical benefit or have caused harm, when used in CHD patients with ventricular arrhythmias (8–11).

There are still remaining questions, however, with respect to other populations or settings in which ICDs might be useful. For example, might people with identified atherosclerosis and one or more risk factors for sudden cardiac death benefit from these devices? And, if so, what is the cost effectiveness? What are the adverse effects, and how do ICDs affect quality of life? Are there other pharmacological agents that might give better results than those that have already been studied? Can the pharmacological agents be evaluated in more responsive populations, or with studies better designed to identify the benefits? How should use of ICDs and drugs be combined? What about other approaches to reducing

351

sudden cardiac death? What is the role of primary prevention of the underlying diseases?

The purpose of this chapter is to describe recently completed, ongoing or planned clinical trials of drugs or devices aimed at suppression of ventricular arrhythmias or their consequences. Only trials that are randomized and phase III/IV (of adequate size to assess clinical outcomes) are presented. All studies deal with populations considered to be at high risk of arrhythmic death or mortality from any cause, having one or more risk factors in addition to evidence of ischemic heart disease or heart failure. The investigators of these studies seek to examine in different populations the effects of treatments (e.g., ICD, amiodarone) proven to be useful in certain high-risk groups. Other pharmacological agents are also being evaluated.

CLINICAL TRIALS OF ICD TREATMENT (Table 1)

Sudden Cardiac Death in Heart Failure: Trial of Prophylactic Amiodarone Versus Implantable Defibrillator (SCD-HeFT)

SCD-HeFT (12) is a three-arm trial comparing amiodarone, ICD, and placebo in patients with CHF [New York Heart Association (NYHA) class II and III] and left ventricular ejection fraction (EF) $\leq$ 0.35. The EF is measured using radionuclide ventriculography, echocardiography, or left ventriculography within 3 months of enrollment. The study will include 2500 patients. Enrollment began in the fall of 1997. The enrollment period is planned to be 2.5 years, with a minimum follow-up of 2.5 years. The primary endpoint is all-cause mortality. Other outcomes being assessed are cardiac and arrhythmic mortality, the incidence of serious, but nonfatal arrhythmias, quality of life, and cost effectiveness. (See Chap. 17 for a further description of the study and its anticipated impact).

Multicenter Automatic Defibrillator Implantation Trial II (MADIT II)

MADIT II will test whether an ICD will increase survival in high-risk CAD patients. Two-hundred patients who are at least a month from their myocardial infarction, have a low ejection fraction ($<$0.30), and have $\geq$10 ventricular premature beats (VPDs)/h on Holter will be randomized to ICD or no ICD, with both groups receiving conventional therapy (13). Outcomes of interest are total mortality, cardiovascular mortality, noncardiovascular mortality, sudden cardiac death, recurrent myocardial infarction, quality of life, and economic assessment. Patient enrollment began in 1997 and is expected to be completed in 1999. Follow-up is a minimum of 2 years. (MADIT II is covered in more detail in Chap. 8).

Table 1 Implantable Cardiac Defibrillator (ICD) Trials

Trial (location)	Intervention groups	Sample size	Key eligibility	Start date	Endpoints
SCD-HeFT (U.S., Canada)	Amiodarone Placebo ICD	2500	CHF, NYHA class II, III EF ≤ 0.35	1997	Total mortality QoL Cost
MADIT II (U.S.)	ICD No ICD	1200	Prior MI EF ≤ 0.30 ≥ 10 VPDs/h	1997	Total mortality QoL Cost
NORDIC (Denmark)	ICD No ICD	400	AMI EF 0.10–0.36 + risk factor	1998	Total mortality QoL
DINAMIT (Canada, Germany)	ICD No ICD	525	AMI EF ≤ 0.35 ↓ HRV	1998	Total mortality QoL Cost
BEST-ICD (Italy)	EPS-guided drug or ICD therapy No ICD	1500	MI EF <0.36 + another risk factor	1998	Total mortality
DEFINITE (U.S.)	ICD No ICD	440	Symptomatic CHF EF ≤ 0.35 NSVT and/or > 10 VPDs/h	1998	Total mortality QoL Cost

BEST-ICD = BEta-blocker STrategy plus Implantable Cardioverter Defibrillator Trial; DEFINITE = Defibrillators in Non-Ischemic Cardiomyopathy Treatment Evaluation; DINAMIT = Defibrillator in Acute Myocardial Infarction Trial; NORDIC = The Nordic Study; SCD-HeFT = Sudden Cardiac Death in Heart Failure Trial; MADIT II = Multicenter Automatic Defibrillator Implantation Trial II.

The Nordic Study

The Nordic Study is assessing the efficacy of the ICD in patients with acute myocardial infarction who are at high risk of sudden death because of reduced EF (0.10–0.36) and at least one other risk factor: the presence of reduced heart rate variability, nonsustained ventricular tachycardia on Holter, atrial fibrillation, or QT-dispersion >110 ms (14). Four hundred patients will be randomized; 200 will have an ICD implanted 8 to 21 days after randomization and 200 controls will not receive an ICD; all patients will receive best medical treatment. The primary endpoint is all-cause mortality, and secondary endpoints are cardiovascular mortality, sudden cardiac death, and quality of life.

Defibrillator IN Acute Myocardial Infarction Trial (DINAMIT)

DINAMIT will assess whether use of an ICD in patients who have survived an acute MI reduces total mortality compared with no ICD. Unless contraindicated, all patients will receive conventional therapy consisting of beta-blockade, aspirin, ACE inhibition, and lipid lowering with HMG-CoA reductase inhibitors (15). Patients are eligible if they are 6 to 31 days after an MI, have EF $\leq$ 35% (measured by radionuclide angiography or echocardiography), and either depressed heart rate variability (standard deviation of sinus RR interval $\leq$ 70 ms) or elevated heart rate (mean RR interval $\leq$ 750 ms) on 24-h Holter. Beginning in April 1998, 525 patients will be enrolled and followed for at least 2 years. Other outcomes of interest are arrhythmic death, quality of life, and economic assessment. Unlike previous trials of the ICD, this study will evaluate the use of the ICD in a broad population that is not at extremely high risk for sudden cardiac death.

BEta-blocker STrategy plus Implantable Cardioverter-Defibrillator Trial (BEST-ICD)

BEST-ICD is a trial comparing electrophysiological (EP)-guided therapy (drug or ICD) with conventional therapy in patients with a recent MI, EF $<$ 0.36, and at least one other risk factor (VPDs $\geq$ 10/h, reduced heart rate variability [standard deviation of normal intervals (SDNN) $<$ 70 ms], or presence of late ventricular potentials) (16). More than 1500 patients will be randomized, three-fifths to the EP-guided therapy arm. In the EP-guided group, those who have suppressible arrhythmias will be treated with the indicated drug; those whose arrhythmias are not suppressed will receive an ICD. Conventional therapy, given to all patients, including those in the EP-guided group, consists of beta-blockers, aspirin, HMG-CoA reductase inhibitors, and ACE-inhibitors. The primary endpoint of the trial is total mortality. Patient enrollment began in 1998; follow-up is for a minimum of 2 years. Although BEST-ICD is looking at a high-risk population, it is considerably broader than the populations already shown to benefit from the ICD.

Defibrillators in Non-Ischemic Cardiomyopathy Treatment Evaluation (DEFINITE)

DEFINITE will compare ICD with standard therapy in 440 patients with cardiomyopathy due to nonischemic causes (17). Patients are eligible for the trial if they have had symptomatic heart failure, left ventricular EF $\leq$ 0.35 measured by any technique, and nonsustained VT and/or $>$ 10 VPDs/h. The primary endpoint is total mortality. Other outcomes are quality of life, cost effectiveness, and cardiac and sudden death. All patients will receive conventional therapy, consisting of digoxin, diuretics, ACE inhibitors (or hydralazine/nitrate), and beta-blockers, if tolerated. DEFINITE will complement SCD-HeFT by evaluating the ICD in patients with heart failure and without previous serious arrhythmic events.

CLINICAL TRIALS OF DRUG TREATMENT (Table 2)

The Multicenter UnSustained Tachycardia Trial (MUSTT)

MUSTT (18) was designed to determine whether antiarrhythmic therapy guided by programmed electrical stimulation in patients with CAD, diminished EF (≤ 0.40), spontaneous nonsustained VT, and inducible VT will reduce the incidence of SCD, compared to treatment without antiarrhythmic drugs or devices. The drugs used include procainamide, quinidine, disopyramide, mexiletine, acebutolol, propafenone, amiodarone, and sotalol. Tocainide and flecainide were not used. The ICD was used as back-up treatment if drug therapy is deemed ineffective by electrophysiological testing. Follow-up of 704 patients enrolled in the trial is completed. (Chapter 16 contains a more detailed description of MUSTT.)

Azimilide Postinfarct Survival Evaluation Trial (ALIVE)

Azimilide is an antiarrhythmic agent that blocks both rapid (I_{kr}) and slow (I_{ks}) potassium channels. ALIVE is a trial of azimilide (75 and 100 mg/day) versus placebo in patients recovering from myocardial infarction (within 6–21 days) who have EF between 0.15 and 0.35. The study, which began enrollment in winter 1998, seeks to enroll 5900 patients and is scheduled to be completed in 2001 (19). This trial will evaluate azimilide's potential for decreasing all-cause mortality in a population at high risk for SCD.

Sotalol in Patients with an ICD

A trial of d,l-sotalol versus placebo in patients with life-threatening arrhythmias, all of whom have had an ICD implanted, was recently reported (20). The rationale for this study was to see if the addition of d,l-sotalol to ICD reduces symptoms. The primary outcome was death or first shock. Another major outcome is quality of life. Sotalol treatment led to a significant 48% reduction in the primary outcome in the 302 patients randomized.

A similar study, Dofetilide in Patients with an ICD, comparing dofetilide with placebo (21) will evaluate ICD discharges and antitachycardia pacing. Of 196 patients screened, 174 have been randomized.

Table 2 Drug Trials

Trial (location)	Intervention groups	Sample size	Key eligibility	Start date	Endpoints
MUSTT (USA, Canada)	EPS-guided antiarrhythmic drugs and ICD	704	$\geq$4 days post-MI NSVT, EF $\leq$ 0.40 and positive EPS	1992	Arrhythmic death or cardiac arrest
ALIVE (Worldwide)	Azimilide Placebo	5900	MI 6–21 days EF 0.15–0.35	1998	Total mortality
Amio-Aqueous (U.S.)	I.V. Amiodarone Lidocaine	225	In-hospital Resistant VT/VF	1994	24-h mortality
Dofetilide with ICD	Dofetilide Placebo	174	ICD for VT/VF	1993	ICD shocks and antitachycardia pacing
Sotalol with ICD	d,1-Sotalol Placebo	302	ICD for VT/VF	1996	Death plus ICD shocks

ALIVE = Azitmilide Postinfarct Survival Evaluation Trial; MUSTT = Multicenter Unsustained Tachycardia Trial.

Amio-Aqueous

Amio-aqueous is a unique formulation of intravenous amiodarone designed to avoid the hypotensive and negative inotropic effects of the solvent ordinarily used to dissolve the drug. Amio-aqueous is being used in a randomized study of intravenous amiodarone versus lidocaine in hospitalized patients with incessant ventricular fibrillation or ventricular tachycardia resistant to external cardioversion/defibrillation (22). The primary endpoint is 24-h survival. Two hundred twenty-five patients have been randomized. Two other studies with this agent are evaluating: (1) hemodynamically unstable ventricular tachycardia and (2) ventricular inducibility in the electrophysiology laboratory.

The Lignocaine/Bretylium Study (CALIBRE)

CALIBRE (23) is sponsored by the European Resuscitation Council and the Resuscitation Council of the United Kingdom. It is a three-arm multicenter trial comparing lidocaine, bretylium, and placebo in patients who are defibrillated because of ventricular fibrillation or pulseless ventricular tachycardia. Adult patients remaining in VF or pulseless VT after resuscitation efforts, including three DC shocks (200 J, 200 J, 360 J according to the European protocol) are eligible. A minimum of 1000 patients will be enrolled. The primary endpoint is return of spontaneous circulation for at least 5 min. Secondary endpoints are survival to 1 h and to 6 weeks or discharge from hospital, whichever is sooner.

SUMMARY

Ongoing clinical trials should answer several important questions about treatment of ventricular arrhythmias. The studies of implantable cardiac defibrillators for primary prevention are being conducted in people at high risk of sudden death, but who have not yet suffered a cardiac arrest or sustained ventricular tachycardia. Thus, we will know whether we should implant defibrillators in (1) survivors of a myocardial infarction who have other factors that place them at high risk, and (2) high-risk patients with heart failure. Additionally, we will have information whether the etiology of the heart failure is an important determinant for defibrillator implantation. Other trials look at the use of electrophysiological testing in the selection of optimal drug therapy, either in comparison with an ICD or in comparison with standard therapy. These trials will help to define the role of EP testing in the treatment of ventricular arrhythmias. Two studies of antiarrhythmic drugs look at the possible benefits of treatment in the setting of patients who have had defibrillators implanted. These provide important information about the adjunctive use of antiarrhythmic drugs in patients who have had an ICD implanted. Finally, despite the generally unpromising or unfavorable results of antiarrhythmic agents in the postmyocardial infarction setting (with the exception of amiodarone and beta-blockers), at least one trial is assessing a new antiarrhythmic drug in a high-risk group of MI patients.

Even if these ongoing trials demonstrate benefits of treatment, sudden cardiac death will remain a major public health problem. There will still be hundreds of thousands of such events each year, and millions of people will need to be treated at great cost and with considerable adverse effects. Therefore, new directions are needed. One new direction involves better identification of those likely to have arrhythmic death (and, equally important, those unlikely to do so) (24, 25). Trials such as AVID and MADIT required the use of defibrillators in patients who had demonstrated susceptibility to serious arrhythmic events, either by having had a cardiac arrest or sustained ventricular tachycardia or nonsuppressibility on EP testing. Although these criteria identify people at very high risk of sudden death (26), they do not identify the majority of patients who will die from an arrhythmic event. Therefore, identification of patients who need an ICD is still imperfect. Unnecessary ICD implantation is costly and can harm some patients unnecessarily. We need to improve selection of patients and our tailoring of the treatments, whether they are devices, surgery, or drugs. Thus, a better understanding of the underlying mechanisms of fatal arrhythmias in individuals will assist in knowing which treatment is best for that individual (27, 28).

Of course, we need to focus more attention toward preventing conditions, such as coronary artery disease and heart failure, that often lead to sudden cardiac death. The concept of pharmacogenetics, though not new, is also being explored with greater interest and capabilities. The use of genetic makeup to characterize patients in clinical trials and assess treatment response could advance the field considerably (29). That factor, together with the improved understanding of the specific arrhythmia mechanisms, will allow for better trial design and more focused interventions.

REFERENCES

1. The Antiarrhythmics Versus Implantable Defibrillators (AVID) Investigators. A comparison of antiarrhythmic-drug therapy with implantable defibrillators in patients resuscitated from near-fatal ventricular arrhythmias. N Engl J Med 1997;337:1576–1583.
2. Moss AJ, Hall WJ, Cannom DS, et al. for the Multicenter Automatic Defibrillator Implantation Trial Investigators. Improved survival with an implantable defibrillator in patients with coronary disease at high risk for ventricular arrhythmia. N Engl J Med 1996;335:1933–1940.
3. Julian DG, Camm AJ, Frangin G, et al. for the European Myocardial Infarct Amiodarone Trial Investigators. Randomized trial of the effect of amiodarone on mortality

in patients with left ventricular dysfunction after recent myocardial infarction: EMIAT. Lancet 1997;349:667–674.

4. Cairns JA, Connolly SJ, Roberts R, Gent M, for the Canadian Amiodarone Myocardial Infarction Arrhythmia Trial Investigators. Randomized trial of outcome after myocardial infarction in patients with frequent or repetitive ventricular premature depolarisations: CAMIAT. Lancet 1997;349:675–682.

5. Doval HC, Nul DR, Grancelli HO, et al. Grupo de Estudio de la Sobrevida en la Insuficiencia Cardiaca en Argentina (GESICA): Randomised trial of low-dose amiodarone in severe congestive heart failure. Lancet 1994;344:493–498.

6. Amiodarone Trials Meta-analysis Investigators. Effect of prophylactic amiodarone on mortality after acute myocardial infarction and in congestive heart failure: meta-analysis of individual data from 6500 patients in randomised trials. Lancet 1997; 350:1417–1424.

7. Singh SN, Fletcher RD, Risher SG et al for the Survival Trial of Antiarrhythmic Therapy in Congestive Heart Failure. Amiodarone in patients with congestive heart failure and asymptomatic ventricular arrhythmia. N Engl J Med 1995;333:77–82.

8. The Cardiac Arrhythmia Suppression Trial (CAST) Investigators. Preliminary Report: effect of encainide and flecainide on mortality in a randomized trial of arrhythmia suppression after myocardial infarction. N Engl J Med 1989;321:406–412.

9. Waldo AL, Camm AJ, DeRuyter H, et al for the SWORD Investigators. Effect of d-sotalol on mortality in patients with left ventricular dysfunction after recent and remote myocardial infarction. Lancet 1996;348:7–12.

10. Teo KK, Yusuf S, Furberg CD. Effects of prophylactic antiarrhythmic drug therapy in acute myocardial infarction. An overview of results from randomized controlled trials. JAMA 1993;270:1589–1595.

11. Bloch-Thomsen PE. Presentation at the American Heart Association's 70th Scientific Session. Orlando, FL, November 12, 1997.

12. Bardy GH, Lee KL, Mark DB, et al. Sudden cardiac death in heart failure: pilot study. PACE 1997;20:1148 (abstract).

13. Myerburg RJ, Castellanos A. Clinical trials of implantable defibrillators. N Engl J Med 1997;337:1621–1623.

14. Bloch-Thomsen PE. Personal communication.

15. Connolly S. Personal communication.

16. Raviele A, Bonso A, Gasparini G, Themistoclakis S. Role of ICD for the primary prevention of sudden death in post-myocardial infarction patients. G Ital Cardiol 1998;28 (suppl 1):511–516.

17. Kadish A. Personal Communication.

18. Buxton AE, Fisher JD, Josephson ME, et al for the MUSTT Investigators. Prevention of sudden death in patients with coronary artery disease: the Multicenter Unsustained Tachycardia Trial. (MUSTT). Prog Cardiovasc Dis 1993;36:215–226.

19. Pratt C. Personal communication.

20. Pacifico A, Hohnloser SH, William JH, et al. Prevention of implantable-defibrillator shocks by treatment with sotalol. N Engl J Med 1999;340:1855–1862.

21. Pratt C. Personal communication.

22. Somberg JC. Personal communication.

23. Chamberlain D. Personal communication.

24. Myerburg RJ, Interian A, Mitrani RM, Kessler KM, Castellanos A. Frequency of sudden cardiac death and profiles of risk. Am J Cardiol 1997;80(5B):10F–19F.

25. Hartikainen JEK, Malik M, Staunton A, Poloniecki J, Camm JA. Distinction between arrhythmic and nonarrhythmic death after acute myocardial infarction based on heart rate variability, signal-averaged electrocardiogram, ventricular arrhythmias and left ventricular ejection fraction. J Am Coll Cardiol 1996;28:296–304.

26. Myerburg RJ, Mitrani R, Interian A, Castellanos A. Interpretation of outcomes of antiarrhythmic clinical trials: design features and population impact. Circulation 1998;97:1514–1521.

27. Domanski MJ, Zipes DP, Schron E. Treatment of sudden cardiac death. Current understandings from randomized trials and future research directions. Circulation 1997;95:2694–2699.

28. Rosen MR. Consequences of the Sicilian Gambit. Eur Heart J 1995;Suppl G:32–36.

29. Linder MW, Prough RA, Valdes R Jr. Pharmacogenetics: a laboratory tool for optimizing therapeutic efficiency. Clin Chem 1997;43(2):254–266.

Index

About the Editors

RAYMOND L. WOOSLEY is Chairman of the Department of Pharmacology, a Professor of Pharmacology and Medicine, and the Director of the General Clinical Research Center at Georgetown University School of Medicine, Washington, D.C. An associate editor of *Clinical Pharmacology and Therapeutics* and the *Journal of Pharmacology and Experimental Therapeutics*, he is the coeditor of nine books, the holder of six patents, and the author or coauthor of over 460 journal articles, book chapters, reviews, editorials, and abstracts. He is a Fellow of the American College of Physicians, the American Heart Association, and the American College of Cardiology, and a member of the American Society for Pharmacology and Experimental Therapeutics. Dr. Woosley received the B.S. degree (1964) in chemistry and biology from Western Kentucky University, Bowling Green, the Ph.D. degree (1967) in pharmacology from the University of Louisville, Kentucky, and the M.D. degree (1973) from the University of Miami, Florida.

STEVEN N. SINGH is a Staff Cardiologist at the Veterans Affairs Medical Center, Washington, D.C., and a Professor of Medicine and Pharmacology at Georgetown University School of Medicine, Washington, D.C. The author or coauthor of over 200 papers, abstracts, book chapters, and editorials, he is a Fellow of the American College of Cardiology and the Council of Clinical Cardiology of the American Heart Association. Dr. Singh received the B.S. (1967) and M.D. (1971) degrees from Howard University, Washington, D.C.